P9-CCI-319

Boards
AND
Wards

for USMLE Steps 2 & 3

FIFTH EDITION

Carlos Ayala, MD, FACS
Lt Col. USAF, MC, FS
Adjunct Assistant Professor of Surgery
Uniformed Services University of
Health Sciences (USUHS)
Chief of ENT/Facial Plastic Surgery
Department of Otolaryngology,
Head and Neck Surgery
Nellis Air Force Base
Las Vegas, Nevada

Brad Spellberg, MD, FIDSA, FACP
Associate Professor of Medicine
David Geffen School of Medicine at UCLA
Division of General Internal Medicine
Associate Program Director,
Internal Medicine Residency
Harbor-UCLA Medical Center
Medical Director, Clinical Research Solutions
Los Angeles Biomedical Research Institute

 Wolters Kluwer | Lippincott Williams & Wilkins
Health
Philadelphia · Baltimore · New York · London
Buenos Aires · Hong Kong · Sydney · Tokyo

Acquisitions Editor: Susan Rhyner
Product Manager: Stacey Sebring
Marketing Manager: Joy Fisher-Williams
Designer: Doug Smock
Compositor: Aptara, Inc.

Fifth Edition

Library of Congress Cataloging-in-Publication Data

Ayala, Carlos, MD.
  Boards and wards for USMLE steps 2 & 3 / Carlos Ayala, Brad Spellberg.
   5th ed.
    p.; cm.
  Rev. ed. of: Boards and wards / Carlos Ayala, Brad Spellberg. 4th ed. 2009.
  Includes bibliographical references and index.
  ISBN 978-1-4511-4406-2 (alk. paper)
  I. Spellberg, Brad. II. Ayala, Carlos, MD. Boards and wards. III. Title.
  [DNLM: 1. Clinical Medicine—Examination Questions. WB 18.2]
  610.76—dc23

                                                        2012004973

DISCLAIMER
Care has been taken to confirm the accuracy of the information present and to describe generally accepted practices. However, the authors, editors, and publisher are not responsible for errors or omissions or for any consequences from application of the information in this book and make no warranty, expressed or implied, with respect to the currency, completeness, or accuracy of the contents of the publication. Application of this information in a particular situation remains the professional responsibility of the practitioner; the clinical treatments described and recommended may not be considered absolute and universal recommendations.

The authors, editors, and publisher have exerted every effort to ensure that drug selection and dosage set forth in this text are in accordance with the current recommendations and practice at the time of publication. However, in view of ongoing research, changes in government regulations, and the constant flow of information relating to drug therapy and drug reactions, the reader is urged to check the package insert for each drug for any change in indications and dosage and for added warnings and precautions. This is particularly important when the recommended agent is a new or infrequently employed drug.

Some drugs and medical devices presented in this publication have Food and Drug Administration (FDA) clearance for limited use in restricted research settings. It is the responsibility of the health care provider to ascertain the FDA status of each drug or device planned for use in their clinical practice.

To purchase additional copies of this book, call our customer service department at **(800) 638-3030** or fax orders to **(301) 223-2320**. International customers should call **(301) 223-2300**.

Visit Lippincott Williams & Wilkins on the Internet: http://www.lww.com. Lippincott Williams & Wilkins customer service representatives are available from 8:30 am to 6:00 pm, EST.

Dedicated to my wife and family, Teresa, Juancarlos, and Yasmin.
To my wonderful mother Lydia Quinones, who gave me the drive to
search for a higher purpose in life.

Carlos Ayala, MD

To all the interns manning the front lines of our hospitals,
and to all the MS IVs who will soon know their pain.

Brad Spellberg, MD

CONTRIBUTORS

Fourth Edition Contributors

Ryan Blenker, MD

James T. Kwiatt, MD

Jay Mepani, MD

Benjamin M. Schneeberger, MD

Fifth Edition Contributors

Joseph Love, DO

Lisa Mihora, MD

Jonathan Ricker, DO

Shawn M. Varney, MD, FACEP

David J. Walick, MD

Yang Xia, MD

PREFACE

Scutted-out medical students and exhausted interns have no time to waste studying for the USMLE Steps 2 and 3 exams. That's where we come in. We cover all the major fields of medicine tested on the USMLE exams: Internal Medicine, Surgery, Obstetrics-Gynecology, Pediatrics, Family Medicine, Psychiatry, Neurology, Dermatology, Radiology, Emergency Medicine, and Medical Ethics/Law. However, in contrast to most review texts, we have targeted each chapter toward clinicians *who are not going into that field of medicine*. Thus, Family Medicine is written for surgeons, Obstetrics-Gynecology is written for psychiatrists, Internal Medicine is written for pediatricians, and so on.

None of you surgeons out there want to spend the 5 minutes you have before nodding off to sleep learning Dermatology for the USMLE Step 2 or 3 exam! Rather, you need a concise review, broad in content but lacking extensive detail, to jar your memory of testable concepts you long ago learned and forgot. Don't waste your precious waking hours poring over voluminous review texts! Remember, sleep when you can sleep. During those few minutes before dozing off in the call room, use a text written by colleagues and designed to help you breeze through the subjects you have little interest in and have forgotten most of, but in which you need to review the most. Like you, we know and live by the old axiom: study 2 months for the USMLE Step 1 exam, 2 days for the Step 2 exam, and bring a Number 2 pencil to the Step 3 exam!

We welcome any feedback you may have about *Boards and Wards*. Please feel free to contact the authors with your comments or suggestions. You can email us at Boards_Wards@yahoo.com or write us at the following address:

Boards and Wards
c/o Lippincott Williams & Wilkins
351 W. Camden Street
Baltimore, MD 21201

Finally, we would also like to thank all the medical students and residents and attendings who have reviewed this new edition and provided their suggestions and comments.

CONTENTS

Contributors v

Preface vii

Abbreviations xiii

List of Tables xv

1. Internal Medicine 1
   Cardiology 1
   Pulmonary 38
   Gastroenterology and Hepatology 56
   Nephrology 70
   Endocrinology 79
   Musculoskeletal 93
   Hematology 111
   Empiric Antibiotic Tx for Specific Infxns 125
   Electrolyte Disorders & Management 135

2. Surgery 138
   Fluid and Electrolytes 138
   Blood Product Replacement 142
   Perioperative Care 145
   Trauma 148
   Burns 154
   Neck Mass Differential 156
   Surgical Abdomen 158
   Esophagus 159
   Gastric Tumors 166
   Hernia 167
   Hepatic Tumors 169
   Gallbladder 169
   Exocrine Pancreas 172
   Small Intestine 175
   Colon 177
   Rectum and Anus 184
   Bariatric Surgery 186
   Breast 189
   Urology 198
   Neurosurgery 202
   Vascular Diseases 208

3. **Obstetrics and Gynecology** 218
   Obstetrics 218
   Gynecology.. 247

4. **Pediatrics** 268
   Development 268
   Infections 268
   Respiratory Disorders................................... 268
   Musculoskeletal... 281
   Metabolic 287
   Genetic and Congenital Disorders....................... 290
   Trauma and Intoxication................................ 299
   Adolescence 303

5. **Family Medicine**....................................... 306
   Headache 306
   Ears, Nose, and Throat 306
   Outpatient Gastrointestinal Complaints................. 318
   Urogenital Complaints................................... 320
   Common Sports Medicine Complaints 331
   Nutrition... 343
   Cancer Screening 347

6. **Psychiatry**... 348
   Introduction 348
   Mood Disorders 349
   Psychosis... 352
   Anxiety Disorders 354
   Personality Disorders................................... 357
   Somatoform and Factitious Disorders 360
   Child and Adolescent Psychiatry 363
   Abuse of Drugs 367
   Miscellaneous Disorders 368
   Sleep... 370

7. **Neurology** 373
   Stroke 373
   Infection and Inflammation............................. 376
   Demyelinating Diseases................................. 378
   Metabolic and Nutritional Disorders 380
   Seizures.. 382
   Degenerative Diseases................................... 385

8. **Dermatology** 389
   Terminology 389
   Topical Steroids.. 396

Infections 396
Common Disorders 399
Cancer 414
Neurocutaneous Syndromes (Phakomatoses) 418
Blistering Disorders 420
Vector–Borne Diseases. 423
Parasitic Infections. 424
Fungal Cutaneous Disorders 428

9. Ophthalmology 431
Eyes. 431

10. Radiology. 452
Helpful Terms and Concepts 452
Common Radiologic Studies 453
An Approach to a Chest X-Ray 453
Common Radiologic Findings 454

11. Emergency Medicine. 471
Toxicology 471
Fish and Shellfish Toxins 473
Bites and Stings. 475
ENT Trauma 476

12. Ethics/Law/Clinical Studies 479
Biostatistics 479
Calculation of Statistical Values 480
Law and Ethics 485
Doctoring 489
Health Care Delivery 492

Appendix 495

Questions 513

Answers 538

Index 563

ABBREVIATIONS

↑ (↑↑)	Increases/High (Markedly Increases/Very High)
↓ (↓↓)	Decreases/Low (Markedly Decreases/Very Low)
→	Causes/Leads to/Analysis shows
⊕	Positive
1°/2°	Primary/Secondary
Abd	Abdominal
BP	Blood Pressure
Bx	Biopsy
c/o	complain of
CA	Carcinoma
CBC	Complete Blood Count
CN	Cranial Nerve
CNS	Central Nervous System
CT	Computed Tomography Scan
Cx	Culture
CXR/X-ray	Chest X-ray/X-ray
Dx/DDx	Diagnosis/Differential Diagnosis
dz	Disease
EKG	Electrocardiogram
GI	Gastrointestinal
H&P	History and Physical
HA	Headache
HIV	Human Immunodeficiency Virus
HTN	Hypertension
Hx/FHx	History/Family History
ICP	Intracranial Pressure
I&D	Incision and Drainage
infxn	Infection
ICU	Intensive Care Unit
IV	Intravenous
IVIG	Intravenous Immunoglobulin

Lab/Labs	Laboratory/Laboratory Tests/Results
N or Nml	Normal
PE	Physical Exam or Pulmonary Embolus
pt(s)	Patient(s)
Px	Prognosis
RBC	Red Blood Cell
Rx	Prescription/Indicated Drug
q#	Every #
Si/Sx/aSx	Sign/Symptom/Asymptomatic
subQ	Subcutaneous
Tx	Treatment/Therapy
Utz	Ultrasound
WBC	White Blood Cell

LIST OF TABLES

1.1   Hypertension Definitions and Treatment Indication 1

1.2   Causes of Secondary Hypertension 2

1.3   Medical Treatment of Hypertension 3

1.4   Angina Treatment 5

1.5   Initiation of Therapy for Hypercholesterolemia 6

1.6   Treatment by Risk Stratification of Unstable Angia (UA) 7

1.7   Risk Stratification for Acute Coronary Syndrome 8

1.8   Cardiomyopathy 31

1.9   Summary of Major Murmurs 33

1.10   Physical Exam Differential Diagnosis for Murmurs 34

1.11   Duke Criteria for Endocarditis Diagnosis 36

1.12   Five Mechanisms of Hypoxemia 38

1.13   Chronic Obstructive Pulmonary Disease (COPD) 41

1.14   Diagnosis and Treatment of Restrictive Lung Disease 43

1.15   Lab Analysis of Pleural Effusions 44

1.16   Parenchymal Lung Cancers 47

1.17   Mediastinal Tumors 49

1.18   Community-acquired Pneumonia (CAP) 54

1.19   Comparison of Inflammatory Bowel Disease 58

1.20   Congenital Hyperbilirubinemia 60

1.21   Hepatitis Diagnosis and Treatment 62

1.22   Ascites Differential Diagnosis 63

1.23   Causes of Portal Hypertension 68

1.24   Laboratory Characteristics of Acute Renal Failure 71

1.25   Renal Tubular Acidosis 72

1.26   Nephrotic Glomerulopathies 74

1.27   Systemic Glomerulonephropathies 75

1.28   Nephritic Glomerulonephropathies 76

1.29   Urinalysis in Primary Glomerula Diseases 77

1.30   Oral Hypoglycemic Agents 83

1.31   Differential Diagnosis of Male Gonadal Disorders 87

1.32   Genetic Hypogonadism 88

1.33   Multiple Endocrine Neoplasia Syndromes 92

1.34 Diagnosis and Treatment of Primary Bone Neoplasms 95
1.35 α-Thalassemia. 114
1.36 β-Thalassemia 115
1.37 Hypoproliferative Anemias 118
1.38 Hemolytic Anemias. 118
1.39 Causes of Platelet Destruction (Thrombocytopenia) 119
1.40 Labs in Platelet Destruction. 120
1.41 Hypercoagulable Diseases. 120
1.42 Myeloproliferative Diseases. 121
1.43 Empiric Antibiotic Treatment of Specific Infections 125
1.44 Hypokalemia. 135
1.45 Hyperkalemia 136
2.1 Common Electrolyte Disorders 140
2.2 Risk of Viral Infection from Blood Transfusions 144
2.3 Goldman Cardiac Risk Index. 146
2.4 Glasgow Coma Scale 152
2.5 Differential Diagnosis of Shock 153
2.6 Correction of Defect in Shock. 153
2.7 Body Surface Area in Burns. 155
2.8 Neck Mass Differential Diagnosis 156
2.9A Right Upper Quadrant Differential Diagnosis 161
2.9B Right Lower Quadrant Differential Diagnosis 162
2.9C Left Upper Quadrant Differential Diagnosis. 163
2.9D Left Lower Quadrant Differential Diagnosis. 163
2.9E Midline Differential Diagnosis 164
2.10 Hernia Definitions. 167
2.11 Ranson's Criteria. 173
2.12 Intracranial Hemorrhage. 202
2.13 CNS Malignancy. 206
3.1 Teratogens 219
3.2 US Food and Drug Administration Drug Categories 220
3.3 Height of Uterus by Gestational Week 220
3.4 Types of Pregnancy-Induced Hypertension 226
3.5 Bishop Score. 237
3.6 Types of Abortions 242
3.7 Comparison of Placenta Previa and Placental Abruption . . . 244
3.8 Phases of the Menstrual Cycle 249

3.9	Risks and Benefits of Oral Contraceptives	250
3.10	Alternatives to Oral Contraceptives	251
3.11	Differential Diagnosis of Vaginitis	253
3.12	Differential Diagnosis of Hirsutism and Virilization	258
3.13	Ovarian Neoplasms	265
4.1	Developmental Milestones	269
4.2	Tanner Stages	269
4.3	The ToRCHS	270
4.4	Viral Exanthems	272
4.5	Pediatric Upper Respiratory Disorders	276
4.6	Pediatric Painful Limp	284
4.7	Types of Juvenile Rheumatoid Arthritis	286
4.8	Differential Diagnosis of Neonatal Jaundice by Time of Onset	289
4.9	Pediatric Toxicology	302
5.1	Summary of Headaches	307
5.2	Treatment of Headache	308
5.3	Causes of Vertigo	310
5.4	Sinusitis	314
5.5	Pharyngitis	316
5.6	Diarrheas	321
5.7	Infectious Causes of Diarrhea	323
5.8	Sexually Transmitted Diseases	325
5.9	Low Back Pain Red Flags	332
5.10	Knee Injuries	341
6.1	DSM-IV Classifications	348
6.2	Prognosis of Psychiatric Disorders	349
6.3	Pharmacologic Therapy for Depression	350
6.4	Diagnosis of Psychotic Disorders	353
6.5	Antipsychotic Drugs	354
6.6	Antipsychotic-Associated Movement Disorders	355
6.7	Specific Personality Disorders	359
6.8	Drug Intoxications and Withdrawal	367
6.9	Sleep Stages	370
7.1	Presentation of Stroke	373
7.2	Cerebrospinal Fluid Findings in Meningitis	376

7.3   Empiric Therapy for Community Acquired
         Meningitis by Age 377
7.4   Bacterial Meningitis 377
7.5   Encephalitis 379
7.6   Seizure Therapy 383
7.7   Anti-Seizure Medications 384
7.8   Dementia versus Delirium.......................... 386
8.1   Use of Topical Steroids........................... 396
8.2   Skin Cancer 414
8.3   Neurocutaneous Syndromes (Phakomatoses) 418
8.4   Fungal Cutaneous Disorders....................... 429
9.1   Palpebral Inflammation........................... 435
9.2   Red Eye.. 437
9.3   Eye-related Trauma.............................. 447
9.4   Opthalmic Medications........................... 449
10.1   Common Radiologic Studies 453
10.2   Common Radiologic Findings...................... 455
12.1   Biostatistics.................................... 479
12.2   Sample Calculation of Statistical Values 481
12.3   Ethical/Legal Terms 486
12.4   Interviewing Techniques.......................... 490

1. INTERNAL MEDICINE

I. Cardiology

A. **HTN** (Table 1.1)

1. **Causes**

   a. Ninety five percent of all HTN is idiopathic, called "**essential HTN**"

   b. Most of 2° HTN causes can be divided into three organ systems and drugs (Table 1.2)

2. **Malignant HTN**

   a. Can be hypertensive urgency or emergency

   b. Hypertensive urgency

      (1) High BP (e.g., systolic >200 or diastolic >110, but numbers vary depending upon source) **without evidence of end-organ damage**

      (2) Tx = oral BP medications with goal of slowly reducing BP over several days—does not require admission to hospital

   c. Hypertensive emergency

      (1) Defined as severe HTN with evidence of end-organ compromise (e.g., encephalopathy, renal failure, congestive heart failure [CHF]/ischemia)

      (2) Si/Sx = mental status changes, papilledema, focal neurologic findings, renal failure, chest pain, evidence of CHF, or microangiopathic hemolytic anemia (hemolysis with schistocytes on smear)

Table 1.1 Hypertension Definitions and Treatment Indication

Condition	BP	Life-Style Modification	Medications
Normal	<120/80	• Encourage	• None
Prehypertension	120/80–139/89	• Yes	• Only if chronic kidney disease or diabetes (goal <130/80)
Stage I hypertension	140/90–159/99	• Yes	• Yes—thiazide first-line
Stage II hypertension	≥160/100	• Yes	• Yes—most require >1 drug

Table 1.2 Causes of Secondary Hypertension

Cardiovascular	• Aortic regurgitation causes **wide pulse pressure** • Aortic coarctation causes HTN in arms with ↓ **BP in legs**
Renal	• **Glomerular dz commonly presents with proteinuria** • **Renal artery stenosis causes refractory HTN** in older men (atherosclerosis) or young women (fibromuscular dysplasia) • Polycystic kidneys
Endocrine	• Hypersteroidism, typically **Cushing's and Conn's syndromes, which cause HTN with hypokalemia** (↑ aldosterone) • Pheochromocytoma causing episodic autonomic Sx • Hyperthyroidism causing **isolated systolic HTN**
Drug induced	• Oral contraceptives, glucocorticoids, phenylephrine, NSAIDs

      (3) **This is a medical emergency and immediate Tx is needed**

      (4) Tx = IV drip with nitroprusside or nitroglycerin (the latter preferred for ischemia), but **do not lower BP by more than one-fourth within the first hour or the pt may stroke**

  3. **HTN Tx**

    a. Lifestyle modifications first line in pts without comorbid dz

      (1) Weight loss, exercise, salt restriction, and quitting alcohol and smoking can each lower BP

      (2) ↓ Fat intake to ↓ risk of coronary artery dz (CAD); HTN is a cofactor

    b. Medications (Table 1.3)

B. **Ischemic Heart Dz (CAD)**

  1. **Risk Factors for CAD**

    a. **Major risk factors (memorize these!!!)**

      (1) Diabetes

      (2) Smoking

      (3) HTN

      (4) Hypercholesterolemia

      (5) FHx

      (6) Age (>45 yrs for men, >55 yrs for women)

      (7) HDL <40 mg/dL

      (8) Chronic renal failure

    b. Smoking is the number one preventable risk factor

  2. **Stable Angina Pectoris**

    a. Caused by atherosclerotic CAD, supply of blood to heart<demand

Table 1.3 Medical Treatment of Hypertension

Indications and goal	1. Failure of lifestyle modifications after 6 mos to 1 yr 2. Immediate use necessary if comorbid organ disease present (e.g., stroke, angina, renal disease) 3. Immediate use in emergent or urgent hypertensive states (e.g., neurologic impairment, ↑ ICP) 4. ≤140/90, unless the patient has chronic renal failure or diabetes mellitus (DM), for which the goal is ≤130/80
First-line Drugs	
No comobid dz	**Thiazide diuretic** (proven safe and effective)
Diabetes	**ACE inhibitors or angiotensin receptor blocker (ARB)** (proven to ↓ vascular and renal dz)
CHF	**ACE inhibitors, ARB, β-blocker, and K-sparing diuretic** (all proven to ↓ mortality)
Myocardial infarction	**β-blocker and ACE inhibitor** (proven to ↓ mortality)
Osteoporosis	**Thiazide diuretics** (↓ Ca^{2+} excretion)
Prostatic hypertrophy	**α-blockers** (treat HTN and BPH concurrently)
Pregnancy	**α-methyldopa** (known safe in pregnancy)
Other Agents	
Dihydropyridine calcium blocker (e.g., amlodipine)	• Second line for essential hypertension and heart failure • First line for coronary vasospasm (Prinzmetal's angina) • Avoid short-acting dihydropyridines during ischemia (↑ mortality)
Diltiazem/verapamil	First line for rate control of atrial fibrillation or flutter (can also use β blocker)
Hydralazine	Combined with isordil, second line for CHF (proven to ↓ mortality but not as effectively as ACE inhibitors)
Minoxidil	• Only for severe, refractory HTN • Must combine with β-blocker to prevent reflex tachycardia and diuretic to counteract edema resulting from aggressive arteriolar vasodilation • Beware of hair growth as a side effect
Clonidine	• Only for refractory HTN, particularly in renal failure or patients withdrawing from illicit substances • CNS depression, fatigue, and dry mouth are common side effects

(continued)

Table 1.3 *Continued*

Contraindications

β-Blockers	**Chronic obstructive pulmonary dz,** due to bronchospasm
ACE inhibitors	**Pregnancy,** due to teratogenicity
ACE inhibitors	**Renal artery stenosis,** due to precipitation of acute renal failure (GFR dependent on angiotensin-mediated constriction of efferent arteriole)
ACE inhibitors	**Renal failure (creatinine >1.5),** due to hyperkalemia morbidity
K⁺-sparing diuretics	**Renal failure (creatinine >1.5),** due to hyperkalemia morbidity
Diuretics	**Gout,** due to causation of hyperuricemia
Diltiazem/verapamil	**CHF,** due to depression of contractility

    b. Si/Sx = precordial pain radiating to left arm, jaw, back, relieved by rest and nitroglycerin, EKG → **ST depression and T-wave inversion** (see Figure 1.2R)

    c. **Classic Sx often not present in elderly and pts with diabetes (neuropathy)**

    d. Dx = clinical, based on Sx, CAD risks; confirm CAD with stress test or angiography

    e. Tx (Tables 1.4 and 1.5)

3. **Acute Coronary Syndrome (ACS)**

    a. ACS occurs when insufficient perfusion occurs to the myocardium because of obstruction in one or more coronary arteries

    b. ACS has a spectrum of severity, ranging from ischemia without infarction (unstable angina) to non-ST-elevation myocardial infarction (NSTEMI) to ST-elevation myocardial infarction (STEMI)

    c. Dx of ACS is based on H&P, EKG, and cardiac enzymes

4. **Unstable Angina**

    a. Sx similar to stable angina but occur more frequently with less exertion and/or **occurs at rest**

    b. Unstable angina is caused by transient clotting of atherosclerotic vessels; clot spontaneously dissolves before infarction occurs

    c. EKG during ischemia typically shows ST depression or T-wave inversions (Figure 1.2R)

Table 1.4 Angina Treatment

Acute	• Sublingual nitroglycerin • Usually acts in 1–2 min • May be taken up to 3 times q3–5 min intervals • If doesn't relieve pain after 3 doses, pt may be infarcting
Chronic prevention	• Isordil (long-acting nitrate) effective in prophylaxis • β-blockers ↓ myocardial O_2 consumption in stress/exertion • Aspirin to prevent platelet aggregation in atherosclerotic plaque • Quit smoking! • ↓ LDL levels, ↑ HDL with diet, ↑ exercise, ↑ fiber intake, stop smoking, lose weight, drug therapy if LDL/HDL are not at goal (see Table 1.5)
Endovascular intervention	Percutaneous transluminal coronary angioplasty (PTCA) • Indicated with failure of medical management • Morbidity less than surgery but has up to 50% restenosis rate • Stent placement, particularly drug eluting stent, greatly reduces restenosis • Platelet GPIIb-IIIa antagonists further reduce restenosis rate
Surgery	Coronary artery bypass graft (CABG) • Indications = failure of medical Tx, 3-vessel CAD, or 2-vessel dz in DM • Comparable mortality rates with PTCA after several years, except in diabetic patients who do better with CABG

    d. Labs: by definition cardiac enzymes are negative in unstable angina

    e. Tx is based on stratification of risk of bad outcome, defined as risk of recurrent unstable angina, infarction, or death 30 days after presentation (Table 1.6)

    f. Once a pt has ruled out for myocardial infarction (MI) with negative enzymes, the pt should undergo risk stratification (Table 1.7)

  5. **NSTEMI**

    a. Sx similar to unstable angina, but pain often lasts ≥20 min without resolving and may only partially respond or not respond to nitroglycerin

    b. EKG similar to unstable angina (ST depression or T-wave inversions)

Table 1.5 Initiation of Therapy for Hypercholesterolemia

Risk[a]	LDL Goal (mg/dL)[b]	LDL at Drug Initiation (mg/dL)
Low = <2 risk factors (10-yr cardiac risk <1%)	<160	>190
Intermediate = ≥2 CAD risk factors (no DM) (10-yr cardiac risk 1–10%)	<130	>160
High = ≥2 CAD risk factors but no known CAD/PVD (10-yr cardiac risk 11–20%)	<100	>130
Highest = Known CAD, PVD, DM, metabolic syndrome (10-yr cardiac risk >20%)	<100, consider <70	>100

Common Drug Options

HMG-CoA Reductase Inhibitors	• First-line for cholesterol reduction, inhibit the rate limiting step in cholesterol synthesis (HMG-CoA reductase) • Most potent reducers of LDL, mildly elevate HDL • Several have been shown to reduce deaths from CAD and stroke • Primary side effect is muscle injury, can lead to rhabdomyolysis • Examples = lovastatin, simvastatin, pravastatin, atorvastatin, fluvastatin
Fenofibrate	• Raises HDL levels, reduces triglycerides
Niacin	• Most effective at lower triglycerides and raising HDL • May be added to HMG-CoA reductase inhibitor if LDL is at goal but HDL remains too low or triglycerides too high • Common side effect is cutaneous flushing, lessened by slow dose titration • Also can worsen gout and diabetic control (↑insulin resistance)
Ezetimibe	• Inhibits cholesterol absorption
Gemfibrozil	• Inhibits VLDL production, primary effect is triglyceride reduction • Used for isolated hypertriglyceridemia • Don't add to statins due to increased risk of rhabdomyolysis

[a]Risks = family Hx CAD, smoking, HTN, age (45 for men, 55 for women), HDL <40; DM automatically goes to high risk; if HDL >60, subtract 1 risk point. If known CAD or peripheral vascular disease (PVD), automatically goes to highest risk category.
[b]If LDL is above goal, immediately initiate diet and exercise.

Table 1.6	Treatment by Risk Stratification of Unstable Angia (UA)[a]		
	Low Risk	**Intermediate Risk**	**High Risk**
Defining factors[b]	• Increased frequency of angina compared to baseline • Rest pain <20 min	• Rest pain ≥20 min now resolved • Nocturnal angina • Pain resolved with nitroglycerin • Symmetric T-wave inversions or ST depressions <1 mm	• Rest pain ≥20 min ongoing • ST depressions ≥1 mm • + Troponon or CK-MB (i.e., NSTEMI) • Presence of acute pulmonary edema or S_3 on exam
Treatment	• Aspirin • O_2 • β-blocker • Sublingual NTG prn	• Add longer-acting nitro drug (i.e., isosorbide dinitrate) • Consider low-molecular-weight heparin	• Add low-molecular-weight heparin • Nitro drip if pain ongoing • Add GPIIb-IIIa antagonist if enzymes positive or ST depressions >1 mm • Clopidogrel can be added for NSTEMI or if stent placed during catheterization

[a]Defined as risk of recurrent UA, myocardial infarction, or death at 30 days after presentation.
[b]This list of defining factors is not inclusive but rather highlights the most "testable" factors on the boards. Note that ST-elevation MI does not fit into this algorithm.

   c. Labs: by definition, cardiac enzymes (i.e., troponin and creatine-MB [CK-MB]) are elevated, and this is how NSTEMI is Dx—both have similar sensitivities and specificities, but CK-MB normalizes 72 hrs after infarction, whereas troponin remains elevated for up to 1 wk
   d. Acute Tx: see Table 1.6

6. **ST Elevation MI**
   a. Infarct usually 2° to acute plaque rupture causing thrombosis in atherosclerotic vessel
   b. Si/Sx = crushing substernal pain, as per angina, but not relieved by rest, ↑ diaphoresis, nausea/vomiting, tachycardia or bradycardia, dyspnea
   c. Dx
      (1) **EKG → ST elevation and Q waves** (Figures 1.1 and 1.2S)

Table 1.7 Risk Stratification for Acute Coronary Syndrome

Test	Sensitivity/Specificity[a]	Comments
Stress treadmill	70%/70%	• Inexpensive • Due to low sensitivity/specificity, only useful for patients with intermediate probability of having CAD
Stress echocardiogram	80%/80%	• Only form of stress test that enables visualization of valve function • Also measures ejection fraction • Can be done with exercise or pharmacologically with dobutamine—pharmacological done for people who cannot exercise but sensitivity is lower
MIBI	80%/80%	• Also measures ejection fraction • Can be done with exercise or pharmacologically with persantine—do not use persantine in patients with asthma
Catheterization	95%/95%	• Gold standard for diagnosis • Provides an anatomical view of the coronaries and estimate of ejection fraction • Can be false negative for partial coronary lesions if the artery undergoes compensatory dilation

[a]Sensitivities and specificities are for finding evidence of coronary artery disease; approximate values shown—studies typically show a range of +/– 5% from values shown.

      (2) Enzymes: troponin I or CK-MB
      (3) Appropriate signs and symptoms with risk factors
   d. Tx = reestablish vessel patency
      (1) Medical Tx = thrombolysis within 6 hrs of the infarct: by using tissue plasminogen activator **(tPA) + heparin** (first line) or streptokinase
      (2) Percutaneous transluminal coronary (PTCA)—may be more effective—can open vessels mechanically or with local administration of thrombolytics
      (3) Coronary artery bypass graft (CABG) is longer-term Tx, rarely used for acute process
   e. Adjuvant medical therapies
      (1) **Number one priority is aspirin! (proven to ↓ mortality)**
      (2) **Number two priority is β-blocker (proven to ↓ mortality)**

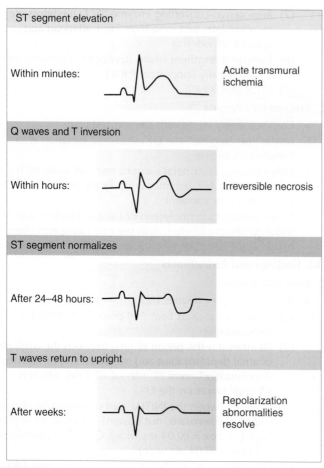

ST segment elevation		
Within minutes:		Acute transmural ischemia
Q waves and T inversion		
Within hours:		Irreversible necrosis
ST segment normalizes		
After 24–48 hours:		
T waves return to upright		
After weeks:		Repolarization abnormalities resolve

FIGURE 1.1

The changing pattern of the EKG in the affected leads during the evolution of a myocardial infarction. (Adapted from Axford JS. *Medicine.* Oxford: Blackwell Science, 1996.)

    (3) Statin drugs to lower cholesterol are essential (**low-density lipoprotein [LDL] must be <100 postinfarct,** proven to ↓ mortality)

    (4) Heparin should be given for 48 hrs postinfarct

    (5) Oxygen (O_2) and morphine for pain control

    (6) Nitroglycerin to reduce both preload and afterload

(7) Angiotensin-converting enzyme (ACE) inhibitors are excellent late- and long-term Tx; ↓ afterload and prevent remodeling

(8) Exercise strengthens heart, develops collateral vessels, ↑ high-density lipoprotein (HDL)

(9) STOP SMOKING!

7. **Prinzmetal's Angina**

a. Coronary artery vasospasm causing rest pain

b. Unlike true "angina," the EKG shows ST elevation with Prinzmetal's angina

c. Differentiating Prinzmetal's angina from an acute MI is challenging at first, but enzymes typically are negative, and ST elevation is only transient

d. Tx is vasodilators (nitroglycerin or calcium blocker), and pts should undergo catheterization because vasospasm often occurs at the site of an atherosclerotic lesion in the coronaries

C. EKG Findings and Arrhythmias

1. Basic EKG Review

a. P-QRS-T complex (Figure 1.2A)

(1) P wave is the sinus beat that precedes ventricular depolarization

(2) PR interval is the period of time between the beginning of atrial depolarization and the beginning of ventricular depolarization—nml PR interval ≤0.2 ms, which is ≤5 small boxes on the EKG

(3) Q wave is when the INITIAL part of ventricular depolarization is downward, not upward—Q wave is nonpathologic (<1 box = <0.04 ms wide), Q wave is pathologic (>1 box = >0.04 ms wide)

(4) QRS represents ventricular depolarization—nml QRS interval = <0.12 ms (3 small boxes wide)

(5) ST segment represents the beginning of ventricular repolarization—should be isoelectric (neither higher nor lower) with the PR segment

(6) T wave represents the bulk of ventricular repolarization—should be upright

b. Rate

(1) Nml sinus node rate is 60–100 bpm

(2) Tachycardia = >100 bpm

(3) Bradycardia = <60 bpm

Text continues on page 25

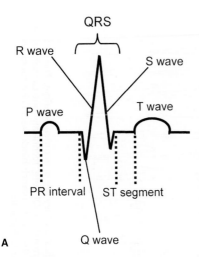

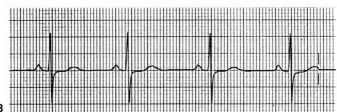

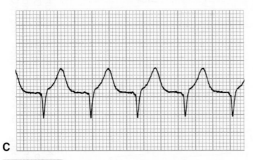

FIGURE 1.2 **P-QRS-T Complex.** *(continued)*

A. Figure of wave form. **B.** Nml sinus rhythm. There is a p before every QRS and a QRS after every p. There are no prolonged intervals or conduction delays. The rate is approximately 60 bpm. **C.** Junctional tachycardia. Note the absence of p waves, indicating no sinus activity. Therefore, the rhythm must be an escape rhythm originating at the AV junction or below. Because the complexes are narrow, this rhythm originates in the junction and not in the ventricle. The rate exceeds 100 bpm (rate is approximately 105 bpm). Therefore, this is a tachycardia originating from the AV junction.

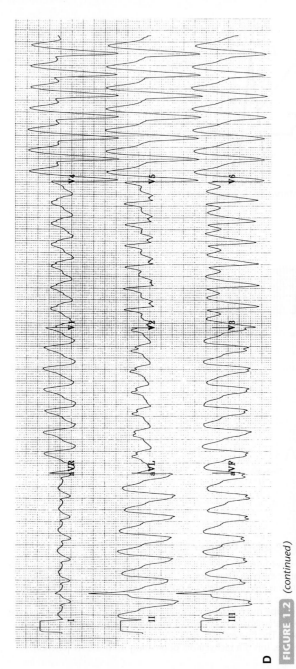

FIGURE 1.2 *(continued)*

D. Ventricular tachycardia. Note lack of p waves, and all complexes are very wide, indicating they are of ventricular origin. The rate is approximately 150 bpm, so this is ventricular tachycardia. Do not miss this on an examination! Of note, technically one cannot be certain that this is not supraventricular tachycardia with a bundle branch block, because the bundle branch block would also cause wide complexes. However, on a step 2 or 3 examination, this EKG will always be ventricular tachycardia.

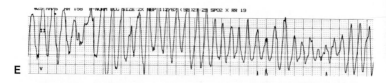

E

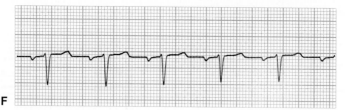

F

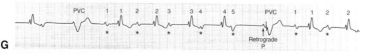

G

FIGURE 1.2 *(continued)*

E. Ventricular fibrillation—torsades de pointes. The wide complexes that vary in amplitude are indicative of ventricular fibrillation. The twisting of the axis and amplitude resulting in increasing and decreasing height, like a ribbon, is consistent with torsades de pointes. **F.** First-degree block. The rhythm is sinus, and the rate is nml. However, the interval between the **beginning** of the p wave and the beginning of the small r wave exceeds 1 large box, meaning that it is >5 mm, or 0.2 ms. This indicates first-degree block. **G.** Second-degree, type 1 (Wenckebach) block. Note how the PR interval becomes progressively longer; that is, the p waves (marked with *asterisks*) become progressively farther apart from each corresponding QRS complex (*numbers above* refer to the same p wave and resulting QRS complex). The fifth p wave occurs during the T wave of the fourth QRS complex, and that p wave is not conducted, so there is no fifth QRS complex. The next complex that appears is actually a premature ventricular contraction (PVC, a ventricular escape beat), with a retrograde p wave in front of it (you know the p wave is retrograde because it is so close to the PVC, and because it is shaped differently from the sinus p waves before and after it). The PVC "resets" the system, and the sinus p waves take over again, with the same increasing PR interval between beats 1 and 2. Incidentally noted is the presence of a bundle branch block (note the rabbit ears in the QRS complexes—more on this to come).

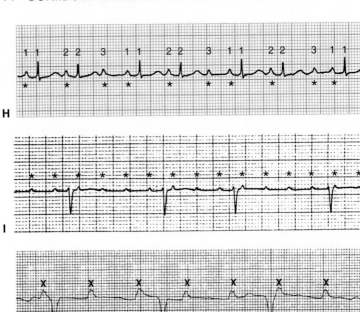

FIGURE 1.2 *(continued)*

H. Second-degree, type 2 (Mobitz) block. P waves again marked by *asterisk,* and *numbers above* refer to paired p waves and QRS complexes. In contrast to Figure 1.2G, note the consistent PR intervals. However, the third p wave in each series is not conducted, resulting in a dropped beat. This is a 3:2 second-degree Mobitz block. **I.** Third-degree block with junctional escape. Note the absence of relationship between the much faster p waves (annotated with *asterisk*) and the slower QRS complexes. By their narrow width and rate (approximately 55), the QRS rhythm is junctional escape. **J.** Third-degree block with ventricular escape. Again there is no relationship between the p waves (annotated with *asterisk*) and the QRS complexes. Here the QRS complexes are very wide and the rate (approximately 40) is slower, indicative of a ventricular escape rhythm.

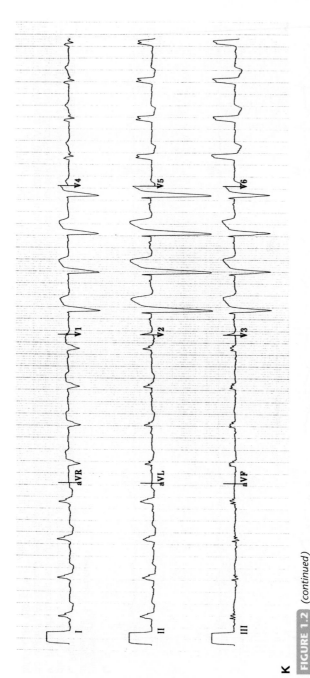

K

FIGURE 1.2 *(continued)*

K. Left bundle branch block (LBBB). This is a classic LBBB EKG. Note the following characteristic features: (i) QRS complex ≥0.12 ms (≥3 small boxes in width); (ii) RSR' (rabbit ears) in leads V5 and V6; (iii) diffuse ST elevation, which is part of the LBBB complex and cannot be used to evaluate risk of MI in the presence of the LBBB.

FIGURE 1.2 (continued)

L. Right bundle branch block (RBBB) + left anterior fascicular block (LAFB) = bifascicular block. This EKG is typical for RBBB: (i) QRS complex >0.12 ms (>3 small boxes in width); (ii) RSR′ pattern (rabbit ears) in leads V_1 and V_2; (iii) deep S wave in lateral leads I, aVL, V_5, and V_6. RBBB often causes a rightward axis. However, in this tracing, there is a left-axis deviation (note that lead I is upright and lead aVF is downward). An unexplained left-axis deviation is diagnostic of LAFB. The combination of block in the RBBB and LAFB is known as bifascicular block.

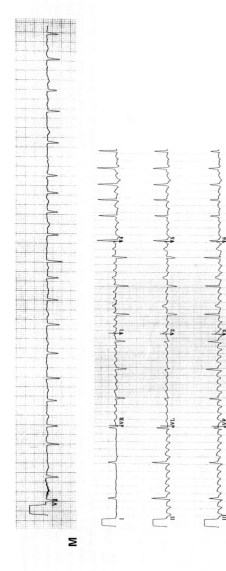

M

N

FIGURE 1.2 *(continued)*

M. Atrial fibrillation. We are no longer dealing with sinus rhythm. Note the absence of p waves and the fact that the QRS complex comes in irregularly irregular frequency, characteristic of atrial fibrillation. N. Atrial flutter. Do not let leads aVR and V_1 fool you. Check out leads II, III, and aVF—the inferior leads. Those look a lot like "sawtooths," don't they? Those are flutter waves, going at a rate of 300 bpm, which is classic for atrial flutter. At the beginning, the ventricular rate is 75 bpm (4:1 block of atrial/ventricular rates). However, note that the ventricular rate speeds up at the end of the tracing (check leads V_4, V_5, V_6). Here, the ventricle is firing at a rate of 150 bpm (2:1 block). This instability in ventricular response to atrial flutter is the reason why this rhythm is more dangerous than atrial fibrillation.

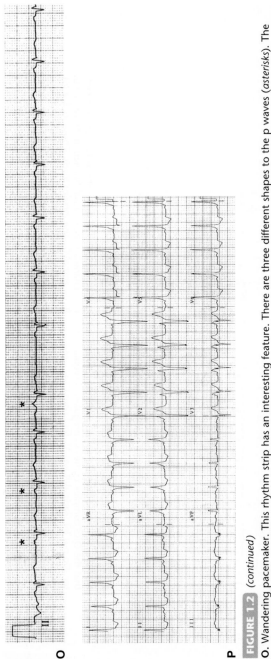

FIGURE 1.2 (continued)

O. Wandering pacemaker. This rhythm strip has an interesting feature. There are three different shapes to the p waves (*asterisks*). The ventricle is being paced by three atrial pacers (probably the SA node and two ectopic pacers). But the ventricular rate is approximately 75 bpm, so this is not a tachycardia. This is a "wandering pacemaker" (slow form of multifocal tachycardia). If the rate were ≥100 bpm, this would be multifocal atrial tachycardia (MFAT). **P.** Wolff–Parkinson–White (WPW) syndrome. The two characteristic features are shown on this tracing: (i) short PR interval (especially clear in leads I and V₁) and (ii) slurring delta wave connecting the P wave to the QRS complex (especially clear in leads I, aVR, aVL, V₄, V₅, V₆). Note also the prominent ST depressions in leads I, II, aVL, and V₄–V₆, highly concerning for anterolateral ischemia.

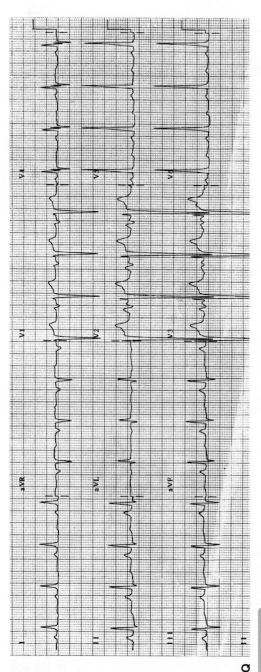

FIGURE 1.2 *(continued)*

Q. Left ventricular hypertrophy (LVH) + left atrial enlargement (LAE) + right atrial enlargement (RAE). R wave in V_5 or V_6 + S wave in V_1 or V_2 ≥35 mm (35 small boxes = 7 large boxes) is diagnostic for LVH. Other LVH criteria (R wave in V_5 ≥25 mm; R wave in aVL ≥11 mm) are not present here, but any one of these criteria is diagnostic, and all do not need to be present. The P waves in lead V_1 are impressively depressed; ≥1 × 1 box depression in the P wave in lead V_1 is diagnostic for LAE. The P waves in lead II are very tall; ≥2.5-mm amplitude of the P wave in lead II is diagnostic for RAE.

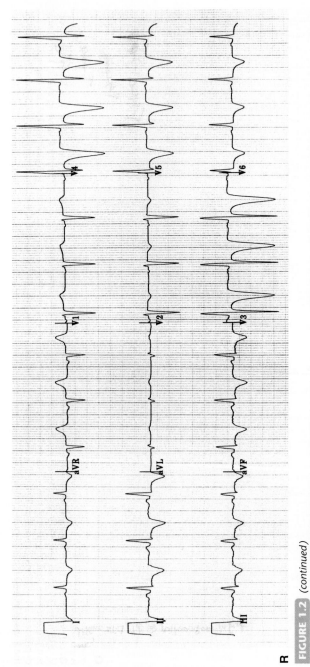

FIGURE 1.2 (continued)

R. Ischemia. Note the deep, symmetric T waves in leads II, III, aVF, V_3–V_6 with ST-segment depression in leads V_3–V_6. This is highly concerning for inferior (II, III, aVF), anterior (V_3–V_4), and lateral (V_5, V_6) ischemia.

R

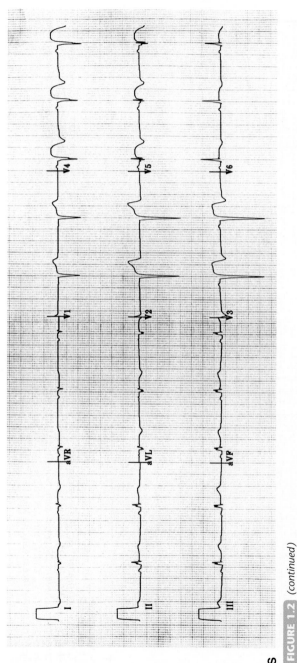

FIGURE 1.2 *(continued)*

S. ST-elevation myocardial infarction (STEMI). Note the prominent ST elevations in leads V_2–V_5. The shape of the ST elevations in leads V_3–V_4 is very much like a "tombstone." You can imagine the letters "RIP" being placed there. This is the classic tombstone sign of STEMI. Note also the prominent Q waves in leads V_1–V_5, demonstrating that the MI occurred a number of hours earlier.

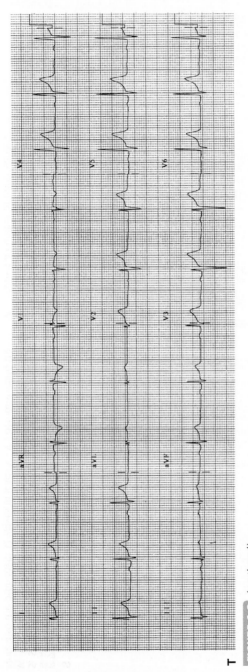

FIGURE 1.2 (continued)

T. "Early repolarization" or "J-point elevation." Not all ST elevations are because of myocardial infarction. The most common cause of ST elevation on EKGs is early repolarization, which is a nml variant that typically is found in young people and in athletes. This tracing was taken from a healthy 29-yr-old man. Note that the ST segments cove gently upward concavely. Draw two dots above the ST segments in leads V_2, V_4, V_5, and V_6 and you will see smiley faces staring back at you, with the dots representing the eyes and the ST segments the lips. The smiley face means no MI.

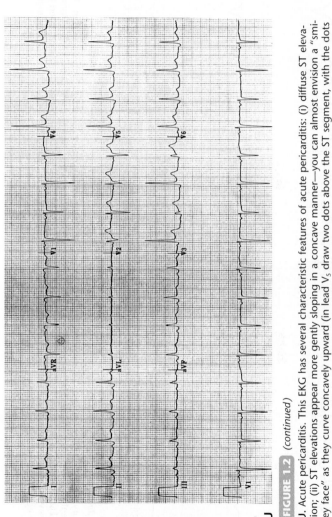

FIGURE 1.2 *(continued)*

U. Acute pericarditis. This EKG has several characteristic features of acute pericarditis: (i) diffuse ST elevation; (ii) ST elevations appear more gently sloping in a concave manner—you can almost envision a "smiley face" as they curve concavely upward (in lead V_5, draw two dots above the ST segment, with the dots being the eyes and the ST segment being the lips); (iii) diffuse PR segment depressions in all leads, with reciprocal PR-segment elevation in aVR; (iv) finally, the classic finding of "electrical alternans" (check leads V_1–V_4, and the rhythm strip at the bottom, which is lead V_1), in which there is a beat-to-beat change in the amplitude of the QRS complex.

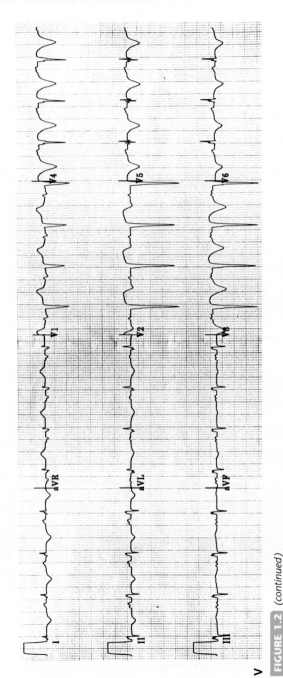

FIGURE 1.2 (continued)

V. Ventricular aneurysm. Yet another cause of ST elevation is a fixed defect in the ventricular wall caused by a prior infarction. This causes the fibrosed segment of the myocardial wall to bulge outward during systole, manifested by ST-segment elevation. EKG is from the same pt whose acute STEMI was shown in Figure 1.2S. This tracing was taken 6 wks after the acute episode, when the pt presented for routine follow-up. Enzymes were checked, and there was no evidence of reinfarction, indicating the likely presence of a ventricular aneurysm, later confirmed by echocardiogram.

c. Rhythm
  (1) Nml sinus rhythm = regular rhythm with a rate of 60–99 where there is a p in front of every QRS and a QRS after every p (Figure 1.2B)
  (2) Junctional rhythm
    (a) Atrioventricular (AV) node starts firing, causing **narrow QRS complexes in the absence of p waves**
    (b) Nml junctional escape rhythm has a rate of 40–60 bpm; junctional rhythm with rate >60 bpm = "accelerated junctional rhythm," junctional rhythm with rate >100 bpm = "junctional tachycardia" (Figure 1.2C)
  (3) Ventricular rhythm
    (a) Ventricle starts firing in the absence of conduction from above
    (b) **Ventricular beats have very wide QRS complexes**
    (c) Nml rate = 20–40 bpm (= ventricular escape rhythm), ventricular rhythm with rate >40 bpm = "accelerated ventricular rhythm," ventricular rhythm with rate >100 bpm = ventricular tachycardia (Figure 1.2D)
    (d) Ventricular fibrillation (v-fib) = chaotic ventricular rhythm (Figure 1.2E); **this is a medical emergency requiring immediate electrical cardioversion!**
    (e) Torsades de pointes ("twisting of the points") = special form of v-fib in which the axis of the waveforms shifts or twists over time, resulting in a ribbon-like pattern (Figure 1.2E)—associated with medications that cause QT prolongation, such as tricyclic antidepressants, antipsychotics, some antiarrhythmics (e.g., quinidine, procainamide), clarithromycin, erythromycin
  (4) Heart blocks
    (a) First-degree AV block—nml sinus rhythm with PR interval ≥0.2 ms (= 5 small boxes or 1 large box; Figure 1.2F)
    (b) Second-degree, type 1 (Wenckebach) block—PR interval elongates from beat to beat until it becomes so long that a beat drops (Figure 1.2G)
    (c) Second-degree, type 2 (Mobitz) block—PR interval fixed, but there are regular nonconducted p waves leading to dropped beats (Figure 1.2H)
    (d) Third-degree block—no relationship between p waves and QRS complexes, typically presents with

junctional escape rhythm (Figure 1.2I) or ventricular escape rhythm (Figure 1.2J)

- (e) Left bundle branch block (LBBB) (Figure 1.2K)
  - (i) QRS complex ≥0.12 ms (≥3 small boxes)
  - (ii) RSR' (rabbit ears) in V5 and V6
  - (iii) Diffuse ST elevation that makes it difficult to diagnose MI
- (f) Right bundle branch block (RBBB) (Figure 1.2L)
  - (i) QRS complex ≥0.12 ms (≥3 small boxes)
  - (ii) RSR' (rabbit ears) in V1 and V2
  - (iii) Deep S waves in lateral leads (I, aVL, V_5, V_6)
- (g) Left anterior fascicular block (LAFB)—presents with an unexplained left-axis deviation (see Figure 1.2L)
- (h) Left posterior fascicular block (LPFB)—presents with an unexplained right-axis deviation
  - (i) Bifascicular block—RBBB + LAFB, appears like RBBB, but axis is leftward instead of rightward (see Figure 1.2L)
- (5) Atrial conduction abnormalities
  - (a) Atrial fibrillation (A-fib)—irregularly irregular QRS complexes with no p waves visible (Figure 1.2M)
  - (b) Atrial flutter–atrial "sawtooth" pattern most prominent in inferior leads, with rate of 200–400 bpm (Figure 1.2N)
  - (c) Atrial ectopy
    - (i) Wandering pacemaker = ≥3 different p waves with a ventricular rate <100 bpm (Figure 1.2O)
    - (ii) Multifocal atrial tachycardia (MFAT) = ≥3 different p waves with a ventricular rate >100 bpm
- (6) Wolff–Parkinson–White syndrome (Figure 1.2P)
  - (a) Caused by a "short-circuit" conducting system that bypasses the AV node and allows re-entrant ventricular tachycardia
  - (b) Short PR interval
  - (c) Delta wave, which appears like a slurring of the upstroke of the r wave
- d. Axis
  - (1) If leads I and aVF are upright, the axis is nml
  - (2) If lead I is upright and aVF is downward, there is a left-axis deviation (axis <−30°)
  - (3) If lead I is downward and aVF is upward, there is a right-axis deviation (axis >90°)

       (4) If leads I and aVF are downward, there is extreme right-axis deviation (axis >180°)

  e. Hypertrophy

       (1) Left atrial enlargement (LAE): >1 × 1 box depression in p wave in lead V_1 (Figure 1.2Q)

       (2) Right atrial enlargement (RAE): >2.5 box height of p wave in lead II (see Figure 1.2Q)

       (3) Left ventricular hypertrophy (LVH): S wave in V_1 + R wave in V_5 or V_6 ≥35 mm OR R wave in V_5 or V_6 ≥25 mm or R wave in lead aVL ≥11 mm (see Figure 1.2Q)

       (4) Right ventricular hypertrophy (RVH): R wave in V_1 >5 mm

  f. Ischemia/infarction

       (1) Ischemia or NSTEMI (subendocardial infarction) presents with deep symmetric T-wave inversions and/or ST depressions ≥1 mm (Figure 1.2R)

       (2) Transmural MI presents with ST elevations = STEMI (Figure 1.2S)

       (3) Differential diagnosis of ST elevations—must distinguish these from STEMI

         (a) Most common cause of ST elevation is "early repolarization" (i.e., "J-point elevation")—concave J point on the tracing is the gentle concave upward slope of the transition from the S wave to the ST segment (Figure 1.2T)

         (b) Pericarditis—characteristics include diffuse ST elevations, diffuse PR depressions, PR elevation in lead aVR, electrical alternans (beat-to-beat change in amplitude of R wave; Figure 1.2U)

         (c) Ventricular aneurysm—characteristics include ST elevations concerning for MI but no symptoms and enzymes negative; echocardiogram confirms the presence of the aneurysm, which occurs at the site of a prior MI (Figure 1.2V)

         (d) Prinzmetal's angina (see Section I.B.6)

2. **Atrial Fibrillation** (see Figure 1.2M)

  a. Most common chronic arrhythmia

  b. Etiologies include ischemia, atrial dilation (often from valve dz), surgery (or any systemic trauma), pulmonary dz, toxicity (e.g., thyrotoxicosis, alcohol intoxication, or withdrawal)

  c. Pulse is **irregularly irregular, classic descriptor of A-fib**

  d. Si/Sx = chest discomfort/palpitations, hypotension/syncope, tachycardia

    e. Complications = diffuse embolization, often to brain, of atrial mural thrombi

    f. Tx

       (1) Rate control with β-blockers, digoxin (not acutely), calcium blockers (e.g., verapamil and diltiazem)

       (2) Convert to nml rhythm (cardioversion) with drugs or electricity

          (a) Drug = IV procainamide (first line), sotalol, or amiodarone

          (b) Electrical → shocks of 100–200 J followed by 360 J

          (c) All pts with A-fib lasting >24 hrs should be anticoagulated with warfarin for 3 wks before electrical cardioversion to prevent embolization during cardioversion

       (3) For recurrence of A-fib post-cardioversion, rate control is the focus—medications to attempt to maintain sinus rhythm add toxicity and do not improve long-term clinical outcome

       (4) Calculate CHADS score to determine if anticoagulation is necessary

          (a) 1 point for **C**HF, **H**TN, **A**ge ≥75 yrs, or **D**iabetes; 2 points for prior **S**troke or TIA

          (b) For 0 points administer aspirin

          (c) For 1 point aspirin or warfarin

          (d) For 2 points or more use warfarin

3. **Atrial Flutter** (see Figure 1.2N)

    a. Atrial tachyarrhythmia that is less stable than A-fib

    b. In flutter, the atrium beats at a **slower** rate than in fibrillation (~250–350 bpm in flutter)

    c. However, the ventricular rate in flutter has the potential to go much faster than the ventricular rate in fibrillation, and flutter is considered a more dangerous, more unstable rhythm—medically slowing the atrial rate can ↑ nodal conduction resulting in an ↑ ventricular rate

    d. **The classic rhythm is an atrial flutter rate of 300 bpm with 2:1 block resulting in a ventricular rate of 150 bpm**

    e. Etiologies and Si/Sx are similar to those of A-fib

    f. Complications include syncope, embolization (as in fibrillation), ischemia, and heart failure

    g. The classic EKG finding in flutter is "sawtooth" pattern on EKG (see Figure 1.2N)

h. Tx

(1) For stable pts slow ventricular rate with diltiazem or β-blockers—avoid use of class I agents such as procainamide, which can result in ↑ ventricular rate as the atrial rate slows

(2) Particularly for patients with low ejection fractions, use digoxin (slow acting so may need to cautiously use diltiazem or β-blocker while waiting for digoxin to kick in)

(3) Cardioversion in a nonemergent setting (e.g., pt is stable) requires anticoagulation for 3 wks prior to prevent embolization

(4) Unstable pts require direct cardioversion, but atrial flutter is easier to convert than fibrillation, so start at 50 J

4. **MFAT**

a. Multiple concurrent pacemakers in the atria, also an irregularly irregular rhythm, usually found in pts with chronic obstructive pulmonary dz (COPD)

b. **EKG → tachycardia with ≥3 distinct P waves present in 1 rhythm strip** (Note: if the pt has ≥3 distinct P waves but is not tachycardic, rhythm = wandering pacemaker)

c. Tx = verapamil; also treat underlying condition

5. **Supraventricular Tachycardia (SVT)**

a. SVT is a "grab bag" of tachyarrhythmias originating "above the ventricle"

b. Pacer can be in atrium or at AV junction, and multiple pacers can be active (MFAT)

c. Very difficult to distinguish ventricular tachycardia from SVT if the pt also has a bundle branch block

d. Tx depends on etiology

(1) Correct electrolyte imbalance, ventricular rate control (digoxin, Ca^{2+}-channel blocker, β-blocker, adenosine) and electrical cardioversion in unstable pts

(2) Attempt carotid massage in pts with paroxysmal SVT

(3) Adenosine breaks >90% of SVT, converting it to sinus rhythm; failure to break a rhythm with adenosine is a potential diagnostic test to rule out SVT

6. **Ventricular Tachycardia (V-tach)** (see Figure 1.2D)

a. Defined as ≥3 consecutive premature ventricular contractions (PVCs)

b. Sustained V-tach lasts a minimum of 30 sec, requires immediate intervention because of risk for onset of v-fib (see later)

    c. If hypotension or no pulse is coexistent → defibrillate and treat as v-fib

    d. Tx depends on symptomatology

      (1) If hypotension or pulseless → emergency electrical defibrillation, 200–300–360 J

      (2) If pt is aSx and not hypotensive, first-line medical Tx is amiodarone or lidocaine, which can convert rhythm to nml

7. **V-fib** (see Figure 1.2E)

    a. Si/Sx = syncope, severe hypotension, sudden death

    b. **Emergent electric countershock is the primary Tx** (very rarely precordial chest thump is effective), converts rhythm 95% of the time (200–300–360 J) if done quickly enough

    c. Second-line Tx is amiodarone or lidocaine

    d. Without Tx, natural course = total failure of cardiac output → death

D. CHF

1. **Etiologies and Definition**

    a. Causes = valve dz, MI (acute and chronic), HTN, anemia, pulmonary embolism (PE), cardiomyopathy, thyrotoxicosis, endocarditis

    b. Definition = cardiac output insufficient to meet systemic demand, can have right-, left-, or both-sided failure

2. **Si/Sx, and Dx**

    a. Left-sided failure Si/Sx due to ↓ cardiac output and ↑ cardiac pressures = **exertional dyspnea, orthopnea, paroxysmal nocturnal dyspnea**, cardiomegaly, rales, S_3 gallop, renal hypoperfusion → ↑ aldosterone production → sodium retention → ↑ total body fluid → worse heart failure

    b. Right-sided failure Si/Sx because of blood pooling "upstream" from R-heart = ↑ jugular venous pressure (JVP), dependent edema, hepatic congestion with transaminitis, fatigue, weight loss, cyanosis

    c. A-fib common in CHF, ↑ risk of embolization

    d. Dx = Si/Sx and echocardiography that reveals ↓ ejection fraction for systolic failure or ↓ cardiac filling from diastolic dysfunction

3. **Tx**

    a. First-line regimen = ACE inhibitor or angiotensin receptor blocker (ARB), β-blocker, diuretics (loop and potassium [K]-sparing)

    b. **ACE inhibitors and ARBs proven to ↓ mortality in CHF**

    c. If pt intolerant of ACE inhibition, use a combination of hydralazine and isosorbide dinitrate, which also ↓ mortality but not as effectively as ACE inhibition

    d. β-blockers

        (1) **Proven to ↓ mortality**

        (2) β-blockers should NEVER be started while the pt is in active failure because they can acutely worsen failure

        (3) Add the β-blockers once the pt is diuresed and on other medicines

    e. **Spironolactone is proven to ↓ mortality in class III or IV CHF**

    f. Loop diuretics (usually furosemide) are almost always used to maintain dry weight in CHF pts

    g. Digoxin does not improve mortality in CHF but does improve Sx and ↓ hospitalizations

    h. Beware of giving loop diuretics without spironolactone (a K^+-sparing diuretic), because in the presence of hypokalemia, digoxin can become toxic at formerly therapeutic doses—digoxin toxicity presents as **SVT with AV block and yellow vision** and can be acutely treated with antidigitalis Fab antibodies (Abs) as well as correction of the underlying potassium deficit

E. **Cardiomyopathy** (Table 1.8)

F. **Valvular Dz**

    1. **Mitral Valve Prolapse (MVP)**

        a. Seen in 7% of population; in vast majority is a benign finding in young people that is aSx and eventually disappears

Table 1.8 Cardiomyopathy

	Dilated	Hypertrophic	Restrictive
Cause	Ischemic, infectious (HIV, Coxsackievirus, Chagas disease), metabolic, drugs (alcohol, doxorubicin, AZT)	Genetic myosin disorder	Amyloidosis, scleroderma, hemochromatosis, glycogen storage dz, sarcoidosis
Si/Sx	R & L heart failure, A-fib, S_3 gallop, mitral regurgitation **Systolic dz**	Exertional syncope, angina, EKG → LVH **Diastolic dz**	Pulmonary HTN, S_4 gallop, EKG → ↓ QRS voltage **Diastolic dz**
Tx	Stop offending agent, once cardiomyopathy onsets, Tx similar to CHF	Implantable cardiac defibrillator to prevent sudden death from arrhythmia	Tx underlying disease if possible

  b. **Murmur: pathologic prolapse → late systolic murmur with midsystolic click (Barlow's syndrome),** predisposing to regurgitation
  c. Dx = clinical, confirm with echocardiography
  d. Tx not required

2. **Mitral Valve Regurgitation (MVR)**
  a. Seen in severe MVP, rheumatic fever, papillary muscle dysfunction (often due to MI) and endocarditis, Marfan's syndrome
  b. Results in dilation of left atrium (LA), ↑ in LA pressure, leading to pulmonary edema/dyspnea
  c. See Table 1.9 for physical findings
  d. Dx = clinical, confirm with echocardiography
  e. Tx = ACE inhibitors, vasodilators, diuretics, consider surgery in severe dz

3. **Mitral Stenosis (MS)**
  a. Almost always because of prior rheumatic fever
  b. ↓ Flow across the mitral valve leads to LAE and eventually to right heart failure
  c. Si/Sx = dyspnea, orthopnea, hemoptysis, pulmonary edema, A-fib
  d. See Table 1.9 for physical findings
  e. Dx = clinical, confirm with echocardiography
  f. Tx
    (1) β-blockers to slow HR, enabling prolongation of flow of blood across the narrowed valve
    (2) Digitalis to slow ventricle in pts with A-fib
    (3) Anticoagulants for embolus prophylaxis
    (4) Surgical valve replacement for uncontrollable dz

4. **Aortic Regurgitation (AR)**
  a. Seen in endocarditis, rheumatic fever, ventricular septal defect (children), congenital bicuspid aorta, 3° syphilis, aortic dissection, Marfan's syndrome, trauma
  b. **There are three murmurs in AR** (Tables 1.9 and 1.10)
  c. AR has numerous classic signs
    (1) **Water Hammer pulse** = wide pulse pressure presenting with forceful arterial pulse upswing with rapid falloff
    (2) **Traube's sign** = pistol-shot bruit over femoral pulse
    (3) **Corrigan's pulse** = unusually large carotid pulsations
    (4) **Quincke's sign** = pulsatile blanching and reddening of fingernails upon light pressure

Table 1.9 Summary of Major Murmurs

Disease	Murmur	Physical Exam
Mitral stenosis	**Diastolic apical rumble** and opening snap	Feel for RV lift 2° to RVH
Mitral valve prolapse	**Late systolic murmur with midsystolic click (Barlow's syndrome)**	Valsalva → click earlier in systole, murmur prolonged
Mitral regurgitation	High-pitched **apical blowing holosystolic murmur radiate to axilla**	Laterally displaced PMI, systolic thrill
Tricuspid stenosis	**Diastolic rumble** often confused with MS	**Murmur louder with inspiration**
Tricuspid regurgitation	High-pitched **blowing holosystolic** murmur at left sternal border	**Murmur louder with inspiration**
Aortic stenosis (AS)	**Midsystolic crescendo-decrescendo murmur at second right interspace, radiates to carotids and apex, with S$_4$ due to atrial kick,** systolic ejection click	**Pulsus parvus et tardus =** peripheral pulses are weak and late compared to heart sounds, systolic thrill second interspace
Aortic sclerosis	Peaks earlier in systole than AS	None
Aortic regurgitation	3 murmurs: • **Blowing early diastolic** at aorta and LSB • **Austin Flint = apical diastolic rumble** like mitral stenosis but no opening snap • Midsystolic flow murmur at base	Laterally displaced PMI, **wide pulse pressure, pulsus bisferiens** (double-peaked arterial pulse): see text for classic physical findings
HCM	Systolic murmur at apex and left sternal border that is poorly transmitted to carotids	**Murmur increases with standing and Valsalva**

LSB, left sternal border; PMI, point of maximum impulse.

(5) **de Musset's sign** = head bobbing caused by carotid pulsations
(6) **Müller's sign** = pulsatile bobbing of the uvula
(7) **Duroziez's sign** = to-and-fro murmur over femoral artery heard best with mild pressure applied to the artery
d. Dx = clinical, confirm by echocardiography

Table 1.10 Physical Exam Differential Diagnosis for Murmurs[a]

Timing	Possible Disease: Differentiating Characteristics			
Midsystolic ("ejection")	**Aortic stenosis/ sclerosis:** crescendo-decrescendo, second right interspace	**Pulmonic stenosis:** second left interspace, EKG → RVH	**Any high low state → "flow murmur": aortic regurgitation** (listen for other AR murmurs), **A-S defect** (fixed split S₂), **anemia, pregnancy, adolescence**	
Late systolic	**Aortic stenosis:** worse dz → later peak	**Mitral valve prolapse:** apical murmur	**Hypertrophic cardiomyopathy:** murmur louder with Valsalva	
Holosystolic	**Mitral regurgitation:** radiates to axilla	**V-S defect:** diffuse across precordium	**Tricuspid regurgitation:** louder with inspiration	
Early diastolic	**Aortic regurgitation:** blowing aortic murmur		**Pulmonic regurgitation:** Graham Steell murmur	
Middiastolic	**Mitral stenosis:** opening snap, no change with inspiration	**Aortic regurgitation** (Austin Flint murmur): apical, resembles MS	**A-S defect:** listen for fixed spit S₂, diastolic rumble	**Tricuspid stenosis:** louder with inspiration
Continuous	**Patent ductus** machinery murmur loudest in back	**Mammary soufflé:** harmless, heard in pregnancy due to ↑ flow in mammary artery	**Coarctation of aorta:** upper/ lower extremity pulse discrepancy	**A-V fistula**

[a]The authors thank Dr. J. Michael Criley and Dr. Richard D. Spellberg for assistance with creation of this table. A-S defect, atrial-septal defect; A-V, arterio-venous; V-S defect, ventricular-septal defect.

e. Tx

   (1) ↓ Afterload with ACE inhibitors or vasodilators (e.g., hydralazine)

   (2) Consider valve replacement if dz is fulminant or refractory to drugs

5. **Aortic Stenosis (AS)**
   a. Frequently congenital, also seen in rheumatic fever; mild degenerative calcification = AS that is a normal part of aging
   b. **Si/Sx** = classic triad of syncope, angina, exertional dyspnea
   c. Dx = clinical, confirm by echocardiography
   d. Tx is surgery for all symptomatic pts who can tolerate it
      (1) Either mechanical or bioprosthesis required; pt anticoagulated chronically after surgery
      (2) Use balloon valvuloplasty of aortic valve for poor surgical candidates
      (3) Pts need endocarditis prophylaxis prior to procedures
      (4) Be cautious with β-blockers or afterload reducers (vasodilators and ACE inhibitors)—peripheral vasculature is maximally constricted to maintain BP, so administration of such agents can cause pt to go into shock

6. **Hypertrophic Cardiomyopathy (HCM)**
   a. Ventricular septum hypertrophies inferior to the aorta
   b. Septal wall impinges upon anterior leaflet (rarely posterior leaflet) of mitral valve during systole, resulting in outflow obstruction—valsalva decreases the obstruction resulting in increased flow across the valve and a louder murmur
   c. Also previously known as hypertrophic obstructive cardiomyopathy and idiopathic hypertrophic subaortic stenosis

7. **Tricuspid and Pulmonary Valve Diseases**
   a. Both undergo fibrosis in carcinoid syndrome
   b. Tricuspid stenosis → **diastolic rumble easily confused with MS, differentiate from MS by ↑ loud with inspiration**
   c. Tricuspid regurgitation → holosystolic murmur differentiated from MS by being louder with inspiration; look for jugular and hepatic systolic pulsations
   d. Pulmonary stenosis → dz of children or in adults with carcinoid syndrome, with midsystolic ejection murmur
   e. Pulmonary regurgitation → develops 2° to pulmonary HTN, endocarditis, or carcinoid syndrome, because of valve ring widening; **Graham Steell murmur** = diastolic murmur at left sternal border, mimicking AR murmur
   f. Tx for stenosis = balloon valvuloplasty; valve replacement rarely done

8. **Endocarditis**
   a. Acute endocarditis usually is caused by *Staphylococcus aureus*

b. Subacute dz (insidious onset, Sx less severe) usually caused by viridans group *Streptococcus* (oral flora), other *Streptococcus* spp., *Enterococcus,* and HACEK bacteria: *Haemophilus, Aggregatibacter* (formerly *Actinobacillus*), *Cardiobacterium, Eikenella, Kingella*

c. Marantic endocarditis is due to CA seeding of heart valves during metastasis—very poor Px, malignant emboli → cerebral infarcts

d. Most common cause of culture-negative endocarditis is antibiotic treatment before drawing blood cultures, other causes = Q fever, Whipple's disease, *Bartonella*

e. Prosthetic valve endocarditis often caused by coagulase negative *S. aureus*

f. Systemic lupus erythematosus (SLE) causes **Libman–Sacks endocarditis**

g. Si/Sx = fevers, splenomegaly, **splinter hemorrhages** in fingernails, **Osler's nodes** (painful red nodules on digits), **Roth spots** (retinal hemorrhages with clear central areas), **Janeway lesions** (dark macules on palms/soles), conjunctival petechiae, brain/kidney/splenic abscesses → focal neurologic findings/hematuria/abd or shoulder pain

h. Dx based upon the Duke criteria (Table 1.11)

i. Tx = prolonged antibiotics, 4–6 wks typically required (2 wks for uncomplicated *S. viridans* endocarditis if aminoglycosides are added to beta-lactam therapy)

j. Empiric Tx often is a combination of a vancomycin for methicillin-resistant *S. aureus* (MRSA), oxacillin for methicillin-susceptible *S. aureus* (MSSA), and third-generation cephalosporin for streptococcal species; then Tx is tailored to the organism cultured from blood

Table 1.11 Duke Criteria for Endocarditis Diagnosis[a]	
Major criteria	1. ⊕ Blood cultures growing of common organisms (e.g., *S. aureus, Strep,* HACEK) 2. ⊕ Echocardiogram (transthoracic 60% sensitive, transesophageal 95% sensitive)
Minor criteria	1. Presence of predisposing condition (i.e., valve abnormality) 2. Fever >38°C 3. Embolic disease (e.g., splenic, renal, hepatic, cerebral) 4. Immunologic phenomena (i.e., Roth spots, Osler's nodes) 5. ⊕ Blood culture but only 1 bottle, or rare organisms cultured

[a]Criteria positive 2 major or 1 major + 3 minor, or 5 minor criteria are met.

k. Surgery required for valve ring abscess, CHF from a dysfunctional valve, multiple systemic emboli occur after initiation of antibiotic Tx, if the organism is very difficult to treat (i.e., vancomycin-resistant enterococci [VRE], multidrug resistant *Pseudomonas, Aspergillus,* etc.), for prosthetic valve endocarditis, or if the vegetation is >1 cm in diameter

9. **Rheumatic Fever/Heart Dz**

   a. Presents usually in 5- to 15-yr-old pts after group A *Streptococcus* infxn

   b. Dx = Jones criteria (two major and one minor)

   c. Major criteria **(mnemonic: J ♥ NES)**

   (1) **J**oints (migratory polyarthritis), responds to nonsteroidal anti-inflammatory drugs (NSAIDs)

   (2) **♥C**arditis (pancarditis, Carey Coombs murmur = mid-diastolic)

   (3) **N**odules (subcutaneous)

   (4) **E**rythema marginatum (serpiginous skin rash)

   (5) **S**ydenham's chorea (face, tongue, upper-limb chorea)

   d. Minor criteria = fever, ↑ erythrocyte sedimentation rate (ESR), arthralgia, long EKG PR interval

   e. In addition to Jones criteria, need evidence of prior strep infxn by either culture or ⊕ antistreptolysin O (ASO) Ab titers

   f. Tx = penicillin

G. **Pericardial Dz**

   1. **Pericardial Fluid**

      a. Pericardial effusion can result from any dz causing systemic edema

      b. Hemopericardium is blood in the pericardial sac, often 2° to trauma, metastatic CA, viral/bacterial infxns

      c. Both can lead to cardiac tamponade

      (1) **Classic Beck's triad: distant heart sounds, distended jugular veins, hypotension**

      (2) **Look for pulsus paradoxus, which is ≥10 mm Hg fall in BP during nml inspiration**

      (3) EKG may show **electrical alternans**, which is beat-to-beat alternating height of QRS complex (see Figure 1.2U)

      d. Dx = clinical, confirm with echocardiography

      e. Tx = immediate pericardiocentesis in tamponade; otherwise, treat the underlying condition and allow the fluid to resorb

2. **Pericarditis**

   a. Caused by bacterial, viral, or fungal infxns, also in generalized serositis 2° to rheumatoid arthritis (RA), SLE, scleroderma, uremia

   b. Si/Sx = retrosternal pain relieved when sitting up, often following upper respiratory infxn (URI), not affected by activity or food, listen for pleural friction rub

   c. **EKG → ST elevation in all leads**, also see PR depression (see Figure 1.2U)

   d. Dx = clinical, confirm with echocardiography

   e. Tx = NSAIDs for viral, antimicrobial agents for more bacterial/fungal dz, pericardiectomy for thickened pericardium after chronic infection

II. Pulmonary

A. **Hypoxemia**

   1. **DDx** (Table 1.12)

   $$PAO_2 = FIO_2 (P_{breath} + P_{H2O}) - (PaCO_2/R)$$

   At sea level: $FIO_2 = 0.21$, $P_{H2O} = 47$, $P_{breath} = 760$:

   $$PAO_2 = 150 - (PaCO_2/R)$$

   $PaCO_2$ is measured by lab analysis of arterial blood, $R = 0.8$

   2. **Causes**

   a. Low inspired FIO_2 most often caused by high altitude

   b. Hypoventilation

   (1) **Hallmark is a rise in CO_2**

   (2) Can be because of hypopnea (↓ respiratory rate) or ↓ vital capacity

Table 1.12 Five Mechanisms of Hypoxemia

Cause	PCO₂	PA-aO₂[a]	Effect of O₂	DLCO	Tx
↓ FIO₂	Nml	Nml	⊕	Nml	O₂
Hypoventilation	↑	Nml	⊕	Nml	O₂
Diffusion impairment	Nml	↑	⊕	↓	O₂
V/Q mismatch	↑/Nml	↑	⊕	Nml	O₂
Shunt	↑/Nml	↑	—	Nml	Reverse cause

[a]PAO_2 gradient (PA-aO₂), defined as PO_2 in **a**lveoli minus PO_2 in **a**rteries.
Normal gradient = 10, ↑ by 5–6 per decade above age 50.

Algorithm 1.1

HYPOXEMIA[a]

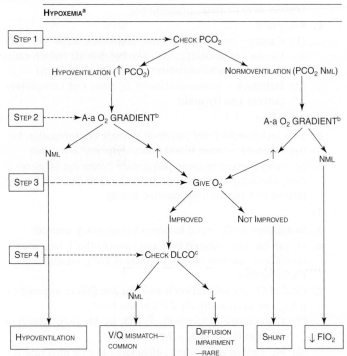

STEP 1 ----------------------------→ CHECK PCO₂

HYPOVENTILATION (↑ PCO₂)   NORMOVENTILATION (PCO₂ NML)

STEP 2 --------→ A-a O₂ GRADIENT[b]   A-a O₂ GRADIENT[b]

NML   ↑   ↑   NML

STEP 3 -------------------------------→ GIVE O₂

IMPROVED   NOT IMPROVED

STEP 4 --------------------------→ CHECK DLCO[c]

NML   ↓

| HYPOVENTILATION | V/Q MISMATCH—COMMON | DIFFUSION IMPAIRMENT—RARE | SHUNT | ↓ FIO₂ |

[a] The authors thank Dr. Arian Torbati for his assistance with this algorithm.

[b] A-a O₂ gradient = difference in alveolar and arterial O₂ concentrations.

[c] DLCO = diffusion limited carbon monoxide, a measurement of diffusion capacity.

    (3) Hypopnea causes = CNS dz (e.g., because of narcotics, trauma, infxn, etc.)

    (4) ↓ Vital capacity causes = chest wall neuromuscular dz (e.g., amyotrophic lateral sclerosis, kyphoscoliosis, etc.), airflow obstruction (e.g., sleep apnea), or any parenchymal lung dz

  c. Diffusion impairment

    (1) Causes = ↑ diffusion path (fibrosis) or ↓ blood transit time through lung (↑ cardiac output, anemia)

    (2) Hallmark = ↓ carbon monoxide diffusing capacity (DLCO)

    (3) DLCO is increased in conditions increasing amount of blood in the lung, for example, polycythemia and pulmonary hemorrhage

    d. Ventilation–perfusion (V/Q) inequality causes = PE, paren-
chymal lung dz (e.g., pneumonia)

    e. R–L shunt

       (1) Causes = pulmonary edema, atelectasis, atrial and ven-
tricular septal defects, and chronic liver dz (which causes
pulmonary arteriovenous malformations to form)

       (2) **Hallmark** = administration of O_2 **does not completely
correct the hypoxia**

3. **Presentation**

    a. Sx = tachycardia (very sensitive; primary compensation for
hypoxia is to ↑ tissue blood flow), dyspnea/tachypnea

    b. Si = rales present in some pulmonary parenchymal disor-
ders, clubbing/cyanosis (not just in lung dz but can be correlated to long-term hypoxemic states)

4. **Tx**

    a. In addition to O_2, need to correct underlying disorder

    b. O_2 can be administered by nasal cannula (NC), face mask,
continuous positive airway pressure (CPAP), intubation/
tracheostomy

    c. Goal of O_2 administration is to ↑ the fraction of inspired O_2
(FIO_2), which is normally 21% at sea level

       (1) General rule: 1 L/min O_2 ↑, FIO_2 by 3% (e.g., giving pt
1 L/min $O_2 \rightarrow FIO_2$ = 24%)

       (2) NC cannot administer >40% FIO_2, even if flow rate is
>7 L/min

       (3) Face mask ↑ maximum FIO_2 to 50% to 60%; nonre-
breather face mask = maximum FIO_2 to >60%

       (4) CPAP = tightly fitting face mask connected to generator
that creates continuous positive pressure, can ↑ maximum FIO_2 to 80%

       (5) Intubation/tracheostomy = maximum FIO_2 to 100%

    d. **Remember that ↑ FIO_2 will not completely correct hypox-
emia caused by R–L shunt!** (Because alveoli are not venti-
lated, and blood will not come in close contact with O_2)

    e. O_2 toxicity seen with FIO_2 >50% to 60% for >48 hrs pres-
ents with neurologic dz and acute respiratory distress syndrome (ARDS)-like findings

B. **COPD** (Table 1.13)

**↓ Forced expiratory volume (FEV)/forced vital capacity (FVC)
and nml/↑ total lung capacity (TLC)**

(FEC at 1 sec/FVC and TLC)

Table 1.13 Chronic Obstructive Pulmonary Disease (COPD)

Disease	Characteristics	Tx
Emphysema (pink puffer)	• **Dilation of air spaces with alveolar wall destruction** • **Smoking is by far the most common cause,** α_1-antitrypsin deficiency causes **panacinar** disease • Si/Sx = hypoxia, hyperventilation, barrel chest, **classic pursed lips breathing,** ↓ breath sounds • CXR → loss of lung markings and **lung hyperinflation** • Dx = clinical	• Ambulatory O_2 including home O_2 • Stop smoking!!! • Bronchodilators • Steroid pulses for acute desaturations • Antibiotics may be considered for fever or change in sputum (purulent)
Chronic bronchitis (blue bloater)	• Defined as **productive cough on most days during ≥3 consecutive mo for ≥2 consecutive yr** • Si/Sx = as per emphysema but **hypoxia is more severe,** plus pulmonary hypertension with right ventricular hypertrophy, distended neck veins, hepatomegaly • Dx clinical, confirmed by lung biopsy → ↑ Reid index (gland layer is >50% of total bronchial wall thickness)	As per emphysema
Asthma	• Bronchial hyperresponsiveness → **reversible bronchoconstriction** due to smooth muscle contraction • Usually starts in childhood, in which case it often resolves by age 12, but can start in adulthood • Si/Sx = episodic dyspnea and **expiratory wheezing, reversible with bronchodilation** • Dx = ≥10% ↑ in FEV with bronchodilator therapy • Status asthmaticus (refractory attack lasting for days, can cause death) is a major complication	• Albuterol/Atrovent inhalers are mainstay • Add inhaled steroids for improved long-term control • Pulse with steroids for acute attacks • Intubate as needed to protect airway

(continued)

Table 1.13	*Continued*	
Disease	**Characteristics**	**Tx**
Bronchiectasis	• Permanent abnormal dilation of broncholes commonly due to cystic fibrosis, chronic infxn (often tuberculosis, fungal infxn, or lung abscess), or obstruction (e.g., tumor) • Si/Sx = foul breath, purulent sputum, hemoptysis, CXR → **tram-track lung markings,** CT → thickened bronchial walls with dilated airways • Dx = clinical with radiologic support	• Ambulatory O_2 • Aggressive antibiotic use for frequent infections • Consider lung transplant for long-term cure

C. **Restrictive Lung Dz and Pleural Effusion** (Tables 1.14 and 1.15)

NML = FEV/FVC and ↓ **TLC** (Figure 1.3)

D. **Pulmonary Vascular Dz**

   1. **Pulmonary Edema and ARDS** (Figure 1.4)

   a. Si/Sx = dyspnea, tachypnea, resistant hypoxia, diffuse alveolar infiltrate

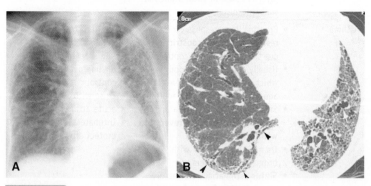

FIGURE 1.3

A. Reticular and honeycomb pattern in a 73-yr-old woman with idiopathic pulmonary fibrosis. Chest radiograph shows asymmetric fine reticular pattern with basal honeycombing. **B.** Computed tomography shows left-sided predominant reticular abnormality with traction bronchiectasis (*white arrows*) and peripheral subpleural rows of honeycomb cysts (*black arrowheads*). (From Crapo JD, Glassroth J, Karlinsky JB, et al. *Baum's textbook of pulmonary diseases,* 7th Ed. Philadelphia, PA: Lippincott Williams & Wilkins, 2004.)

Table 1.14   Diagnosis and Treatment of Restrictive Lung Disease

Disease	Characteristics	Tx
↓ Lung tissue	• Causes = atelectasis, airway obstruction (tumor, foreign body), surgical excision	• Ambulate pt • Incentive spirometer to encourage lung expansion • Remove foreign body/tumor
Parenchymal disease	• Causes = inflammatory (e.g., vasculitis and sarcoidosis), idiopathic pulmonary fibrosis, chemotherapy (the killer **B's**, **b**usulfan and **b**leomycin), amiodarone, radiation, chronic infections (TB, fungal), and toxic inhalation (e.g., asbestos and silica) • Dx = clinical, biopsy to rule out infection	• Antibiotics for chronic infection • Steroids for vasculitis, sarcoidosis, and toxic inhalations
Interstitial fibrosis	• Chronic injury caused by asbestos, oxygen toxicity, organic dusts, chronic infection (e.g., TB, fungi), idiopathic pulmonary fibrosis, and collagen-vascular dz • CXR → **"honeycomb" lung** (Figure 1.4)	• Ambulatory O_2 • Steroids for collagen-vascular dz • Add PEEP to reduce FIO_2 for O_2 toxicity
Extrapulmonary disease	• Neuromuscular dz (e.g., multiple sclerosis, kyphoscoliosis, amyotrophic lateral sclerosis, Guillain–Barré, spinal cord trauma) • ↑ Diaphragm pressure (e.g., pregnancy, obesity, ascites)	Supportive

Pleural effusion	• ↑ Fluid in the pleural space, transudative or exudative
	• Presents on CXR with blunting of the costophrenic angle and causes dullness to percussion, decreased tactile fremitus, and decreased breath sounds on exam
	• Transudate
	  ◊ **Low protein content** due to ↓ oncotic pressure
	  ◊ Causes = CHF, nephrotic syndrome, hepatic cirrhosis
	• Exudate
	  ◊ High protein content due to ↑ hydrostatic pressure
	  ◊ Causes = malignancy, pneumonia ("parapneumonic effusion"), collagen-vascular dz, pulmonary embolism
		Thoracentesis (see later)

Table 1.15 Lab Analysis of Pleural Effusions

Study	Transudate	Exudate
Protein	≤3 g/dL (≤0.5 of serum)	>3 g/dL[a] (>0.5 of serum)
LDH	≤200 IU/L (≤0.6 of serum)	>200 IU/L[a] (>0.6 of serum)
pH	≥7.2	<7.2 (if ≤7.0 = empyema)
Gram stain	No organisms	Any organism → parapneumonic
Cell count	WBC ≤1,000	WBC >1,000 (lymphocytes → TB)
Glucose	≥50 mg/dL	<50 mg/dL → infxn, neoplasm, collagen-vascular dz
Cholesterol	<50 mg/dL—This can distinguish a true transudate from a pseudoexudate, which is a transudate (e.g., from CHF) that is converted into the appearance of an exudate by diuresis, leading to artificially increased concentration of protein and LDH in the fluid—cholesterol is not increased by diuresis	>50 mg/dL
Amylase	↑ in pancreatitis, esophageal rupture, malignancy	
RF	Titer >1:320 → highly indicative for rheumatoid arthritis	
ANA	Titer >1:160 → highly indicative for SLE	

[a]Either of these findings rules out transudative effusion, rules in exudative effusion.

   b. Differential for pulmonary edema
     (1) **If pulmonary capillary wedge pressure <12** = ARDS
     (2) **If pulmonary capillary wedge pressure >15** = cardiogenic
   c. Tx = O_2, diuretics, positive end-expiratory pressure (PEEP) ventilation
   d. Purpose of PEEP
     (1) Helps prevent airway collapse in a failing lung
     (2) Expands alveoli for better diffusion, resulting in maintained lung volume (↑ functional residual capacity) and ↓ shunting

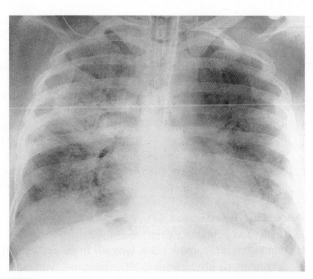

Adult respiratory distress syndrome (ARDS). There is widespread consolidation of the lungs. This pt had experienced extensive trauma to the limbs. (From Berg D. *Advanced clinical skills and physical diagnosis.* Oxford: Blackwell Science, 1999, with permission.)

2. **PE**
   a. Ninety-five percent of emboli are from leg deep venous thrombosis (DVT)
   b. Si/Sx = swollen, painful leg, sudden dyspnea/tachypnea, tachycardia, hemoptysis—**often no Sx at all; most emboli are clinically silent**
   c. Risk factors = **Virchow's triad** = endothelial cell trauma, **stasis, hypercoagulable states** (e.g., nephrotic syndrome, antiphospholipid syndrome, disseminated intravascular coagulation [DIC], tumor, postpartum amniotic fluid exposure, antithrombin III deficiency, protein C or S deficiency, factor V Leiden deficiency, oral contraceptives, smoking)
   d. PE can cause lung infarctions, presenting with pleuritic chest pain, hemoptysis, and "Hampton's hump" on CXR, a wedge-shaped opacification at distal edges of lung fields
   e. EKG findings
      (1) Classically (but rarely) → S wave in I, Q in III, inverted T in III ($S_I Q_{III} T_{III}$)
      (2) **Most common finding is simply sinus tachycardia**

  f. Dx = leg US to check for DVT, **spiral CT of chest and ventilation/perfusion (V/Q) scan best to rule out PE,** pulmonary angiography (gold standard)

  g. Tx = prevention of subsequent emboli with low-molecular-weight heparin, fondaparinux (factor X selective inhibitor), heparin drip, or inferior vena cava (IVC) filter, use tPA thrombolysis in PE with hemodynamic compromise

  h. Patients require ≥3 mos of anticoagulation with warfarin for a provoked PE with reversible cause; ≥6–12 mos for first unprovoked PE with no identified reversible cause (consider even longer if low risk of bleeding); chronic, possibly lifelong for recurrent episode or an irreversible underlying cause

 3. **Pulmonary Hypertension**

  a. Defined as pulmonary pressure ≥¼ systemic

  b. Primary dz is idiopathic (rare, typically in young women)

  c. Secondary dz occurs from COPD, collagen-vascular dz, interstitial restrictive diseases, CHF, or HIV

  d. Si/Sx: dyspnea, severe hypoxia, right heart failure

  e. Dx = echocardiogram, confirm with heart catheterization

  f. Tx = home O_2 and try intravenous or inhaled prostacyclin or endothelin antagonist

E. **Respiratory Tract CA**

 1. **Epidemiology**

  a. **#1 cause of CA deaths and second most frequent CA**

  b. Can only be seen on X-rays if >1 cm in size; usually by that time they have already metastasized, **so X-rays are not a good screening tool**

  c. Si/Sx = cough, hemoptysis, hoarseness (recurrent laryngeal nerve paralysis), weight loss, fatigue, recurrent pneumonia

 2. **Parenchymal Lung CA** (Table 1.16)

 3. **Other CA Syndromes**

  a. **Superior sulcus tumor (Pancoast tumor)** (Figure 1.5A)

   (1) **Horner's syndrome** (ptosis, miosis, anhydrosis) by damaging the sympathetic cervical ganglion in the lower neck (Figure 1.5B), often associated with Pancoast tumor

   (2) **Superior vena cava (SVC) syndrome** = obstructed SVC → facial swelling, cyanosis, and dilation of veins of head and neck

Table 1.16 Parenchymal Lung Cancers

Cancer	Characteristics

Adenocarcinoma	• **Most frequent lung CA in nonsmokers**
	• **Presents in subpleura and lung periphery**
	  ◊ Presents in preexisting scars, "scar cancer"
	  ◊ Carcinoembryonic antigen (CEA) ⊕, used to follow Tx, not for screening due to poor specificity

Bronchoalveolar carcinoma	• Subtype of adenocarcinoma **not related to smoking** • **Presents in lung periphery**
Large cell carcinoma	• **Presents in lung periphery** • Highly anaplastic, undifferentiated cancer • Poor prognosis
Squamous cell carcinoma	• **Central hilar masses arising from bronchus** • **Strong link to smoking** • **Causes hypercalcemia due to secretion of PTHrp** (parathyroid hormone-related peptide)

Small cell (oat cell) carcinoma	• **Usually has central hilar location**
	• **Often already metastatic at Dx, very poor Px**
	• **Strong link to smoking (99% are smokers)**
	• Associated with Lambert–Eaton syndrome
	• Causes numerous endocrine syndromes
	  ◊ ACTH secretion (cushingoid)
	  ◊ Secretes ADH, causing SIADH

Bronchial carcinoid tumors	• Carcinoid syndrome = serotonin (5-HT) secretion • **Si/Sx = recurrent diarrhea, skin flushing, asthmatic wheezing, and carcinoid heart dz** • Dx by ↑ 5-HIAA metabolite in urine • Tx = methysergide, a 5-HT antagonist
Lymphangio leiomyomatosis	• Neoplasm of lung smooth muscle → cystic obstructions of bronchioles, vessels, and lymph • **Almost always seen in menstruating women** • Classic presentation = **pneumothorax** • Tx = progesterone or lung transplant

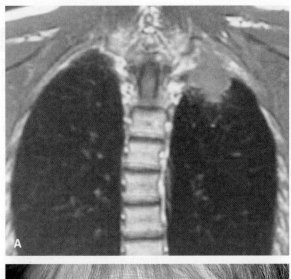

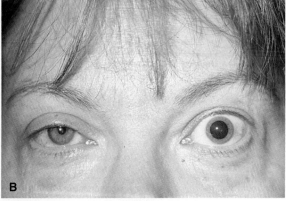

FIGURE 1.5

A. Pancoast tumor. This CA of the lung can be seen invading the root of the neck on this coronal MRI scan (T1-weighted). **B.** Horner's syndrome. The right eye has ptosis and miosis (compare pupil size with the dilated left pupil). (From Tasman W, Jaeger E. *The Wills eye hospital atlas of clinical ophthalmology,* 2nd Ed. Baltimore: Lippincott Williams & Wilkins, 2001.)

> b. Small cell CA can cause a **myasthenia gravis (MG)-like condition known as the Lambert–Eaton syndrome** because of induction of Abs to tumor that cross-reacts with presynaptic calcium (Ca) channel

Table 1.17 Mediastinal Tumors (Figure 1.6)

Anterior[a]	Middle	Posterior
Thymoma	Lymphoma	Neuroblastoma
Thyroid tumor	Pericardial cyst	Schwannoma
Teratoma	Bronchial cyst	Neurofibroma
Terrible lymphoma		
Tx = excision for all, add radiation/chemotherapy as needed		

[a]The four T's.

    c. Renal cell CA metastatic to lung can cause 2° polycythemia by ectopic production of erythropoietin (EPO)

F. **Mediastinal Tumors** (Table 1.17; Figure 1.6)

G. **Tuberculosis (TB)**

  1. **Primary TB**

    a. Classically affects lower lobes (bacilli deposited in dependent portion of lung during inspiration)

    b. Usually aSx

    c. **Classic radiologic finding is "Ghon complex"** = calcified nodule at primary focus ⊕ calcified hilar lymph nodes

  2. **Secondary (Reactivation) TB**

    a. Reactivates in **apical lung** due to ↑ O_2 tension in upper lobes

    b. Si/Sx = insidious fevers, night sweats, weight loss, cough, hemoptysis, upper lobe infiltration, scarring, and/or cavities on CXR (Figure 1.7)

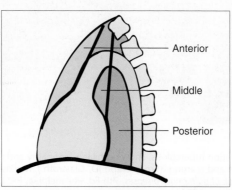

FIGURE 1.6 **Mediastinal compartments.**

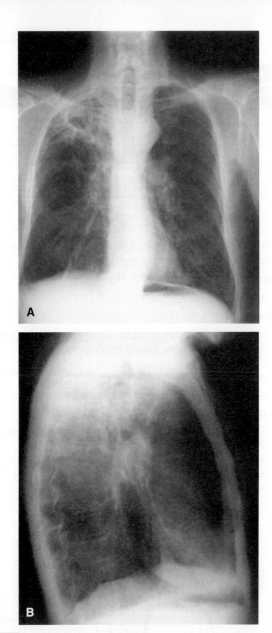

FIGURE 1.7

CXR in reactivation tuberculosis, showing hilar adenopathy and right upper lobe cavitation and scarring. (From Crapo JD, Glassroth J, Karlinsky JB, et al. *Baum's textbook of pulmonary diseases,* 7th Ed. Philadelphia, PA: Lippincott Williams & Wilkins, 2004.)

c. Risk factors = HIV, imprisonment, homelessness, malnourishment, geography (immigrants from Latin America, Africa, Eastern Europe, Asia except for Japan are all high risk)

3. **Miliary (Disseminated) TB**
   a. An acute, hematogenous **dissemination involving any organ**
   b. Often in pts with immune deficiency
   c. Pts appear acutely ill and toxic on top of chronic illness
   d. CXR shows a fine, millet seedlike appearance (i.e., micronodular infiltrates) throughout all the lung fields (Figure 1.8)

4. Classic Chronic Extrapulmonary Reactivation Syndromes
   a. Pott's dz = TB of spine; presents with multiple compression fractures
   b. Scrofula = TB causing massive cervical lymphadenopathy

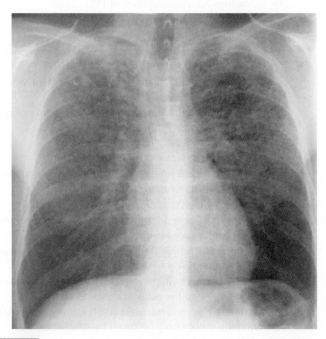

FIGURE 1.8

CXR showing miliary tuberculosis of the lung. (From Crapo JD, Glassroth J, Karlinsky JB, et al. *Baum's textbook of pulmonary diseases,* 7th Ed. Philadelphia, PA: Lippincott Williams & Wilkins, 2004.)

    c. Terminal ideal inflammation and colitis; mimicking Crohn's disease

    d. Serous dz = chronic lymphocyte-predominant effusions of pleural space, pericardial space (associated with chronic constrictive pericarditis), or peritoneum (lymphocyte-predominant ascites)

    e. Meningitis = chronic, lymphocyte predominant pleocytosis in cerebrospinal fluid (CSF)

5. **Dx and Tx**

    a. Latent infxn

      (1) Defined by positive purified protein derivative (PPD) or interferon-γ (IFN-γ) production in peripheral blood tests (e.g., QuantiFERON test)

      (2) No Si/Sx of active dz and no active dz on CXR

      (3) PPD and blood IFN-γ tests are **screening tests for latent infxn,** not Dx tests for active TB

      (4) Guidelines for interpretation of PPD

        (a) ≥5-mm induration is positive if the pt:

          (i) Has HIV

          (ii) Has been in close contact with someone with active TB

          (iii) Has fibrotic changes on CXR consistent with old TB

          (iv) Is taking immunosuppressive medicines (e.g., >15 mg/day of prednisone for >1 mo, cyclosporine, etc.)

        (b) ≥10-mm induration is positive if the pt:

          (i) Is a recent immigrant from a high-risk country (most developing countries)

          (ii) Is an injection drug user

          (iii) Works or resides in a prison/jail, nursing home, health care facility, or homeless shelter

          (iv) Has a chronic debilitating illness such as renal failure, CA, or DM

        (c) ≥15-mm induration is positive test if the pt does not meet any of the above categories

      (5) Tx of latent infxn is isoniazid (INH) × 9 mos (alternate regimens should only be given by specialists)

    b. Active infxn

      (1) To reiterate: **PPD is not intended as a Dx test for active TB**—it is commonly falsely negative in pts with active dz, and a ⊕ test only indicates latent infxn, not

active dz; thus, it is neither sensitive nor specific for active dz

(2) Active infxn is Dx based on three components: clinical assessment, CXR, and sputum (or other body fluid if extrapulmonary dz is considered)

  (a) Clinical indicators of active dz include subacute/chronic cough, night sweats, weight loss, hemoptysis, etc.

  (b) CXR indicators of active dz include upper lobe infiltrates or scarring and cavitary lesions in a pt with Sx

  (c) Sputum for acid-fast staining and culture is the Dx study of choice

(3) Tx

  (a) Start regimen with four drugs: INH, rifampin, ethambutol, and pyrazinamide

  (b) Narrow regimen based on sensitivities of culture organism

  (c) If drug resistance is a concern, start with a minimum of six drugs, at least one of which is injectable

  (d) Treat for a minimum of 6 mos for lung dz, typically longer for extrapulmonary dz

  (e) Tx should be given by specialists in TB care

H. Pneumonia

1. Community-Acquired Pneumonia (CAP)

  a. Can affect healthy outpts or those with chronic dz

  b. See Table 1.18 for typical and atypical causes

  c. Si/Sx = cough, dyspnea, tachypnea, fever, rales on exam

  d. Dx

  (1) Dx = CXR showing pneumonia in the presence of appropriate Si/Sx

  (2) Sputum Gram stain and culture

  (3) Blood cultures are no longer generally recommended due to low yield—do get them for patients sick enough to require ICU admission

  (4) Check an HIV test in all pts with CAP as a matter of routine

  e. Tx

  (1) Empiric Tx is with either:

    (a) A third-generation cephalosporin (e.g., ceftriaxone/cefotaxime) plus either doxycycline or a second-generation macrolide (e.g., clarithromycin or azithromycin); OR

Text continues on page 56

Table 1.18 Community-acquired Pneumonia (CAP)

Organism	Characteristics
Typical Bacterial CAP	
Streptococcus pneumoniae	• **Most commonly identified cause of CAP** • **HIV patients have 100-fold increased risk** • Also increased risk in the elderly and in alcoholics, asplenic patients, and patients with B-cell/Abs deficiencies • Fever, cough, chest pain, may have severe shaking rigors
Haemophilus influenzae	• Less common in the era of vaccination against this bacterium
Moraxella catarrhalis	• Presents with mild to moderate CAP
Klebsiella pneumoniae	• Typically presents in an alcoholic or diabetic • Often with hemoptysis, classically find a bulging upper lobe consolidation, often with cavitation, "current jelly" thick red hemoptysis
Staphylococcus aureus	• A rare cause of CAP (more common in children) • Can cause pneumonia during or after influenza infection • In some parts of the country, methicillin-resistant *S. aureus* (MRSA) is causing CAP even in patients without prior influenza • Causes a severe, necrotizing pneumonia
Atypical CAP	
Legionella pneumonia	• Can cause very severe CAP, requiring ICU care • A hallmark is concurrent CAP + diarrhea • Often with high LDH (>400) and low serum sodium • Send urine *Legionella* antigen to diagnose
Mycoplasma pneumonia	• The classic cause of "walking pneumonia," mild but nagging for weeks • Classically seen in teenagers or young adults living in close quarters, e.g., college dormitory, military barracks, summer camp, etc. • Associated with cold agglutinins and hemolysis, and with erythema multiforme
Chlamydophila pneumoniae	• Typically causes mild CAP
Chlamydia psittaci	• Causes psittacosis, mild to moderate CAP • Contracted from birds (often parrots), and the birds may also show signs of illness (ruffled feathers)
Fungal Pneumonia	
Pneumocystis jiroveci	• Still called PCP (*Pneumocystis* pneumonia) • Almost always in an HIV patient—can be seen in patients on corticosteroids

Table 1.18	*Continued*

Organism	Characteristics

Fungal Pneumonia (continued)

	• Insidious onset of dry cough/dyspnea, bilateral infiltrates, not pleural effusions, high LDH almost always seen • Dx → bronchoscopy, BAL sample silver stain • Tx → TMP-SMX, add prednisone if PO$_2$ <70 or A-a gradient ≥35
Coccidioides immitis	• "San Joaquin Valley Fever," major risks = travel to SW desert (e.g., California, Arizona, New Mexico, Texas), imprisonment, ↑ incidence after earthquakes • Filipinos and African-Americans have ↑ rate disseminated dz • Dx by serum Abs test, or rarely culture or biopsy • Tx = fluconazole
Histoplasma capsulatum	• Seen in the Midwest and south, particularly in the areas of the Ohio/Mississippi River valleys • Can acquire from exposure to bat or bird dung • Typically asymptomatic • Can cause severe reactivation disease in patients with HIV or other immunosuppressives (e.g., corticosteroids) • Tx = itraconazole or amphotericin
Blastomyces dermatitidis	• Rare cause of pneumonia, seen in areas overlapping *Histoplasma,* but a denser endemicity in the St. Lawrence River valley • Can cause acute, fulminant pneumonia in immunocompromised host • Can cause chronic, scarring pneumonia over years • Often associated with skin lesions • Tx = amphotericin
Cryptococcus neoformans	• Causes pneumonia in immunocompromised, often HIV or steroids • Can appear like pneumocystis pneumonia in an AIDS patient, can also cause focal consolidation, nodules, or cavities • Always perform LP to determine if meningitis is co-existent • Tx is fluconazole or amphotericin

Anaerobes

Typically oral flora	• "Aspiration pneumonia," typically seen in patients with altered mental status, on drugs, status post seizure, etc. • Presents with foul smelling sputum, abscess seen on CXR • Treat with clindamycin or metronidazole + cephalosporin

Viral

Influenza	• The most common cause of viral pneumonia • Particular problem in the elderly or immunocompromised • Initiation of amantadine, oseltamivir, or zanamivir within the first 48 hrs can shorten duration and lessen severity of disease

(b) Monotherapy with a respiratory fluoroquinolone (e.g., levofloxacin, moxifloxacin, gatifloxacin, gemifloxacin); OR

(c) For patients in the ICU, may also give cephalosporin plus fluoroquinolone

(2) If the pt has been recently exposed to antibiotics, consider adding broader coverage for drug-resistant pathogens (e.g., *Pseudomonas*)

(3) Narrow Tx based on culture results

(4) See Table 1.18 for Tx of fungal, viral, or anaerobic pneumonia

2. Health Care-Associated Pneumonia (HCAP) and Hospital-Acquired Pneumonia (HAP)

a. HCAP caused by both community and hospital pathogens, whereas HAP only by hospital pathogens

b. For hospital pathogens, need to cover for resistant gram-negative rods (GNR), such as *Pseudomonas* and *Acinetobacter,* and MRSA

c. Dx is also by chest X-ray, but it is critical to obtain sputum Gram stain/culture or bronchoscopy to target antibiotics to appropriate organism

d. Tx is with broad spectrum gram-negative and gram-positive agents, typically vancomycin plus (ceftazidime or piperacillin–tazobactam or a carbapenem, etc.)

III. Gastroenterology and Hepatology

A. **Gastroesophageal Dz**

1. Dyspepsia (see Chapter 5 III.A) and GERD (see Chapter 5 III.B)

2. **Chronic Gastritis (Atrophic Gastritis)**

a. Type A (fundal) = autoimmune (pernicious anemia)

b. Type B (antral) because of *Helicobacter pylori (H.p.),* NSAIDs, herpes, cytomegalovirus (CMV)

c. Si/Sx = usually aSx, may cause pain, nausea/vomiting, anorexia, upper GI bleeding manifested as coffee grounds emesis or hematemesis

d. Dx = upper endoscopy

e. *H. pylori* Dx

(1) By urease breath test, serology, biopsy (CLO test)

(2) Serology will be persistently positive, so does not distinguish active versus previous disease

  (3) Proton pump inhibitors can cause false-negative urease breath test and CLO test on biopsy

f. Tx depends on etiology

  (1) Tx *H. pylori* with proton pump inhibitor + 2 antibiotics (e.g., amoxicillin + clarithromycin)

  (2) If drug induced, stop offending agent (usually NSAIDs), add proton pump inhibitor

  (3) Pernicious anemia Tx = vitamin B_{12} replenishment

  (4) Stress ulcer (especially in ICU setting), prophylax and treat with IV proton pump inhibitor

3. **Gastric Ulcer (GU)**

  a. *H. pylori* found in 70% of GU ulcers; 10% caused by ulcerating malignancy

  b. Si/Sx = gnawing/burning pain in midepigastrium, **worse with food intake;** if ulcer erodes into artery can cause hemorrhage and peritonitis, may be guaiac positive

  c. Dx = endoscopy with Bx to confirm not malignant, *H. pylori* testing as above

  d. Tx = proton pump inhibitors and antibiotics for *H. pylori*

4. **Eosinophilic Esophagitis**

  a. Esophageal inflammatory condition related to food allergies, most prevalent in young Caucasian males age 30–45 yrs

  b. Si/Sx = Presents with frequent dysphagia and food impaction, commonly associated with asthma, atopy, food allergies, and eczema

  c. Dx = Endoscopic biopsy (>15–20 eosinophils per high power field in proximal and distal esophagus), may see furrowing of esophageal lining.

  d. Tx = Dilation, PPI therapy, allergy eval, and fluticasone

B. **Small Intestine**

 1. **Duodenal Ulcer (Peptic Ulcer)**

  a. *H. pylori* found in 90% of duodenal ulcers

  b. Smoking and excessive alcohol intake ↑ risk

  c. Sx/Si = burning or gnawing epigastric pain 1–3 hrs postprandial, **relieved by food/antacids;** pain typically awakens pt at night; melena

  d. Dx = endoscopy, upper GI series if endoscopy is unavailable

  e. Tx = as for GU above, quit smoking

    f. Sequelae

      (1) Upper GI bleed

        (a) Usually see hematemesis, melena, or (rarely) hematochezia if briskly bleeding ulcer

        (b) Dx with endoscopy

        (c) Tx = endoscopic coagulation or sclerosant; surgery rarely necessary

      (2) Perforation

        (a) Change in pain pattern is suspicious for perforation

        (b) Plain abd films and CT scan may show free air

        (c) Tx is emergency surgery

2. **Crohn's Dz (Inflammatory Bowel Dz)** (Table 1.19)

    a. Can affect any part of GI from mouth to rectum, but usually includes the intestines and often spares the rectum (in contrast to ulcerative colitis)

    b. Si/Sx = abd pain, diarrhea, malabsorption, fever, stricture causing obstruction, fistulae; see below for extraintestinal manifestations

    c. Dx = colonoscopy with Bx of affected areas → transmural inflammation, **noncaseating granulomas, cobblestone mucosa, skip lesions, creeping fat on gross dissection is pathognomonic**

Table 1.19 Comparison of Inflammatory Bowel Disease

	Ulcerative Colitis	Crohn's Disease
Location	Isolated to colon	Anywhere in GI tract
Lesions	Contiguously proximal from colon	Skip lesions, disseminated
Inflammation	Limited to mucosa/submucosa	Transmural
Neoplasms	Very high risk for development	Lower risk for development
Fissures	None	Extend through submucosa
Fistula	None	Frequent: can be enterocutaneous
Granulomas	None	Noncaseating are characteristic
Extraintestinal manifestations	Seen in both: • Arthritis, iritis, erythema nodosum, pyoderma gangrenosum • Sclerosing cholangitis = chronic, fibrosing, inflammation of biliary system leading to cholestasis and portal hypertension	

d. Tx
   (1) First line for colonic disease is aminosalicylate (e.g., mesalamine, sulfasalazine)
   (2) Steroids for acute exacerbation/breakthrough flairs
   (3) Immunotherapy
      (a) Azathioprine and mercaptopurine to try to prolong disease remission
      (b) Anti–tumor necrosis factor (TNF) therapy with infliximab, adalimumab, certolizumab, anti-TNF Abs

3. **Carcinoid Syndrome**
   a. APUDoma (**a**mine **p**recursor **u**ptake and **d**ecarboxylate)
   b. Occurs most frequently in the appendix
   c. Carcinoid syndrome results from carcinoid liver metastases that secrete serotonin (5-HT)
   d. Si/Sx = flushing, watery diarrhea and abd cramps, bronchospasm, right-sided heart valve lesions
   e. Dx = ↑ levels of urine 5-hydroxyindoleacetic acid (5-HIAA)
   f. Tx = somatostatin and methysergide

C. **Large Intestine**
   1. **Ulcerative Colitis (Inflammatory Bowel Dz)** (Table 1.19)
      a. Idiopathic autoinflammatory disorder of the colon
      b. Always starts in rectum and spreads proximal
      c. If confined to rectum = ulcerative proctitis, a benign subtype
      d. Si/Sx = bloody diarrhea, colicky abd pain, can progress to generalized peritonitis, watch for toxic megacolon
      e. Dx = colonoscopy with bx → crypt abscess with numerous polymorphonuclear leukocytes (PMNs), friable mucosal patches that bleed easily
      f. Tx depends on site and severity of dz
         (1) Distal colitis → topical mesalamine and corticosteroids
         (2) Moderate colitis (above sigmoid) → oral steroids, mesalamine/sulfasalazine, infliximab
         (3) Severe colitis → IV steroids, cyclosporine, and surgical resection if unresponsive
         (4) Fulminant colitis (rapidly progressive) → broad-spectrum antibiotics

D. **Liver**
   1. Jaundice
      a. Visible when serum bilirubin exceeds 2 mg/dL

Table 1.20 Congenital Hyperbilirubinemia		
Syndrome	**Characteristics**	**Tx**
Gilbert	• Mild defect of glucoronyl transferase in 5% of population • Si/Sx = ↑ serum **unconjugated bilirubin** → jaundice in stressful situations and during fasting, completely benign	None required
Crigler–Najjar	• Genetic deficiency of glucuronyl transferase → ↑ serum **unconjugated bilirubin** • Type 1 = severe, presents in neonates with markedly ↑ bilirubin levels → death from kernicterus by age 1 • Type 2 = mild, pts suffer no severe clinical deficits	Phenobarbital
Dubin–Johnson	• ↑ **Conjugated bilirubin** due to defective bilirubin excretion • Si/Sx = jaundice, liver turns black, no serious sequelae	None required
Rotor	• ↑ **Conjugated bilirubin** similar to Dubin–Johnson • Defect is in bilirubin storage, not excretion	None required

b. Congenital hyperbilirubinemia (Table 1.20)
c. Hemolytic anemias
   (1) Excess production → ↑ unconjugated bilirubin
   (2) Si/Sx = as per any anemia (weakness, fatigue, etc.), others depend on etiology of hemolytic anemia (see Hematology)
   (3) Dx = ⊕ Coombs test, ↓ haptoglobin, ⊕ urine hemosiderin
   (4) Tx depends on etiology (see Hematology)
d. Intrahepatic cholestasis (hepatocellular)
   (1) May be because of viral hepatitis or cirrhosis
   (2) May be because of drug-induced hepatitis (acetaminophen, methotrexate, oral contraceptives, phenothiazines, INH, fluconazole, etc.)
   (3) Dx = ↑ transaminases, liver Bx to confirm hepatitis
   (4) Tx = cessation of drugs, or supportive for viral infxn
e. Extrahepatic
   (1) Myriad causes include choledocholithiasis (but not cholelithiasis), CA of biliary system or pancreas, cholangitis,

biliary cirrhosis—increased alkaline phosphatase predominates, AST/ALT variably elevated for these conditions

(2) 1° biliary cirrhosis (see Section 3 later)

(3) 2° biliary cirrhosis from long-standing biliary obstruction due to any cause

(4) Sclerosing cholangitis

   (a) Primary sclerosing cholangitis is an idiopathic inflammatory condition in which bile ducts are destroyed, leading to fibrosis and hepatic cirrhosis

   (b) Strong correlation exists between primary sclerosing cholangitis and ulcerative colitis

   (c) Many pts are aSx and are diagnosed by an isolated abnormal alkaline phosphatase on laboratories, while some pts present with pruritus and jaundice

   (d) Increased risk of bile duct cancer

   (e) Eventually liver failure develops with transaminitis and hyperbilirubinemia

   (f) Dx made by endoscopic retrograde cholangio-pancreaticoduodenoscopy (ERCP) or magnetic resonance CP (MRCP) showing "beads on a string" appearance of the bile ducts

   (g) 2° sclerosing cholangitis can be because of chronic infxns (often in the setting of HIV), drugs, etc.

   (h) Tx = ursodiol to control itching symptoms, ultimately liver transplantation required

(5) Si/Sx of acquired jaundice = acholic stools (pale), urinary bilirubin, fat malabsorption (which can lead to vitamin deficiencies of A, D, E, and K, with resulting symptoms), pruritus, ↑ serum cholesterol, xanthomas

(6) Dx may require abd CT or ERCP to rule out malignancy or obstruction of bile pathway

(7) Tx depends on etiology

2. **Hepatitis**

   a. General Si/Sx = jaundice, abd pain, diarrhea, malaise, fever, ↑ aspartate aminotransferase (AST), and alanine aminotransferase (ALT)

   b. Dx and Tx (Table 1.21)

3. **1° biliary cirrhosis**

   a. Autoimmune disorder usually seen in women

   b. Si/Sx = jaundice, pruritus, hypercholesterolemia, fat-soluble vitamin deficiencies

Table 1.21	Hepatitis Diagnosis and Treatment
Type	**Characteristics**
Fulminant	• Complications of acute hepatitis, progresses over <4 wks • Can be 2° to viral hepatitis, drugs (INH), toxins, and some metabolic disorders, e.g., Wilson's dz • AST/ALT in the thousands plus elevated PT and hepatic encephalopathy • Tx = urgent liver transplantation
Ischemic (shock liver)	• AST/ALT in the thousands very rapidly • Can occur after any significant episode of hypotension

Viral	• HAV → fecal-oral transmission, transient flu-like illness
	• HBV and HCV → blood transmission, HBV also sex and vertical → chronic hepatitis
	• 5%–10% of HBV and >50% of HCV infxn → chronic
	• Dx = serologies (Figure 1.9) and ↑ ALT and AST—ratio ≅ 1:1
	  ◊ HBV surface antigen = active infection
	  ◊ Anti-HBV surface antibody = immunity
	  ◊ Anti-HBV core antibody = exposed, not necessarily immune
	  ◊ HBV e antigen = highly infectious
	  ◊ HCV antibody = exposure, not immune
	• Tx
	  ◊ HAV: supportive
	  ◊ HBV: antivirals (lamivudine, emtricitabine, adefovir, telbivudine, entecavir)
	  ◊ HCV: IFN + ribavirin, several antivirals near approval as of 2011

Granulomatous	• Causes = TB, fungal (e.g., *Coccidioides*, *Histoplasma*), sarcoidosis, brucella, rickettsia, syphilis, leptospirosis • Dx = liver biopsy • Tx = anti-TB, antifungals, antibiotics, or steroids (sarcoidosis)

Alcoholic	• Most common form of liver disease in the United States
	• Si/Sx = as per other hepatitis with specific alcohol signs = palmar erythema, Dupuytren's contractures, spider angiomas, gynecomastia, caput medusae
	• DX = clinical ↑ AST and ALT, with AST/ALT = 2:1 is highly suggestive
	• This is an inflammatory disease and can present with systemic inflammatory response, marked fever and leukocytosis, difficult to distinguish from sepsis
	• Tx
	  ◊ Benzodiazepines for withdrawal
	  ◊ If the patient meets the discriminant function, add steroids or pentoxyphylline
	  ◊ Discriminant function = 4.6 * (prothrombin time minus the control prothrombin time) + total bilirubin: if this totals ≥32, drug therapy is indicated

Table 1.21	Continued
Type	Characteristics
Autoimmune	• Type I occurs in young women, ⊕ ANA, ⊕ anti-smooth muscle Ab
	• Type II occurs mostly in children, linked to Mediterranean ancestry, ⊕ anti–liver-kidney-muscle (anti-LKM) antibody
	• Si/Sx as for any other hepatitis
	• Tx = prednisone

HAV, hepatitis A virus; HBV, hepatitis B virus; HCV, hepatitis C virus.

   c. Dx = clinical ⊕ serology (**antimitochondrial Ab test is 90% sensitive**), confirm with bx

   d. Tx = liver transplant, otherwise supportive (e.g., ursodiol for pruritus)

4. **Cirrhosis**

   a. Most commonly because of alcoholism or chronic hepatitis B virus (HBV) or hepatitis C virus (HCV) infxn; also 1° biliary cirrhosis, other chronic hepatic dz (e.g., sclerosing cholangitis, Wilson's dz, hemochromatosis, etc.)

   b. Si/Sx = purpura and bleeding ↑ and prothrombin time (PT)/ partial thromboplastin time (PTT), jaundice, ascites 2° to ↓ albumin and portal HTN, spontaneous bacterial peritonitis (SBP), encephalopathy, asterixis

   c. Ascites differential (Table 1.22)

   d. SBP

     (1) Usually low protein ascites

     (2) Si/Sx can be very subtle, in some cases even without abd pain; fever is variable—all patients with new onset

Table 1.22	Ascites Differential Diagnosis	
	Portal Hypertension	No Portal Hypertension
Serum/ascites albumin gradient (SAAG)	≥1.1 g/dL	<1.1 g/dL
Causes	Cirrhosis, alcoholic hepatitis, nephrosis, Budd–Chiari, CHF	Pancreatic dz, TB, peritoneal mets, idiopathic
Other labs	Ascites total protein >2.5 → heart dz Ascites total protein ≤2.5 → liver dz	Amylase ↑ in pancreatic dz

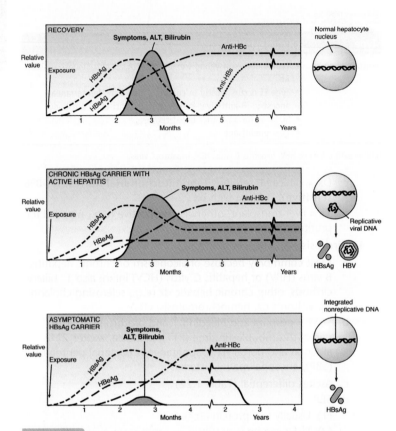

FIGURE 1.9

Typical serologic events in three distinct outcomes of hepatitis B. (*Top panel*) In most cases, the appearance of anti-HBs ensures complete recovery. Viral DNA disappears from the nucleus of the hepatocyte. (*Middle panel*) In about 10% of cases of hepatitis B, HBs antigenemia is sustained for longer than 6 mos, because of the absence of anti-HBs. Pts in whom viral replication remains active, as evidenced by sustained high levels of HBeAg in the blood, develop active hepatitis. In such cases, the viral genome persists in the nucleus but is not integrated into host DNA. (*Lower panel*) Pts in whom active viral replication ceases or is attenuated, as reflected in the disappearance of HBeAg from the blood, become aSx carriers. In these individuals, fragments of the HBV genome are integrated into the host DNA, but episomal DNA is absent. (From Rubin E, Farber JL. *Pathology*, 3rd Ed. Philadelphia, PA: Lippincott Williams & Wilkins, 1999.)

or acute increase in ascites need to have paracentesis to rule out SBP

    (3) Common organisms include *Escherichia coli, Klebsiella, Enterococcus,* and *Streptococcus pneumoniae*

    (4) Tx = ceftriaxone or cefotaxime, plus IV albumin to maintain renal perfusion pressure

  e. Encephalopathy

    (1) Because of ↑ levels of toxins, likely related to ammonia, but ammonia levels do not correlate well with encephalopathy

    (2) Flapping tremor of the wrist upon extension (asterixis)

    (3) Tx of encephalopathy is to lower ammonia levels

      (a) Lactulose metabolized by bacteria, acidifies the bowel, $NH_3 \rightarrow NH_4^+$, which cannot be absorbed

      (b) Neomycin or rifaximin kills bacteria-making NH_3 in gut

    (4) Watch for Wernicke–Korsakoff's encephalopathy (triad = confusion [largely confabulation], ataxia, ophthalmoplegia)

  f. Alcohol withdrawal has four phases—any given pt can go through any of these phases but does not have to go through all of them, and the phases occurring during a prior withdrawal episode are predictive for what will happen the next time withdrawal occurs

    (1) Tremor—occurs within hours of last drink, so it is the first sign of withdrawal

    (2) Seizure—occurs several hours to approximately 48 hrs after the last drink; seizures can be fatal and are best Tx with benzodiazepines, not standard antiseizure medicines

    (3) Hallucinosis—occurs 48–72 hrs after the last drink; this is NOT delirium tremens (DTs), but rather is simply auditory or tactile hallucinations, also best Tx with benzodiazepines

    (4) DTs—at approximately 72 hrs after the last drink, the autonomic instability that defines DTs begins with dangerous tachycardia and hypertension and can be accompanied by each of the other three phases (tremor, seizure, hallucinosis)—the autonomic instability is also best Tx with benzodiazepines

  g. Tx of inpatient alcoholics

    (1) IV thiamine and B_{12} supplements to correct deficiency (very common)

    (2) Give IV glucose, fluids, and electrolytes

    (3) Correct any underlying coagulopathy

    (4) Benzodiazepine for prevention and Tx of DTs

    (5) If patient meets discriminant function (4.6 × (patient's PT minus control PT) + total bilirubin ≥32) add corticosteroids or pentoxifylline to reduce inflammation and improve survival

5. **Nonalcoholic steatohepatitis (NASH)**

    a. Common cause of unexplained transaminitis, asymptomatic for prolonged periods but can lead to cirrhosis

    b. Typically occurs in middle-aged, obese patients with hypercholesterolemia, and many have diabetes—however, cases can occur in younger patients who are not obese with normal cholesterol

    c. Dx is clinical based on excluding other causes, confirmed by biopsy

    d. Tx is weight loss and normalize cholesterol, no other specific treatment

6. **Hemochromatosis**

    a. Hemochromatosis most commonly due to autosomal recessive mutation in the *HFE* gene, resulting in excessive absorption of iron from the gut

    b. Results in iron accumulation in heart causing CHF, liver causing hepatitis and then cirrhosis, pancreas causing DM, skin causing bronze-like darkening of the skin (hence the term "bronze diabetes" for hemochromatosis), and arthritis (typically MCP of the hand), disease usually becomes apparent in adults

    c. Cirrhosis due to hemochromatosis very commonly leads to hepatocellular carcinoma

    d. Dx = iron studies (showing high iron saturation, Fe/TIBC >50%, very high ferritin >1,000), liver biopsy

    e. Tx = regular phlebotomy

7. **Wilson's Disease (also see Chapter 7 IV.D)**

    a. Disorder of excess copper storage in tissues

    b. Si/Sx = chronic hepatitis or cirrhosis in a teenager or young adult (typically 20s), copper-colored Kayser–Fleischer rings (see Figure 7.2), psychiatric or neurological disorders (can present with acute psychotic break or speech and movement disorders), can present with or lead to fulminant hepatic failure

    c. Dx = clinical + reduced ceruloplasmin level

d. Tx = copper chelation with penicillamine and liver transplantation if caught too late

8. **Hepatic Abscess**

   a. Caused by (in order of frequency in the US) bacteria, parasites (usually amebic) or fungal

   b. Bacterial abscesses usually result from direct extension of infxn from gallbladder, hematogenous spread via the portal vein from appendicitis of diverticulitis, or via the hepatic artery from distant sources such as from a pneumonia or bacterial endocarditis

   c. Organisms in pyogenic hepatic abscesses are usually of enteric origin (e.g., *E. coli, Klebsiella pneumoniae, Bacteroides,* and *Enterococcus*)—recently, *Klebsiella* with a special thick capsule has spread from Asia to the United States and causes multiple loculated, complex liver abscesses, as well as metastatic seeding of other sites plus sepsis syndrome

   d. Amebic abscess caused by *Entaemoeba histolytica,* and in the United States is almost always seen in young Hispanic males

   e. Si/Sx = high fever, malaise, rigors, jaundice, epigastric or right upper quadrant (RUQ) pain and referred pain to the right shoulder

   f. Labs → leukocytosis, anemia, liver function tests may be nml or ↑

   g. Dx = US or CT scan

   h. Tx

      (1) Antibiotics to cover anaerobes (e.g., metronidazole) + Gram negatives (e.g., ceftriaxone, piperacillin, fluoroquinolone, etc.)

      (2) Percutaneous or surgical drainage

      (3) For amebic abscesses (caused by *E. histolytica*) use metronidazole—drainage is not indicated for amebic abscess unless the abscess is adjacent to the pericardium (to prevent fatal rupture into the pericardium)

   i. Complications = intrahepatic spread of infxn, sepsis, and abscess rupture

   j. Mortality of hepatic abscesses is 15%, higher with coexistent malignancy

9. Portal HTN

   a. Defined as portal vein pressure >12 mm Hg (nml = 6–8 mm Hg)

   b. Si/Sx = ascites, hepatosplenomegaly, variceal bleeding, encephalopathy

Table 1.23 Causes of Portal Hypertension		
Prehepatic	**Intrahepatic**	**Posthepatic**
• Portal vein thrombosis • Splenomegaly • Arteriovenous fistula	• Cirrhosis • Schistosomiasis • Massive fatty change • Nodular regenerative hyperplasia	• Idiopathic portal hypertension • Granulomatous dz (e.g., tuberculosis, sarcoidosis)	• Severe right-sided heart failure • Hepatic vein thrombosis (Budd–Chiari syndrome) • Constrictive pericarditis • Hepatic veno-occlusive disease

c. Can be presinusoidal, intrahepatic, or postsinusoidal in nature (Table 1.23)

d. Dx = endoscopy and angiography (variceal bleeding) and US (dilated vessels) (Figure 1.10)

e. Tx

(1) Acute variceal bleeding controlled by endoscopic banding

(2) If continued bleeding, use Sengstaken–Blakemore tube to tamponade bleeding

(3) Pharmacotherapy = IV infusion of octreotide to lower portal pressures

(4) Long term → propranolol once varices are identified (↓ bleeding risk but effect on long-term survival is variable)

(5) Many patients with variceal bleeds are infected (the infection increases portal pressures, resulting in the bleed), so antibiotics are typically given and a search for infection should be made

(6) Decompressive shunts—most efficacious way of stopping bleeding

(7) **Indication for liver transplant is end-stage liver dz, not variceal bleeding**

10. Budd–Chiari syndrome

a. Rarely congenital, usually acquired thrombosis occluding hepatic vein or hepatic stretch of IVC

b. Associated with hypercoagulability (e.g., polycythemia vera, hepatocellular or other CA, pregnancy, etc.)

c. Sx = acute onset of abd pain, jaundice, ascites

d. Hepatitis quickly develops, leading to cirrhosis and portal HTN

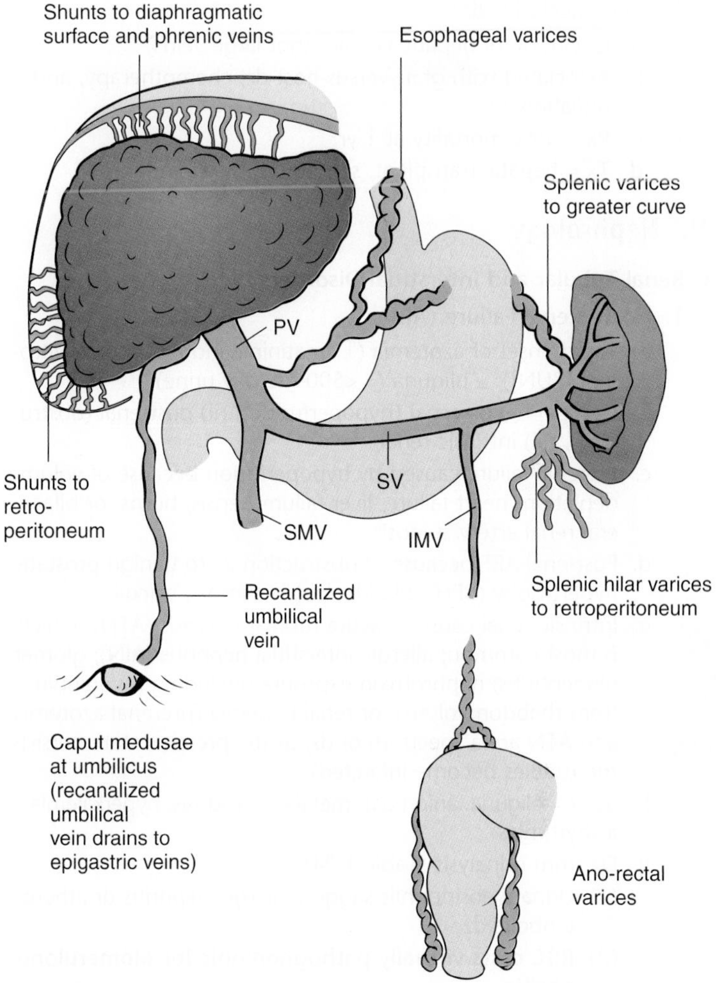

FIGURE 1.10

Sites of occurrence of portal–systemic communications in pts with portal hypertension. IMV, inferior mesenteric vein; PV, portal vein; SMV, superior mesenteric vein; SV, splenic vein.

e. Dx = RUQ US

f. Tx = anticoagulation, thrombectomy or clot lysis, transjugular intrahepatic portosystemic shunt, or liver transplant

g. Px poor; less than one-third of pts survive at 1 yr

11. Veno-occlusive dz
   a. Occlusion of hepatic venules (not large veins)
   b. Associated with graft-versus-host dz, chemotherapy, and radiation Tx
   c. Px = 50% mortality at 1 yr
   d. Tx = hepatic transplant, sometimes is self-limiting

IV. Nephrology

A. **Renal Tubular and Interstitial Disorders**
   1. **Acute Renal Failure (ARF)**
      a. Rapid onset of azotemia ($\uparrow$ creatinine and blood urea nitrogen [BUN]), ± oliguria (= <500 mL/day urine)
      b. Causes = (i) prerenal (hypoperfusion), (ii) postrenal (obstruction), (iii) intrinsic renal
      c. Prerenal failure caused by hypoperfusion because of volume depletion, heart failure, liver failure, sepsis, burns, or bilateral renal artery stenosis
      d. Postrenal ARF because of obstruction $2°$ to benign prostatic hypertrophy (BPH), bladder/pelvic tumors, calculi
      e. Intrinsic renal causes = acute tubular necrosis (ATN), which is most common; allergic interstitial nephritis (AIN); glomerulonephritis; nephrotoxin exposure (including myoglobin from rhabdomyolysis); or renal ischemia (prerenal azotemia and ATN are a spectrum of dz; as the prerenal state persists the tubules become infarcted)
      f. Si/Sx = oliguria, anion gap metabolic acidosis, hyperkalemia → arrhythmias
      g. Dx from urinalysis (Table 1.24)
         (1) Urinary eosinophils suggest allergic nephritis or atheroembolic dz
         (2) **RBC casts virtually pathognomonic for glomerulonephritis**
         (3) Muddy brown casts in urine are typical of ATN
      h. Tx
         (1) IV fluids to maintain urine output, diurese to prevent volume overload
         (2) Closely monitor electrolyte abnormalities
         (3) Indications for dialysis: recalcitrant volume overload status, critical electrolyte abnormalities, unresponsive metabolic acidosis, toxic ingestion, uremia

Table 1.24 Laboratory Characteristics of Acute Renal Failure

Test/Index	Prerenal	Postrenal	Renal
Urine osmolality	>500	<350	<350
Urine Na	<20	>40	>20
FE_{Na}[a]	<1%	>4%	>2%
FE_{UREA}[b]	≤35%		>50%
BUN/creatinine	>20	>15	<15

[a]FE_{Na} = (Urine/Serum sodium)/(Urine/Serum creatinine)—this is not reliable if the patient is taking a diuretic.
[b]FE_{UREA} = (Urine/Serum urea)/(Urine/Serum creatinine), this is reliable even if the patient is taking a diuretic.

2. **ATN**
   a. Most common cause of ARF, falls into the intrinsic renal category
   b. ATN causes = persistent prerenal state of any cause, rhabdomyolysis → myoglobinuria, direct toxins (e.g., amphotericin, aminoglycosides, radiocontrast dyes)
   c. Three phases of injury: (i) prodromal, (ii) oliguric, (iii) post-oliguric
   d. Tx = resolution of precipitating cause, IV fluids to maintain urinary output, monitor electrolytes, diurese as needed to prevent fluid overload

3. **Drug-Induced AIN**
   a. β lactam antibiotics, sulfonamides, diuretics, and NSAIDs are the most frequent causes
   b. Si/Sx = pyuria, maculopapular rash, eosinophilia, proteinuria, hematuria, oliguria, flank pain, fever, eosinophiluria
   c. Dx = clinical, improvement following withdrawal of offending drug can help confirm dx, but sometimes the dz can be irreversible
   d. Tx = removal of underlying cause, consider corticosteroids for allergic dz

4. **Renal Tubule Functional Disorders**
   a. Renal tubular acidosis (RTA) (Table 1.25)
   b. Diabetes insipidus (DI)
      (1) ↓ antidiuretic hormone (ADH) secretion (central) or ADH resistance (nephrogenic)

Table 1.25 Renal Tubular Acidosis[a]

Type	Characteristic	Urinary pH
Type I	• **Distal tubular defect** of urinary H^+ gradient • Seen in amphotericin nephrotoxicity	>5.5
Type II	• **Proximal tubule failure** to resorb HCO_3 • Classic causes include acetazolamide, nephrotic syndrome, multiple myeloma, Fanconi's syndrome	>5.5 early, then → <5.5 as acidosis worsens
Type IV	• ↓ **aldosterone** → hyperkalemia and hyperchloremia • Usually due to ↓ secretion **(hypereninemic hypoaldosteronism)**, seen in diabetes, interstitial nephritis, NSAID use, ACE inhibitors, and heparin • Also due to aldosterone resistance, seen in urinary obstruction and sickle cell dz	<5.5

[a]There is no RTA III for historical reasons.

    (2) Si/Sx = polyuria, polydipsia, nocturia, urine-specific gravity <1.010, urine osmolality (U_{osm}) ≤200, serum osmolality (S_{osm}) ≥300

    (3) Central DI

        (a) 1° (idiopathic) or 2° (acquired via trauma, infarction, granulomatous infiltration, fungal, or TB infxn of pituitary)

        (b) Tx = Desmopressin acetate (DDAVP) (ADH analogue) nasal spray

    (4) Nephrogenic DI

        (a) 1° dz is X-linked, seen in infants, may regress with time

        (b) 2° dz usually do to drugs (lithium, demeclocycline), rarely due to sickle cell, amyloid, multiple myeloma

        (c) Tx = ↑ water intake, sodium restriction

    (5) **Dx** = water deprivation test

        (a) Hold all water, administer vasopressin

        (b) Central DI: U_{osm} after deprivation no greater than S_{osm}, but ↑ ≥10% after vasopressin

        (c) Nephrogenic DI: U_{osm} after deprivation no greater than S_{osm}, and vasopressin does not ↑ U_{osm}

  c. Syndrome of inappropriate antidiuretic hormone (SIADH)

    (1) Etiologies

        (a) CNS dz: trauma, tumor, Guillain–Barré, hydrocephalus

  (b) Pulmonary dz: pneumonia, tumor (usually small cell CA), abscess, COPD
  (c) Endocrine dz: hypothyroidism, Conn's syndrome
  (d) Drugs: NSAIDs, antidepressants, chemotherapy, diuretics, phenothiazine, oral hypoglycemics
(2) Dx = hyponatremia with U_{osm} >300 mmol/kg
(3) Tx
  (a) If euvolemic, water restriction is first line
  (b) If euvolemic and no response to water restriction (i.e., serum sodium does not ↑), consider 3% saline or prescribe conivaptan, which is a vasopressin receptor antagonist
  (c) If hypovolemic, prescribe nml saline
  (d) **Beware of central pontine myelinolysis with rapid correction of hyponatremia**

5. **Chronic Renal Failure**
  a. Always associated with azotemia of renal origin
  b. Uremia is <u>not</u> just a synonym for azotemia—uremia is a biochemical and clinical syndrome of the following characteristics
    (1) Azotemia (i.e., elevated serum creatinine and/or BUN)
    (2) Acidosis because of accumulation of sulfates, phosphates, organic acids
    (3) Hyperkalemia because of inability to excrete K+ in urine
    (4) Fluid volume disorder (early cannot concentrate urine, late cannot dilute)
    (5) Hypocalcemia because of lack of vitamin D production
    (6) Anemia because lack of EPO production
    (7) Hypertension $2°$ to activated renin–angiotensin axis
  c. Si/Sx = anorexia, nausea/vomiting, dementia, convulsions, eventually coma, bleeding because of platelet dysfunction, fibrinous pericarditis, which can lead to tamponade
  d. Dx = renal US → small kidneys in chronic dz, anemia from chronic lack of EPO, diffuse osteopenia
  e. Tx = salt and water restriction, diuresis to prevent fluid overload, dialysis to correct acid–base or severe electrolyte disorders

B. **Glomerular Dz**

1. **Nephrotic Syndrome**
  a. Si/Sx = proteinuria >3.5 g/day, generalized edema (anasarca), lipiduria with hyperlipidemia, marked ↓ serum albumin, hypercoagulation (e.g., DVT)

Table 1.26 Nephrotic Glomerulopathies

Disease	Characteristics
Minimal change disease (MCD)	• Classically seen in young children • EM shows fusion of podocyte foot processes • Tx = prednisone, disease is very responsive, Px is excellent
Focal segmental glomerulosclerosis	• Clinically similar to MCD, but occurs in adults with refractory HTN • Usually idiopathic, but heroin, HIV, diabetes, sickle cell are associated • The idiopathic variant typically presents in young, hypertensive males • Tx = prednisone + cyclophosphamide, dz is refractory, Px poor
Membranous glomerulonephritis	• Most common primary cause of nephritic syndrome in adults • Slowly progressive disorder with ↓ response to steroid treatment seen • Causes of this disease are numerous ◊ Infections include HBV, HCV, syphilis, malaria ◊ Drugs include gold salts, penicillamine (note, both used in RA) ◊ Occult malignancy ◊ SLE (10% of patients develop) • Tx = prednisone ± cyclophosphamide, 50% → end-stage renal failure
Membranoproliferative glomerulonephritis	• Disease has 2 forms ◊ Type I often slowly progressive ◊ Type II more aggressive, often have an autoantibody against C3 convertase "C3 nephritic factor" → ↓ serum levels of C3 • Tx = prednisone ± plasmapheresis or interferon-α, Px very poor
Systemic diseases	See Table 1.27

   b. Dx of type made by renal bx

   c. General Tx = protein restriction, salt restriction and diuretic Tx for edema, HMG-CoA reductase inhibitor for hyperlipidemia

   d. Nephrotic glomerulopathies (Table 1.26)

   e. Systemic glomerulopathies (Table 1.27)

Table 1.27	Systemic Glomerulonephropathies
Disease	**Characteristic Nephropathy**

Diabetes	• Most common cause of end-stage renal disease in United States
	• Early manifestation is microalbuminuria
	  ◊ ACE inhibitors ↓ progression to renal failure if started early
	  ◊ Strict glycemic and hypertensive control also ↓ progression
	• Biopsy shows pathognomonic Kimmelstiel–Wilson nodules
	• As dz progresses only Tx is renal transplant

HIV	• Usually seen in HIV acquired by intravenous drug abuse • Presents with focal segmental glomerulonephritis • Early Tx with antiretrovirals may help kidney disease
Renal amyloidosis	• Dx → birefringence with Congo red stain • Tx = transplant, dz is refractory and often recurrent
Lupus	
Type I	• No renal involvement visible by histopathology
Type II	• **Mesangial disease** with focal segmental glomerular pattern • Tx not typically required for kidney involvement
Type III	• **Focal proliferative disease** • Tx = aggressive prednisone ± cyclophosphamide
Type IV	• **Diffuse proliferative disease,** the most severe form of lupus nephropathy • Presents with a combination of nephritic/nephritic disease • Classic light microscopy (LM) → wire-loop abnormality • Tx = prednisone + cyclophosphamide, transplant may be required
Type V	• **Membranous disease,** indistinguishable from other 1° membranous GNs • Tx = consider prednisone, may not be required

2. **Nephritic Syndrome**
   a. Results from diffuse glomerular inflammation
   b. Si/Sx = acute onset hematuria (smoky-brown urine), ↓ glomerular filtration rate (GFR) resulting in azotemia (↑ BUN and creatinine), oliguria, hypertension, and edema
   c. Nephritic glomerulopathies (Table 1.28)
3. **Urinalysis in primary glomerular dz** (Table 1.29)
C. **Renal Artery Stenosis**
   1. **Classic dyad** = sudden hypertension with low K⁺ (pt not on diuretic)

Table 1.28 Nephritic Glomerulonephropathies

Disease	Characteristics
Poststreptococcal (postinfectious) glomerulonephritis (PSGN/PIGN)	• Prototype of nephritic syndrome (acute glomerulonephritis) • Classically follows infection with group A β-hemolytic streptococci (*S. pyogenes*) but can follow infxn by virtually any organism, viral or bacterial • Lab → urine red cells and casts, azotemia, ↓ serum C3, ↑ ASO titer (for strep infection) • **Immunofluorescence → coarse granular IgG or C3 deposits** • Tx typically not needed, dz usually self-limiting

Crescentic (rapidly progressive) glomerulonephritis	• Nephritis progresses to renal failure within weeks or months
	• May be part of PIGN or other systemic diseases
	• Goodpasture's disease
	  ◊ **Disease causes glomerulonephritis with pneumonitis**
	  ◊ **Presents with positive anti-glomerula basement membrane (anti-GBM) antibody**
	  ◊ **90% pts present with hemoptysis,** only later get glomerulonephritis
	  ◊ **Classic immunofluorescence → smooth, linear deposition of IgG**
	• Tx = prednisone and plasmapheresis, minority → end-stage renal dz

Berger's disease (IgA nephropathy)	• **Most common worldwide nephropathy** • Due to IgA deposition in the mesangium • Si/Sx = recurrent hematuria with low-grade proteinuria • Whereas PIGN presents weeks after infection, **Berger's presents concurrently or within several days of infection** • 25% of pts slowly progress to renal failure, otherwise harmless • Tx = prednisone for acute flares, will not halt dz progression
Henoch–Schönlein purpura (HSP)	• Also an IgA nephropathy, but almost always presents in children • Presents with abdominal pain, vomiting, hematuria and GI bleeding • **Classic physical finding = "palpable purpura" on buttocks and legs in kids** • Often follows respiratory infection • Tx not required, dz is self-limiting

Table 1.28	Continued
Disease	**Characteristics**
Multiple myeloma	• ↑ Production of light chains → tubular plugging by Bence-Jones proteins • 2° hypercalcemia also contributes to development of "myeloma kidney" • Myeloma cells can directly invade kidney parenchyma • Defect in normal antibody production leaves pt susceptible to chronic infections by encapsulated bacteria (e.g., *S. pneumoniae*) → chronic renal failure • Tx is directed at underlying myeloma

2. Causes are atherosclerotic plaques and fibromuscular dysplasia
   a. Fibromuscular dysplasia is fibrous and muscle stenosis of renal artery
   b. Causes renovascular HTN seen most commonly in women during their reproductive years
   c. Beware of dissecting aneurysms of affected arteries
3. Screening Dx = oral captopril induces ↑ renin
4. Dx confirmed with angiography
5. Tx = surgery versus angioplasty

D. **Urinary Tract Obstruction**
   1. **General Characteristics**
      a. Most common causes in children are congenital
      b. Most common causes in adults are BPH and stones
      c. Obstruction → urinary stasis → ↑ risk of urinary tract infxn (UTI)

Table 1.29	Urinalysis in Primary Glomerula Diseases		
	Nephrotic Syndrome	**Nephritic Syndrome**	**Chronic Disease**
Proteinuria	↑↑↑↑	±	±
Hematuria	±	↑↑↑↑	±
Cells	—	⊕ RBCs ⊕ WBCs	±
Casts	**Fatty casts**	**RBC and granular casts**	**Waxy and pigmented granular casts**
Lipids	Free fat droplets, oval fat bodies	—	—

2. **Nephrolithiasis**
   a. Calcium pyrophosphate stones
      (1) Eighty percent to eighty-five percent of stones are **radiopaque,** associated with hypercalciuria, CT scan the best diagnostic test to find stones
      (2) Hypercalciuria can be idiopathic or due to because of ↑ intestinal calcium absorption, ↑ 1° renal calcium excretion, or hypercalcemia
      (3) Fifty percent **associated with idiopathic hypercalciuria**
      (4) Tx = vigorous hydration, loop diuretics if necessary
   b. Ammonium magnesium phosphate stones ("struvite stones")
      (1) Second most common form of stones, are **radiopaque**
      (2) Most often because of urease ⊕ *Proteus* or *Staphylococcus saprophyticus*
      (3) Can form large staghorn or struvite calculi
      (4) Tx = directed at underlying infxn
   c. Uric acid stones
      (1) Fifty percent of pts with stones have hyperuricemia
      (2) 2° to gout or ↑ cell turnover (leukemia, myeloproliferative dz)
      (3) Stones are **radiolucent**
      (4) Tx = alkalinize urine, treat underlying disorder
   d. Si/Sx of stones = urinary colic = sharp, 10/10 on the pain scale, often described as the worst pain in the pt's life, radiates from back → anterior pelvis/groin
   e. Tx = vigorous hydration, loop diuretics as needed; urology consult for large stones that won't spontaneously pass

E. **Tumors of the Kidney**
   1. **Renal Cell CA**
      a. Most common renal malignancy, most commonly occurs in male smokers aged 50–70 yrs
      b. **Hematogenously disseminates by invading renal veins or the vena cava**
      c. Si/Sx = hematuria, palpable mass, flank pain, fever, 2° polycythemia
      d. Can be associated with von Hippel–Lindau syndrome
      e. Tx = resection, systemic interleukin-2 immunotherapy, poor Px

   2. **Wilms Tumor**
      a. Most common renal malignancy of childhood, incidence peaks at 2–4 yrs

b. Si/Sx = palpable flank mass (often huge)
c. Can be part of **WAGR** complex = **W**ilms' tumor, **A**niridia, **G**enitourinary malformations, mental motor **R**etardation
d. **Also associated with hemihypertrophy of the body**
e. Tx = nephrectomy plus chemotherapy and/or radiation

V. Endocrinology

A. Hypothalamic Pituitary Axis

1. **Prolactinoma**
   a. Si/Sx = headache, diplopia, CN III palsy, impotence, amenorrhea, gynecomastia, galactorrhea, $\uparrow$ androgens in females $\rightarrow$ virilization
   b. Fifty percent **cause hypopituitarism, caused by mass effect of the tumor**
   c. Dx = MRI/CT confirmation of tumor
   d. Tx
      (1) First line = dopamine agonist (e.g., bromocriptine)
      (2) Large tumors or refractory $\rightarrow$ transsphenoidal surgical resection
      (3) Radiation Tx for nonresectable macroadenomas

2. **Acromegaly**
   a. Almost always because of pituitary adenoma secreting growth hormone
   b. Childhood secretion prior to skeletal epiphyseal closure $\rightarrow$ gigantism
   c. If secretion begins after epiphyseal closure $\rightarrow$ acromegaly
   d. Si/Sx = adult whose glove, ring, or shoe size acutely $\uparrow$, coarsening of skin/facial features; prognathism; voice deepening; joint erosions; peripheral neuropathies because of nerve compression
   e. Dx = $\uparrow$ insulin-like growth factor-1 and/or MRI/CT confirmation of neoplasm
   f. Tx = surgery or radiation to ablate the enlarged pituitary; octreotide (somatostatin analogue) second line for refractory tumors

B. Diabetes

1. **Type I Diabetes**
   a. Autoinflammatory destruction of pancreas $\rightarrow$ insulin deficiency

b. Si/Sx = polyphagia, polydipsia, polyuria, weight loss in child or adolescent, can lead to diabetic ketoacidosis (DKA) when pt is stressed (e.g., infxn)

c. Dx = see type II later for criteria

d. Tx = **insulin replacement required—oral hypoglycemics will not work**

e. Complication of type I diabetes = DKA

f. Si/Sx of DKA = **Kussmaul hyperpnea** (deep and labored breathing), **abd pain, dehydration, ⊕ anion gap,** low bicarbonate (may be close to normal in mild DKA because dehydration results in a contraction alkalosis that counteracts the mild metabolic acidosis, but anion gap will always be elevated), urine/blood ketones, hyperkalemia, hyperglycemia, beware of mucormycosis = fatal fungal infxn seen in diabetics (often in DKA), presents with proptosis, periorbital edema, vision loss, late stages develop necrotic eschars of palate and nasopharynx

g. Dx of DKA

  (1) Dx requires three things

    (a) Diabetes mellitus (DKA can occur in either type 1 or type 2, but type 1 at higher risk) and

    (b) Ketosis (blood and urine ketones, blood hydroxybutyrate) and

    (c) Anion gap metabolic acidosis

  (2) Alternative diagnoses if all three conditions are not present

    (a) Starvation ketosis results in mild ketosis (seen mostly in the urine) without acidosis, results from insufficient caloric intake, often in alcoholics, but can also be seen in diabetics who have nausea from various causes (e.g., gastroparesis)—the key distinction from DKA is that there is no significant anion gap acidosis

    (b) Diabetes out of control—glucoses may be high, but there is no anion gap acidosis

h. DKA Tx

  (1) **1° Tx = FLUIDS**

    (a) Patients are typically very dehydrated—liters of normal saline to restore euvolemia followed by half normal saline

    (b) Due to the sodium load from rehydration, patients may develop a mild non-gap hyperchloremic metabolic acidosis as the underlying gap acidosis resolves,

so the bicarbonate may not rise much about 18–20—
this is of no significance as long as the gap closes

(2) **2° = K⁺ and insulin**

- (a) Iv insulin drip is required to stop the acidosis
    - (i) Insulin is to shut off acid production, not for hyperglycemia per se, and the insulin must be continued until the gap closes and the ketones disappear irrespective of the glucose level
    - (ii) If the glucose level falls below 200 mg/dL and the acidosis has not resolved, administer dextrose in the IV until the acidosis has resolved and the insulin drip is stopped
    - (iii) When the gap is closed, ketones are gone, and the patient is ready to eat (nausea resolved), administer SQ insulin, feed the patient, and turn the drip off
- (b) Administer K in the IV unless the patient's serum K is very high
    - (i) Patients typically have normal to slightly elevated serum K levels, but they are typically severely total body potassium depleted, because the serum level is artificially elevated by dehydration, and because acidosis causes K efflux from cells, so intracellular K levels are depleted
    - (ii) Therefore, add K to the patients IV fluids if the serum K is below ~5
- (c) Patients are typically depleted of other electrolytes as well, so measure Mg and phos—can administer Mg if depleted, phos typically does not require repletion unless the level is below ~1.5 mg/dL

2. **Type II Diabetes**
   a. Peripheral insulin resistance—a metabolic dz, not autoinflammatory
   b. Usually adult onset, because of residual insulin production, patients are less likely than those with type 1 DM to develop DKA and more prone to developing hyperglycemic nonketotic coma
   c. Si/Sx
      (1) Acute = dehydration, polydipsia/polyphagia/polyuria, fatigue, weight loss
      (2) Subacute = infxns (e.g., yeast vaginitis, mucormycosis, *S. aureus* boils)

(3) Chronic (Figure 1.10)
  (a) Macrovascular = stroke, CAD
  (b) Microvascular = retinitis, nephritis
  (c) Neuropathy = ↓ sensation, paresthesias, glove-in-hand burning pain, autonomic insufficiency
d. Dx of any diabetes (type I or II)
  (1) Random plasma glucose >200 with Sx *or*
  (2) Fasting glucose >125 *or*
  (3) Two-hour oral glucose tolerance test glucose >200 with or without Sx *or*
  (4) Hemoglobin A1c (HgA1c) >6.5%
  (5) Impaired glucose tolerance (IGT) is a prediabetic state
    (a) Defined as 2-hr oral glucose tolerance test glucose of 140–199 or a fasting glucose of 100–125
    (b) Many patients will progress to DM, recommend weight loss and exercise to prevent
e. Tx
  (1) Oral hypoglycemics first line for mild to moderate hyperglycemia (Table 1.30)
  (2) Dz refractory to oral hypoglycemics requires insulin
  (3) Diet and nutrition education
  (4) ACE inhibitors slow progression of nephropathy
f. Monitoring: glycosylated hemoglobin A_{1c} (HbA_{1c})
  (1) Because of serum half-life of hemoglobin, HbA_{1c} is a marker of the prior 3 mos of therapeutic regimen
  (2) **Tight glucose control has been shown to reduce complications and mortality in type 1 (insulin-dependent DM) and type 2 (noninsulin-dependent DM),** thus HbA_{1c} is a crucial key tool to follow efficacy and compliance of diabetic Tx regimens
  (3) HbA_{1c} <7% (or 6.5% depending on source) is recommended
g. Complication = hyperosmolar hyperglycemic nonketotic coma (HHNK)
  (1) 2° to hypovolemia, precipitated by acute stress (e.g., infxn, trauma)—these patients typically are profoundly dehydrated because they do not get acidosis, which would have prompted severe symptoms and much earlier presentation to the hospital, so these patients can have out of control glucose for many

Table 1.30	Oral Hypoglycemic Agents
Class	**Characteristics**
Biguanide (metformin)	• First line for obese diabetics because it promotes weight loss • Works by upregulating insulin receptors and inhibiting gluconeogenesis • Because it is not a stimulator of insulin secretion, it does not promote weight gain and it is much less likely to cause hypoglycemia • Secreted by the kidneys so contraindicated in renal failure, and relatively contraindicated in CHF—accumulation of the drug in either setting can lead to profound lactic acidosis (be careful with iodinated contrast induced renal failure as well, hold metformin for the procedure)
Sulfonylureas (glipizide, glyburide, glimepiride, gliclazide)	• Act by stimulating insulin secretion, so can induce weight gain and hypoglycemia • Hypoglycemia can be prolonged (particularly with first-generation drugs which are rarely used now), requiring a day or more of iv D5W
Thiazolidinediones (rosiglitazone, pioglitazone)	• Increase tissue sensitivity to insulin • Can cause salt retention leading to peripheral volume expansion leading to CHF—contraindicated in CHF • Rosiglitazone also linked to increased risk of myocardial infarction
α-glucosidase inhibitors (acarbose)	• Block carbohydrate uptake from the intestines • Major side effect is gassiness and bloating, rarely used
Meglitinides (repaglinide, nateglinide)	• Stimulate insulin secretion only in the presence of glucose • Risk of hypoglycemia lower
Peptide analogues	• Exanetide and liraglutide are injectible peptide mimickers of glucagon-like peptide 1 (GLP-1), the so-called GLP-1 agonists, which stimulate insulin secretion, typically used as adjunctive therapy with other oral agents • Sitagliptin and saxagliptin are oral agents that inhibit dipeptidyl peptidase-4 (DPP-4), which normally degrades endogenous GLP-1, so the inhibitors prolong endogenous GLP-1 activity, resulting in insulin secretion
Amylin analog (pramlintide)	• An injectible analogue of the hormone amlyn, which inhibits glucagon secretion • It can be added to insulin or other oral hypoglycemic agents for either Type 1 or Type 2 DM

days to weeks and are more volume depleted than DKA patients

(2) Glucose often >1,000 mg/dL, no acidosis, ⊕ renal failure, and confusion

(3) Tx = rehydrate (may require 10 L), insulin drip; mortality is higher than for DKA, and may result from cerebral edema due to significant changes in sodium and water levels during therapy

C. Adrenal Disorders

1. Cushing's Syndrome

a. Usually iatrogenic (cortisol Tx) or because of pituitary adenoma = Cushing's dz; rarely because of adrenal hyperplasia, ectopic adrenocorticotropic hormone (ACTH)/corticotropin-releasing hormone (CRH) production

b. Si/Sx (Figure 1.11) = **buffalo hump, truncal obesity, moon facies, striae,** hirsutism, hyperglycemia, hypertension, purpura, amenorrhea, impotence, acne

c. Dx = 24-hr urine cortisol and low-dose dexamethasone suppression test

d. Tx

(1) Excision of tumor with postoperative glucocorticoid replacement

(2) Mitotane (adrenolytic), ketoconazole (inhibits P450), metyrapone (blocks adrenal enzyme synthesis), or aminoglutethimide (inhibits P450) for nonexcisable tumors

2. Adrenal Insufficiency

a. Can be 1° (Addison's dz) or 2° (↓ ACTH production by pituitary)

b. Addison's dz

(1) Causes = autoimmune (most common), granulomatous dz, infarction, HIV, DIC (Waterhouse–Friderichsen syndrome)

(2) **Waterhouse–Friderichsen** = hemorrhagic necrosis of adrenal medulla during the course of meningococcemia

(3) Si/Sx = fatigue, anorexia, nausea/vomit, constipation, diarrhea, salt craving (pica), hypotension, **hyponatremia, hyperkalemia**

(4) **Dx = hyperpigmentation, ↑ ACTH, ↓ cortisol response to ACTH**

c. **2° Dz → NO hyperpigmentation, ↓ ACTH,** ↑ cortisol response to ACTH

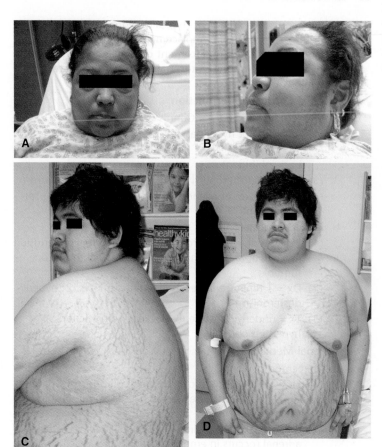

FIGURE 1.11

A, and **B.** Typical cushingoid "moon face" associated with excessive cortico-steroid use or production. (Courtesy of Mark Silverberg, MD.) **C,D.** Moon face, truncal obesity, buffalo hump, and purple striae seen here are all associated with Cushing's syndrome. (Courtesy of Bronson Terry, MD. All photos from Greenberg MI, Hendrickson RG, Silverberg M, et al. *Greenberg's text-atlas of emergency medicine.* Philadelphia, PA: Lippincott Williams & Wilkins, 2004, with permission.)

    d. Acute adrenal crisis
      (1) Because of stress (e.g., surgery or trauma), usually in setting of Tx chronic insufficiency or withdrawal of Tx
      (2) Can occur in pituitary apoplexy (infarction)

e. Tx = cortisol replacement (typically hydrocortisone in the acute setting), ↑ replacement for times of illness or stress—**must taper replacement off slowly to allow hypothalamic-pituitary-adrenal (HPA) axis to restore itself**

3. **Adrenal Cortical Hyperfunction**

   a. 1° hyperaldosteronism = Conn's syndrome

      (1) Adenoma or hyperplasia of zona glomerulosa

      (2) Si/Sx = **HTN**, ↑ **Na**, ↑ **Cl**, ↓ **K, alkalosis**, ↓ renin (feedback inhibition)

      (3) Dx = ↑ aldosterone, ↓ renin, CT → adrenal neoplasm

      (4) Tx = excision of adenoma—bilateral hyperplasia → spironolactone

   b. 2° hyperaldosteronism

      (1) Because of ↑ renin production 2° to renal hypoperfusion (e.g., CHF, shock, renal artery stenosis), cirrhosis, or tumor

      (2) Dx = ↑ renin (renin levels differentiate 1° vs. 2° hyperaldosteronism)

      (3) Tx = underlying cause, β-blocker or diuretic for hypertension

4. **Adrenal Medulla**

   a. Pheochromocytoma

      (1) Si/Sx = HTN (episodic or chronic), **diaphoresis, palpitations,** tachycardia, headache, nausea/vomit, flushing, dyspnea, diarrhea

      (2) **Rule of 10:** 10% malignant, 10% bilateral, 10% extraadrenal (occurs in embryologic cells that reactivate outside the adrenal gland)

      (3) Dx = ↑ urinary catecholamines, CT scan of adrenal showing neoplasm

      (4) Tx

         (a) Surgical excision after preoperative administration of α-blockers

         (b) Ca^{2+} channel blockers for hypertensive crisis

         (c) Phenoxybenzamine or phentolamine (α-blockers) for inoperable dz

         (d) Metastatic disease can be treated with Iodine 131-metaiodobenzylguanidine (I-MIBG)

Table 1.31	Differential Diagnosis of Male Gonadal Disorders
Disease	**Characteristics**
Klinefelter's syndrome	• XXY chromosome inheritance, variable expressivity • Often not Dx until puberty, when ↓ virilization is noted • Si/Sx = tall, eunuchoid, with small testes and gynecomastia, ↓ testosterone, ↑ LH/FSH from lack of feedback • **Dx = buccal smear analysis for presence of Barr bodies** • Tx = testosterone supplement
XYY syndrome	• Si/Sx = may have mild mental retardation, severe acne, ↑ incidence of violence and antisocial behavior • Dx = karyotype analysis • Tx = none
Testicular feminization syndrome	• Defect in the dihydrotestosterone, receptor → female external genitalia with sterile, undescended testes • Si/Sx = appear as females but are sterile and the vagina is blind-ended, testosterone, estrogen, and LH are all ↑ • Dx = history, physical exam, genetic testing • Tx = none
5-α-Reductase deficiency	• Si/Sx = ambiguous genitalia until puberty, then a burst in testosterone overcomes lack of dihydrotestosterone → external genitalia become masculinized, **testosterone and estrogen are normal** • Dx = genetic testing • Tx = testosterone supplements

FSH, follicle-stimulating hormone; LH, luteinizing hormone.

D. **Gonadal Disorders**
   1. **Male Gonadal Axis (see OB-Gyn for Female Axis)** (Table 1.31)
   2. **Hypogonadism of Either Sex** (Table 1.32)
E. **Thyroid**
   1. **Hyperthyroidism**
      a. Si/Sx of hyperthyroidism = tachycardia, **isolated systolic hypertension,** tremor, A-fib, anxiety, diaphoresis, weight loss with ↑ appetite, insomnia/**fatigue,** diarrhea, **exophthalmus, heat intolerance**
      b. Graves dz

Table 1.32 Genetic Hypogonadism

Disease	Characteristics
Congenital adrenal hyperplasia (CAH)	• Defects in steroid synthetic pathway causing either virilization of females or fail to virilize males • 21-α-hydroxylase deficiency causes 95% of all CAH • Severe dz presents in infancy with ambiguous genitalia and salt loss (2° to ↓↓ aldosterone) • Less severe variants → minimal virilization and salt loss, and can have Dx delayed for several years • Tx = replacement of necessary hormones
Prader–Willi syndrome	• Paternal imprinting (only gene from dad is expressed) • Si/Sx = presents in infancy with floppy baby, **short limbs,** obesity due to gross hyperphagia, nasal speech, retardation, **classic almond-shaped eyes with strabismus** • Dx = clinical or genetic analysis • Tx = none
Laurence–Moon–Biedl syndrome	• Autosomal recessive inheritance • Si/Sx = obese children, **normal craniofacial appearance,** may be retarded, **are not short, have polydactyly** • Dx = clinical or genetic • Tx = none
Kallmann's syndrome	• Autosomal dominant hypogonadism with anosmia (cannot smell) • Due to ↓ production/secretion of GnRH by hypothalamus • Dx by lack of circulating LH and FSH • Tx = pulsatile GnRH to cause virilization

GnRH, gonadotropin-releasing hormone.

(1) Diffuse, autoimmune goiter, causes 90% of US hyperthyroid cases

(2) Seen in young adults, is eight times more common in female pts than male pts

(3) **Si/Sx include two findings only seen in hyperthyroid because of Graves' dz: infiltrative ophthalmopathy and pretibial myxedema**

(4) **Infiltrative ophthalmopathy** = exophthalmus not resolving when thyrotoxicosis is cured, because of autoAb-mediated damage (Figure 1.12)

(5) **Pretibial myxedema**

    (a) Brawny, pruritic, nonpitting edema usually on the shins

    (b) Often spontaneously remits after months to years

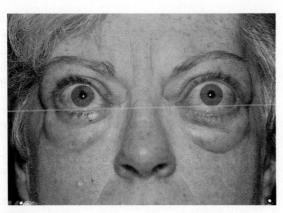

FIGURE 1.12

Exophthalmos in Grave's dz. (From Tasman W, Jaeger E. *The Wills eye hospital atlas of clinical ophthalmology,* 2nd Ed. Baltimore: Lippincott Williams & Wilkins, 2001.)

      (6) Dx confirmed with thyroid-stimulating immunoglobulin (TSI) test (autoAb binds to thyroid receptor, activating it, which is the cause of the dz)

  c. Plummer's dz (toxic multinodular goiter)

      (1) Because of multiple foci of thyroid tissue that cease responding to T_4 feedback inhibition, more common in older people

      (2) Dx = multiple thyroid nodules felt in gland, confirm with radioactive iodine uptake tests → hot nodules with cold background

  d. Thyroid adenoma because of overproduction of hormone by tumor in the gland

  e. Subacute thyroiditis (giant cell or de Quervain's thyroiditis)

      (1) Gland inflammation with spilling of hormone from the damaged gland

      (2) Can be painful (typically following a viral URI) or painless (because of drug toxicity—e.g., amiodarone or lithium, or autoimmune—which can be seen postpartum)

      (3) Painful dz presents with **jaw/tooth pain**, can be confused with dental dz, ↑ ESR

      (4) **Presents initially with hyperthyroidism but later turns into hypothyroidism as thyroid hormone is depleted from the inflamed gland**

  (5) Is typically self-limited within weeks or months as the
       viral or autoimmune cause burns itself out, so thyroid
       replacement is not necessary

  (6) Tx with aspirin or with cortisol in very severe dz

  f. Tx for all forms of hyperthyroidism (not necessary for sub-
      acute thyroiditis)

  (1) Propylthiouracil or methimazole induces remission in
       1 mo to 2 yrs (up to 50% of time); lifelong Tx not
       necessary unless dz relapses

  (2) Radioiodine is first line for Graves' dz: radioactive iodine
       is concentrated in the gland and destroys it, resolving
       the diffuse hyperthyroid state

  (3) If the above Tx fail → surgical excision (of adenoma or
       entire gland)

  g. Thyroid storm is the most extreme manifestation of hyper-
      thyroidism

  (1) Because of exacerbation of hyperthyroidism by surgery
       or infxn

  (2) Si/Sx = high fever, dehydration, cardiac arrhythmias,
       high-output cardiac failure, transaminitis, coma, 25%
       mortality

  (3) Tx

       (a) β-blockers and IV fluids are first priority to restore
            hemodynamic stability

       (b) Give propylthiouracil (PTU) to inhibit iodination of
            more thyroid hormone

       (c) After PTU on board, give iodine compounds,
            which will feedback inhibit further thyroid
            hormone release—make sure the PTU is on
            board first, or the iodine can cause an initial ↑
            in hormone release before it feedback suppresses
            release

       (d) Thyroid storm can precipitate adrenal crisis so
            consider stress dose hydrocortisone

2. **Hypothyroidism**

  a. Causes include Hashimoto's and subacute thyroiditis

  b. Si/Sx = **cold intolerance,** weight gain, **low energy,** husky
      voice, mental slowness, constipation, thick/coarse hair, puffi-
      ness of face/eyelids/hands **(myxedema),** loss of lateral third
      of eyebrows, prolonged relaxation phase of deep tendon
      reflexes (Figure 1.13)

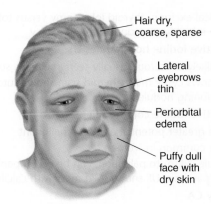

Hair dry,
coarse, sparse

Lateral
eyebrows
thin

Periorbital
edema

Puffy dull
face with
dry skin

FIGURE 1.13

Myxedema. The pt with severe hypothyroidism (myxedema) has a dull, puffy facies. The edema, often particularly pronounced around the eyes, does not pit with pressure. The hair and eyebrows are dry, coarse, and thinned. The skin is dry. (From Bickley LS, Szilagyi P. *Bates' guide to physical examination and history taking*, 8th Ed. Philadelphia, PA: Lippincott Williams & Wilkins, 2003).

   c. Hashimoto's dz
      (1) Autoimmune lymphocytic infiltration of the thyroid gland
      (2) **8:1 ratio in women to men,** usually between ages of 30 and 50
      (3) **Dx confirmed by antithyroid peroxidase (anti-TPO) or antimicrosomal Abs**
      (4) Tx = lifelong synthroid
   d. Subacute thyroiditis—see E.1.f. above
   e. Myxedema coma
      (1) **The only emergent hypothyroid condition**—spontaneous onset or precipitated by cold exposure, infxn, analgesia, sedative drug use, respiratory failure, or other severe illness
      (2) Si/Sx = stupor, coma, seizures, hypotension, hypoventilation
      (3) Tx = IV levothyroxine, cortisol, mechanical ventilation, and treat any infections aggressively with antibiotics
F. **Thyroid Malignancy**
   1. **Solitary dominant thyroid nodule**
      a. Dx by fine-needle aspiration

      b. Surgical excision, thyroid lobectomy versus total thyroidec-
tomy if highly suspicious for malignancy

2. **Radioactive iodine hot nodules** US
   a. Less likely cancerous, usually seen in elderly, soft to palpation
   b. US shows cystic mass; thyroid scan shows autonomously
      functioning nodule

3. **Radioactive iodine cold nodule**
   a. Has a greater potential of being malignant
   b. More common in women
   c. Nodule is firm to palpation, can be accompanied by vocal
      cord paralysis; US shows solid mass with calcifications

4. **Papillary CA**
   a. Most common CA of thyroid
   b. Good Px, 85% 5-yr survival, spread is indolent via lymph
      nodes
   c. Pathologically have ground-glass Orphan Annie nucleus and
      psammoma bodies (with calcifications)
   d. Bilateral thyroid lobe spread is common
   e. Tx = surgical excision followed by radioactive iodine

5. Medullary CA
   a. Has intermediate Px
   b. CA of parafollicular "C" cells that are derived from the
      ultimobranchial bodies (cells of branchial pouch 5)
   c. Secretes calcitonin; can Dx and follow dz with this blood assay

6. Follicular CA
   a. Commonly results in blood-borne metastases to bone and
      lungs
   b. Tx = surgical excision followed by radioactive iodine

7. **Anaplastic CA** has one of the poorest Px of any CA (0%
   survival at 5 yrs)

G. **Multiple Endocrine Neoplasia Syndromes** (Table 1.33)

Table 1.33 Multiple Endocrine Neoplasia Syndromes

Type I (Wermer's syndrome)	**The 3 (4) Ps: P**ituitary (**P**rolactinoma most common), **P**arathyoid, **P**ancreatoma
Type IIa (Sipple's syndrome)	Pheochromocytoma, medullary thyroid CA, parathyroid hyperplasia or tumor
Type IIb (Type III)	Pheochromocytoma, medullary thyroid CA, mucocutaneous neuromas, particularly of the GI tract

VI. Musculoskeletal

A. Metabolic Bone Dz

1. **Osteoporosis**
   a. Because of **postmenopausal (↓ estrogen)**, physical inactivity, high cortisol states (e.g., Cushing's dz, exogenous), hyperthyroidism, Ca^{2+} deficiency
   b. Si/Sx = typically aSx until fracture occurs, particularly of hip and vertebrae
   c. Dx = **Dual Energy X-ray Absortiometry (DEXA) scan** showing ↓ bone density compared with general population
   d. Tx
      (1) Bisphosphonates first line, proven to ↓ risk of fracture and slow or stop bone degeneration
      (2) Estrogens highly effective at stimulating new bone growth and preventing fractures, but long-term side effects (i.e., CA and heart dz risks) limit their use
   e. **Every pt with osteoporosis should take calcium to keep dietary intake ≥1.5 g/day**

2. **Rickets/Osteomalacia**
   a. Vitamin D deficiency in children = rickets; in adults = osteomalacia
   b. Si/Sx in kids (rickets) = **craniotabes** (thinning of skull bones), **rachitic rosary** (costochondral thickening looks like string of beads), **Harrison's groove** (depression along line of diaphragmatic insertion into rib cage), **Pigeon breast** = pectus carinatum (sternum protrusion)
   c. In adults, the dz mimics osteoporosis
   d. Dx = X-ray → radiolucent bones, can confirm with vitamin D
   e. Tx = vitamin D supplementation

3. **Scurvy**
   a. Vitamin C deficiency → ↓ osteoid formation
   b. Si/Sx = subperiosteal hemorrhage (painful), **bleeding gums,** multiple ecchymoses, osteoporosis, **"woody leg" from soft-tissue hemorrhage**
   c. Dx = clinical
   d. Tx = vitamin C supplementation

4. **Paget's Bone Dz (Osteitis Deformans)**
   a. Idiopathic ↑ activity of both osteoblasts and osteoclasts, usually in elderly

b. Si/Sx = **diffuse fractures and bone pain,** most commonly involves spine, pelvis, skull, femur, tibia; **high-output cardiac failure;** ↓ **hearing**

c. Dx = ↑↑ **alkaline phosphatase,** ⊕ bone scans, X-rays → sclerotic lesions

d. Tx = bisphosphonates first line, calcitonin second line

e. Complications = pathologic fractures, hypercalcemia and kidney stones, spinal cord compression in vertebral dz, osteosarcoma in long-standing dz

B. **Nonneoplastic Bone Dz**

1. **Fibrous Dysplasia**

a. Idiopathic replacement of bone with fibrous tissue

b. Three types = (i) monostotic, (ii) polystotic, (iii) McCune–Albright's

c. McCune–Albright's syndrome

(1) Syndrome of hyperparathyroidism, hyperadrenalism, and acromegaly

(2) **Dx** = polystotic fibrous dysplasia, precocious puberty, café-au-lait spots

d. Tx = supportive surgical debulking of deforming defects

2. **Osteomyelitis**

a. Caused by bacterial infxn of bone; *S. aureus* most common cause, but any bacterium can cause, as can certain fungi

b. **Pts with sickle cell dz get** *Salmonella; IV drug abusers get* ***Pseudomonas***

c. Si/Sx = painful inflammation of bone, with chronic or recurrent periods of drainage of pus through skin

d. Dx = **X-ray** → **periosteal elevation, can lag onset of dz by weeks;** MRI is gold-standard, can confirm with cultures of deep bone Bx

e. Tx = surgical débridement + weeks to months of antibiotics

C. **Bone Tumors**

1. Dx/Tx of primary bone neoplasms (Table 1.34)

2. Multiple myeloma

a. Malignant clonal neoplasm of plasma cells producing whole Abs (e.g., IgM, IgG, etc.), light chains only, or very rarely no Abs (just ↑ B cells)

b. Seen in pts >40 yrs; African-American pts have 2:1 incidence

c. **Si/Sx** = bone pain worse with movement, lytic bone lesions on X-ray (Figure 1.14), pathologic fractures, **hypercalcemia,** renal failure, anemia, frequent infxns by encapsulated

Table 1.34 Diagnosis[a] and Treatment of Primary Bone Neoplasms

Tumor	Pt Age[b]	Characteristics
Osteochondroma	<25	• Benign, usually in males • Seen at distal femur and proximal tibia
Giant cell	20–40	• Benign, epiphysical ends of long bones (>50% in knee) • X-ray → **soap bubble** sign • Often recurs after excision • Tx = excision and local irradiation
Osteosarcoma	10–20	• #1 primary bone malignancy • Seen at distal femur and proximal tibia • 2- to 3-fold ↑ alkaline phosphatase • **X-ray → Codman's triangle** = periosteal elevation due to tumor and **"sun burst" sign** = lytic lesion with surrounding speculated periostitis (Figure 1.15) • Tx = excision and local irradiation
Ewing's sarcoma	<15	• Young boys, metastasizes very early • Si/Sx mimic osteomyelitis (Figure 1.14) • Presents with "onion skin" appearance on x-ray • Tx = chemotherapy

[a]Diagnoses all confirmed with bone biopsy.
[b]Peak age of onset.

bacteria, ↓ **anion gap** (Abs positively charged, unseen cations make anion gap appear ↓)

d. **Hyperviscosity syndrome** = stroke, retinopathy, CHF, ESR >100

e. **Bence-Jones proteinuria**

f. Light-chain deposition causes renal amyloidosis

g. Dx

(1) Serum protein and urine protein electrophoresis (SPEP and UPEP)

(2) Both → tall electrophoretic peak called "M-spike" due to ↑ Ab (Figure 1.15)

(3) SPEP → M-spike if clones make whole Ab

(4) UPEP → spike if clones make light chains only

(5) **Either SPEP or UPEP will almost always be ⊕**

(6) Dx = ⊕ SPEP/UPEP and any of (i) ↑ plasma cells in bone marrow, (ii) osteolytic bone lesions, OR (iii) Bence-Jones proteinuria

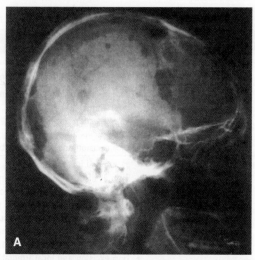

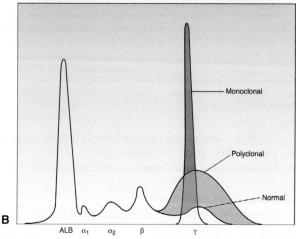

FIGURE 1.14

A. Multiple myeloma. A radiograph of the skull shows numerous punched-out radiolucent areas. (Image from Rubin E, Farber JL. *Pathology,* 3rd Ed. Philadelphia, PA: Lippincott Williams & Wilkins, 1999.) **B.** Serum protein electrophoretic patterns. Abnormal serum protein electrophoretic patterns are contrasted with a nml pattern. In polyclonal hypergammaglobulinemia, which is characteristic of benign reactive processes, there is a broad-based ↑ in immunoglobulins because of immunoglobulin secretion by myriad discrete reactive plasma cells. In monoclonal gammopathy, which is characteristic of monoclonal gammopathy of unknown significance or plasma cell neoplasia, there is a narrow peak, or spike, because of the homogeneity of the immunoglobulin molecules secreted by a single clone of aberrant plasma cells. (Image from Rubin E, Farber JL. *Pathology,* 3rd Ed. Philadelphia, PA: Lippincott Williams & Wilkins, 1999.)

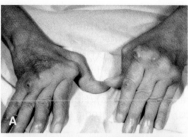
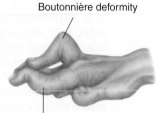

Boutonnière deformity

B Swan neck deformity

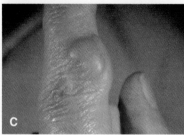

FIGURE 1.15

A. Rheumatoid arthritis. The hands of a pt with advanced arthritis show swelling of the metacarpophalangeal joints and the classic ulnar deviation of the fingers. (Image from Rubin E, Farber JL. *Pathology,* 3rd Ed. Philadelphia, PA: Lippincott Williams & Wilkins, 1999.) **B.** As the arthritic process continues and worsens, the fingers may show "swan neck" deformities (i.e., hyperextension of the proximal interphalangeal joints with fixed flexion of the distal interphalangeal joints). Less common is a boutonniere deformity (i.e., persistent flexion of the proximal interphalangeal joint with hyperextension of the distal interphalangeal joint). (From Bickley LS, Szilagyi P. *Bates' guide to physical examination and history taking,* 8th Ed. Philadelphia, PA: Lippincott Williams & Wilkins, 2003.) **C.** Rheumatoid nodule. A pt with rheumatoid arthritis has a mass on a digit. (Image from Rubin E, Farber JL. *Pathology,* 3rd Ed. Philadelphia, PA: Lippincott Williams & Wilkins, 1999.)

    h. Tx
        (1) Radiation given for isolated lesions, chemotherapy for metastatic dz
        (2) Bone marrow transplantation (BMT) may prolong survival
        (3) Palliative care important for pain
    i. Px poor despite Tx

D. Arthropathies and Connective Tissue Disorders
    1. **RA**
        a. Autoimmune dz of unknown etiology → **symmetric inflammatory arthritis**

b. Female/male = 3:1, pts are commonly **HLA-DR4 ⊕**

c. Si/Sx = **symmetric arthritis worse in morning** affecting knees, feet, metacarpophalangeal **(MCP)** and proximal interphalangeal **(PIP)** joints (Figure 1.15A), flexion contractures → ulnar deviation of digits (Figure 1.15A), swan neck and boutonniere deformity of hand (Figure 1.15B), subcutaneous nodules (present in <50% of pts) (Figure 1.15C), pleural effusions (serositis), anemia of chronic dz

d. Labs

  (1) Rheumatoid factor (RF) = IgM anti-IgG

    (a) Present in >70% of pts with RA but may appear late in dz course

    (b) **Not specific for RA**, can be ⊕ in any chronic inflammatory state and may be present in 5% to 10% of healthy geriatric pts

  (2) Anti cyclic citrullinated peptides (CCP) is much more specific, 95% specific and 70% sensitive for RA

e. Dx = clinical plus serologies

f. Tx

  (1) NSAIDs are first line, methotrexate second line

  (2) TNF antagonists markedly improve symptoms, even in pts refractory to standard Tx—always check a PPD before starting anti-TNF therapy, administer INH if positive, and monitor closely during treatment for infections including standard bacterial infections, TB, and fungal infections

  (3) Other disease-modifying agents include hydroxychloroquine, leflunomide, azathioprine, cyclosporine

2. **SLE**

a. Systemic autoimmune disorder, female/male ratio = 9:1

b. Si/Sx = fever, polyarthritis, skin lesions, splenomegaly, hemolytic anemia, thrombocytopenia, serositis (e.g., pleuritis and pericarditis), Libman–Sacks endocarditis, renal dz, skin rashes, thrombosis, neurologic disorders

c. Labs

  (1) **Antinuclear antibody (ANA) sensitive** (>98%) but not specific

  (2) **Anti–double-stranded DNA (anti–ds-DNA) Abs 99% specific but not sensitive**

  (3) Anti-Smith (anti-Sm) Abs are highly specific but not sensitive

  (4) Anti-Ro Abs are ⊕ in 50% of ANA-negative lupus

(5) Antiribosomal P and antineuronal Abs correlate with risk for cerebral involvement of lupus (lupus cerebritis)

(6) Antiphospholipid autoAbs cause false ⊕ lab tests in SLE

   (a) **Pts with SLE frequently have false ⊕** rapid plasma regain/Venereal Dz Research Laboratory test (**RPR/ VDRL) tests for syphilis**

   (b) Pts with **SLE frequently have ↑ PTT (lupus anticoagulant Ab)**

      (i) PTT is falsely ↑ because the lupus anticoagulant Ab binds to phospholipid that initiates clotting in the test tube

      (ii) **Despite the PTT test and the name lupus anticoagulant Ab, pts with SLE are THROMBOGENIC because antiphospholipid Abs cause coagulation in vivo**

d. Mnemonic for SLE diagnosis: **DOPAMINE RASH**

   (1) **D**iscoid lupus = circular, erythematous macules with scales (Figure 1.16)

   (2) **O**ral aphthous ulcers (can be nasopharyngeal as well)

   (3) **P**hotosensitivity

   (4) **A**rthritis (typically hands, wrists, knees)

   (5) **M**alar rash = classic butterfly macule on cheeks

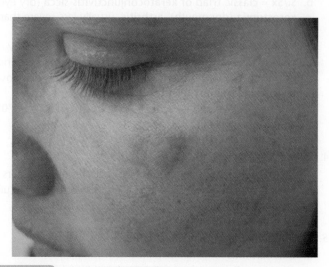

FIGURE 1.16
Circular plaque lesion of discoid lupus on the cheek.

(6) Immunologic criteria = anti–ds-DNA, anti-Sm Ab, anti-Ro Ab, anti-La

(7) Neurologic changes = psychosis, personality change, seizures

(8) ESR rate ↑ (NOT 1 of the 11 criteria but is a frequent lab finding)

(9) Renal dz → nephritic or nephrotic syndrome

(10) ANA⊕

(11) Serositis (pleurisy, pericarditis)

(12) Hematologic dz = hemolytic anemia, thrombocytopenia, leukopenia

e. Drug-induced SLE

(1) Drugs = procainamide, hydralazine, phenytoin, sulfonamides, INH

(2) Labs → antihistone Abs, differentiating from idiopathic SLE

f. Tx = NSAIDs, hydroxychloroquine, prednisone, cyclophosphamide depending on severity of dz

g. Px = variable; 10-yr survival is excellent; **renal dz is a poor Px indicator**

3. **Sjögren's Syndrome (SS)**

a. Autoinflammatory disorder associated with **HLA-DR3**

b. Si/Sx = **classic triad of keratoconjunctivitis sicca** (dry eyes), **xerostomia** (dry mouth), **arthritis,** usually less severe than pure RA

c. Systemic Si/Sx = pancreatitis, fibrinous pericarditis, CN V sensory neuropathy, RTA, 40-fold ↑ in lymphoma incidence

d. Dx = Concomitant presence of two of the triad is diagnostic, consider salivary gland Bx

e. Labs → ANA ⊕, anti-Ro/anti-La Ab ⊕ ("SSA/SSB Abs"), 70% are RF ⊕

f. Tx = steroids, cyclophosphamide for refractory dz

4. **Behçet's Syndrome**

a. Multisystem inflammatory disorder that chronically recurs

b. Si/Sx = painful oral and genital ulcers, also arthritis, vasculitis, neurologic dz

c. Tx = prednisone during flare-ups

5. **Seronegative Spondyloarthropathy**

a. Osteoarthritis

(1) **Noninflammatory arthritis** caused by joint wear and tear

(2) Most common arthritis, results in wearing away of joint cartilage

(3) Si/Sx = pain and crepitation upon joint motion, ↓ range of joint motion, can have radiculopathy because of cord impingement

(4) **X-ray → osteophytes (bone spurs) and asymmetric joint space loss**

(5) Physical exam → **Heberden's nodes** (distal interphalangeal joint [DIP] swelling 2° to osteophytes) and **Bouchard's nodes** (PIP swelling 2° to osteophytes) (Figure 1.17)

(6) **Note: RA affects MCP and PIP joints, while osteoarthritis affects PIP and DIP joints**

(7) Tx = NSAIDs, muscle relaxants, joint replacement (third line)

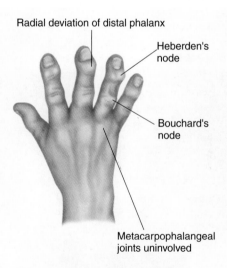

Radial deviation of distal phalanx

Heberden's node

Bouchard's node

Metacarpophalangeal joints uninvolved

FIGURE 1.17

Osteoarthritis (degenerative joint dz). Nodules on the dorsolateral aspects of the distal interphalangeal joints (Heberden's nodes) are because of the bony overgrowth of osteoarthritis. Usually hard and painless, they affect the middle-aged or elderly pts and often, although not always, are associated with arthritic changes in other joints. Flexion and deviation deformities may develop. Similar nodules on the proximal interphalangeal joints (Bouchard's nodes) are less common. The metacarpophalangeal joints are spared. (From Bickley LS, Szilagyi P. *Bates' guide to physical examination and history taking*, 8th Ed. Philadelphia, PA: Lippincott Williams & Wilkins, 2003.)

(8) **Isometric exercise to strengthen muscles around joint has been shown to improve Sx**

b. Ankylosing spondylitis

(1) Rheumatologic dz usually in **HLA-B27** ⊕ male pts (male/female ratio = 3:1)

(2) Si/Sx = sacroiliitis, spinal dz → complete fusion of adjacent vertebral bodies causing **"bamboo spine"** (Figure 1.18), uveitis, heart block

(3) **If sacroiliac joint is not affected, it is not ankylosing spondylitis**

(4) Dx = X-ray signs of spinal fusion and negative RF

(5) Tx = NSAIDs and strengthening of back muscles

c. Reactive Arthritis

(1) Usually seen in male pts; **approximately three-fourths of these pts are HLA-B27⊕**

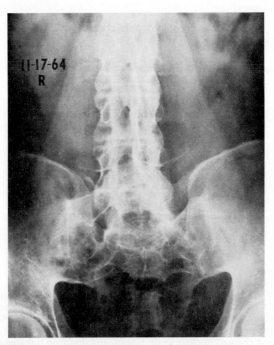

FIGURE 1.18

X-ray changes of spine (classic "bamboo spine"). (From Gold DH, Weingeist TA. *Color atlas of the eye in systemic disease.* Baltimore, MD: Lippincott Williams & Wilkins, 2001.)

    (2) Presents with nongonococcal **urethritis** (often chlamydial), **conjunctivitis, reactive arthritis,** and **uveitis**—mnemonic, "can't see, can't pee, can't climb a tree"

    (3) Classic dermatologic Sx = **circinate balanitis** (serpiginous, moist plaques on glans penis) and **keratoderma blennorrhagicum** (crusting papules with central erosion, looks like mollusk shell)

    (4) Tx = macrolide (for *Chlamydia* coverage) plus NSAIDs for arthritis

  d. Psoriatic arthritis

    (1) Presents with **nail pitting and DIP** joint involvement

    (2) Occurs in up to 10% of pts with psoriasis

    (3) Psoriatic flares may exacerbate arthritis and vice versa

    (4) Tx = ultraviolet light for psoriasis and immunosuppressives (methotrexate, TNF antagonists, cyclosporine) for arthritis

  e. Inflammatory bowel dz can cause seronegative arthritis

  f. Disseminated gonococcal infxn can cause **monoarticular** arthritis

6. **Scleroderma (Progressive Systemic Sclerosis [PSS])**

  a. Systemic fibrosis affecting virtually every organ, female/male ratio = 4:1

  b. Skin tightening of face causing classic facial appearance (Figure 1.19)

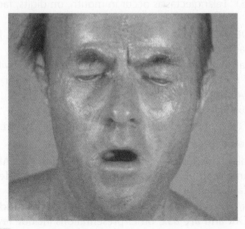

FIGURE 1.19

Classic scleroderma facies with skin tightening. (With permission from Clements PJ, Furst DE. *Systemic sclerosis.* Baltimore, MD: Williams & Wilkins, 1996.)

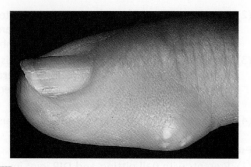

FIGURE 1.20

Calcinosis. Subcutaneous and periarticular calcium deposits may be extremely painful. (From Axford JS, Callaghan CA. *Medicine,* 2nd Ed. Oxford: Blackwell Science, 2004, with permission.)

   c. Can be diffuse dz (PSS) or more benign CREST syndrome

   d. **Si/Sx of CREST syndrome**

     (1) **C**alcinosis = subcutaneous calcifications, often in fingers (Figure 1.20)

     (2) **R**aynaud's phenomenon, often the initial symptom

     (3) **E**sophageal dysmotility because of lower esophageal sphincter sclerosis → reflux

     (4) **S**clerodactyly = fibrosed skin causes immobile digits

     (5) **T**elangiectasias occur in mouth, on digits, face, and trunk

   e. Other Sx = flexion contractures, biliary cirrhosis, lung/cardiac/renal fibrosis

   f. Labs = ⊕ ANA in 95%; anti–Scl-70 has ↓ sensitivity but ↑ specificity; anticentromere is 80% sensitive for CREST syndrome

   g. Dx = clinical

   h. Tx = immunosuppressives for palliation; none are curative

7. **Sarcoidosis**

   a. Idiopathic, diffuse dz presenting in 20s to 40s, **African-American pts are three times more likely to develop than Caucasian pts**

   b. Si/Sx = **50% of pts present with incidental finding on CXR and are aSx;** other presentations include fevers, chills, night sweats, weight loss, cough, dyspnea, rash, arthralgia, blurry vision (uveitis)

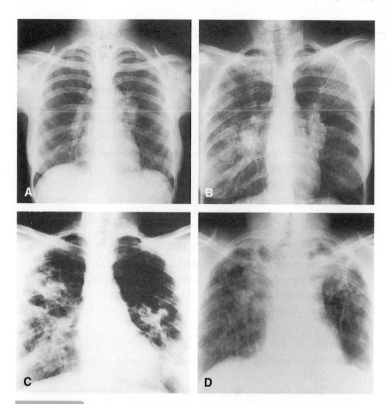

FIGURE 1.21

X-rays illustrating the different stages of sarcoidosis. **A.** Stage I. Bilateral hilar adenopathy and paratracheal adenopathy with nml lung fields. **B.** Stage II. Bilateral hilar adenopathy with interstitial lung field involvement. **C.** Stage III. Lung field involvement only. **D.** Stage IV. Severely fibrotic lungs with volume loss and cyst formation. (From Crapo JD, Glassroth J, Karlinsky JB, et al. *Baum's textbook of pulmonary diseases,* 7th Ed. Philadelphia, PA: Lippincott Williams & Wilkins, 2004.)

   c. **CXR has several stages of dz** (Figure 1.21)
      (1) Stage I = **bilateral hilar adenopathy**
      (2) Stage II = hilar adenopathy with infiltrates
      (3) Stage III = lung involvement only
      (4) Stage IV = chronic scarring
   d. Can affect ANY organ system
      (1) CNS → CN palsy, classically CN VII (can be bilateral)
      (2) **Eye → uveitis (can be bilateral), requires aggressive Tx**

(3) Cardiac → heart blocks, arrhythmias, constrictive pericarditis

(4) Lung → typically a restrictive defect

(5) GI → ↑ AST/ALT; CT → granulomas in liver, cholestasis

(6) Renal → nephrolithiasis because of hypercalcemia

(7) Endocrine → DI

(8) Hematologic → anemia, thrombocytopenia, leukopenia

(9) Skin → various rashes, including erythema nodosum

  e. Dx is clinical; **noncaseating granulomas on bx is very suggestive**

  f. Labs → 50% of pts have ↑ ACE level

  g. Tx = prednisone (first line), but 50% of pts spontaneously remit, so only Tx if (i) eye/heart involved, or (ii) dz does not remit after mos

8. **Mixed Connective Tissue Dz (MCTD)**

  a. Commonly onsets in women in teens and 20s

  b. Si/Sx = overlapping SLE, scleroderma, and polymyositis but **characterized by ⊕ anti-U1 RNP Ab**

  c. Dx = anti-U1 RNP Ab

  d. Tx = steroids, azathioprine

9. **Gout**

  a. **Monoarticular arthritis** because of urate crystal deposits in joint

  b. **Gout develops after 20–30 yrs of hyperuricemia, often precipitated by sudden changes in serum urate levels** (gout in teens → 20s likely genetic)

  c. **Most people with hyperuricemia never get gout**

  d. ↑ Production of uric acid can be genetic or acquired (e.g., alcohol, hemolysis, neoplasia, psoriasis)

  e. Underexcretion of urate via kidney (<800 mg/dL urine urate) can be idiopathic or because of kidney dz, drugs (aspirin, diuretics, alcohol)

  f. Si/Sx of gout = painful monoarticular arthritis affecting distal joints (often first metatarsophalangeal joint = **podagra** [Figure 1.22A]); chronic dz leads to tophaceous gout with destruction of joints (Figure 1.22B)

  g. Dx = **clinical triad of monoarticular arthritis, hyperuricemia, ⊕ response to colchicine,** confirm with needle tap of joint → crystals

  h. Acute Tx = colchicine and NSAIDs (not aspirin)

  i. Px = some people never experience more than one attack; those that do → chronic tophaceous gout, with significant

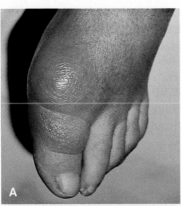
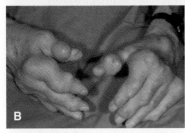
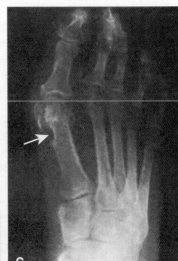

FIGURE 1.22

A. Podagra of acute gout. **B.** Chronic tophaceous gout. (Image from Rubin E, Farber JL. *Pathology,* 3rd Ed. Philadelphia, PA: Lippincott Williams & Wilkins, 1999.) **C.** "Rat-bite" (*white arrow*) appearance of chronic tophaceous gout on X-ray. (Reprinted with permission from Barker LR, Burton JR, Zieve, PD. *Principles of ambulatory medicine,* 4th Ed. Baltimore: Williams & Wilkins, 1995:935.)

      joint deformation (**classic rat-bite appearance to joint on X-ray**—Figure 1.22C) and toothpaste-like discharge from joint

   j. Maintenance Tx
     (1) Do not start unless pt has more than one attack
     (2) Overproducers → allopurinol (inhibits xanthine oxidase)
     (3) Underexcreters → probenecid/sulfinpyrazone
     (4) **Always start while pt still taking colchicine, because sudden ↓ in serum urate precipitates an acute attack**
   k. Pseudogout
     (1) Caused by calcium pyrophosphate dihydrate (CPPD) crystal deposition in joints and articular cartilage (chondrocalcinosis)

(2) Mimics gout very closely; seen in persons age 60 or older; often affects larger, more proximal joints

(3) Can be 1° or 2° to metabolic dz (hyperparathyroidism, Wilson's dz, diabetes, hemochromatosis)

(4) Dx → microscopic analysis of joint aspirate

(5) Tx = colchicine and NSAIDs

l. Microscopy

(1) **Gout → needle-like negatively birefringent yellow crystals** (Figure 1.23A)

(2) **"P"seudogout → "P"ositively birefringent blue crystals** (Figure 1.23B)

10. Septic Arthritis

a. Monoarticular arthritis in a sexually active pt usually because of *Neisseria gonorrhoeae*

b. Otherwise, the most common cause is *S. aureus,* with *Streptococcus* spp. and GNR less common

c. Septic arthritis must be distinguished from gout and pseudogout, which can present similarly

d. Dx = joint fluid Gram stain, culture, swabbing all orifices for *N. gonorrhoeae,* and sending fluid for crystals

e. Joint fluid WBC count in pyogenic septic arthritis (e.g., *S. aureus, Streptococcus,* GNR) typically is >50,000; in arthritis caused by *N. gonorrhoeae* it is often <50,000

f. Tx = antibiotics targeted either at *N. gonorrhoeae* or *Staphylococcus, Streptococcus,* and GNR depending on Gram stain and culture (GS/Cx) results

11. Polymyalgia Rheumatica

a. Inflammatory condition that typically occurs in elderly women (age >50)

b. Si/Sx = painful muscle tenderness in the neck, shoulders, and upper back relieved by NSAIDs or steroids

c. Dx = demographics (elderly, typically but not exclusively female) and invariably a very high ESR (>100)

d. Beware, often associated with temporal arteritis

e. Tx is prednisone taper

E. **Muscle Dz**

1. **General**

a. Dz of muscle are divided into two groups: neurogenic and myopathic

b. Neurogenic dz → **distal weakness, no pain, fasciculations present**

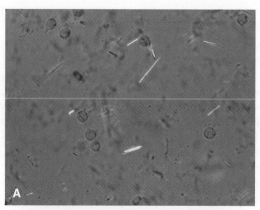

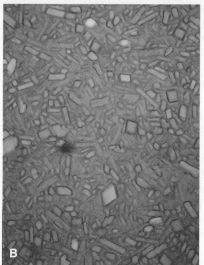

FIGURE 1.23

A. Gout. Synovial fluid microscopy under compensated polarized light showing the slender, needle-shaped, negatively birefringent urate crystals. The axis of slow vibration is from *bottom left* to *top right.* (From Axford JS. *Medicine.* Oxford: Blackwell Science, 1996, with permission.) **B.** Calcium pyrophosphate dehydrate crystals (extracted from synovial fluid), which are pleomorphic, rectangular, and weakly positively birefringent. The axis of slow vibration is from *bottom left* to *top right.* (From Axford JS. *Medicine.* Oxford: Blackwell Science, 1996, with permission.)

    c. Myopathic dz → **proximal weakness, ± pain, no fascicula-tions**

2. **Duchenne's Muscular Dystrophy**
   a. **X-linked** lack of dystrophin
   b. Si/Sx commence at age 1 yr with **progressive proximal weakness and wasting,** ↑ creatine phosphate kinase (CPK), **calf hypertrophy,** waddling gait, Gower's maneuver (pts pick themselves off the floor by using arms to help legs)
   c. Tx = supportive
   d. Px = death occurs in 10s–20s, most often because of pneumonia
   e. Becker's dystrophy is similar but less severe dz

3. **Polymyositis and Dermatomyositis**
   a. Autoinflammatory dz of muscles and sometimes skin (dermatomyositis)
   b. Female/male = 2:1; occurs in young children and geriatric populations
   c. Si/Sx = symmetric weakness/atrophy of proximal limb mus-cles, muscle aches, dysphonia (laryngeal muscle weakness), dysphagia
   d. Dermatomyositis presents with above as well as with **peri-orbital heliotropic** purple rash and **shawl sign** (rash over shoulders, upper back, and V-shaped around neck line); also look for **Gottron's papules,** which are purple papules over the DIP and MCP joints of hand, and **periungal (i.e., around the nail bed) telangiectasias**
   e. Both polymyositis and dermatomyositis are associated with malignancy, both at the time of diagnosis of the myositis and also higher risk for future malignancies
   f. Dx = ANA ⊕, anti-Jo-1 Abs ⊕, ↑ creatine kinase, muscle Bx → inflammatory changes
   g. Tx = steroids, methotrexate, or cyclophosphamide for resistant dz

4. **Myasthenia Gravis (MG)**
   a. AutoAbs block the postsynaptic acetylcholine receptor
   b. Most common in women in 20s–30s or men in 50s–60s
   c. **Associated with thymomas, thyroid, and other autoim-mune dz (e.g., lupus)**
   d. Sx = **muscle weakness worse with use,** diplopia, dyspha-gia, proximal limb weakness, can progress to cause respira-tory failure

e. Dx = trial of edrophonium (the so-called Tensilon test) →
immediate ↑ in strength, confirm with electromyelography
→ repetitive stimulation ↓ action potential

f. DDx

(1) **Lambert–Eaton syndrome**

(a) AutoAb to **pre**synaptic Ca channels seen with small
cell lung CA

(b) Differs from MG in that Lambert–Eaton → ↓
reflexes, autonomic dysfunction (xerostomia, impotence), and **Sx improve with muscle use (action
potential strength ↑ with repeated stimulation)**

(2) Aminoglycosides can worsen MG or induce mild MG Sx
in critically ill pts

g. Tx = anticholinesterase inhibitors (e.g., pyridostigmine) first
line

(1) Steroids, cyclophosphamide, azathioprine for ↑ severe
dz

(2) Plasmapheresis temporarily alleviates Sx by removing
the Ab

(3) Resection of thymoma can be curative

VII. Hematology (Figure 1.24)

A. **Anemia**

1. **Microcytic Anemias (MCV <80)**

a. **Result from ↓ hemoglobin (Hb) production or impaired
Hb function**

b. Iron deficiency anemia

(1) **Must find the cause of iron deficiency**

(2) Epidemiology

(a) Number one anemia in the world; hookworms are
the number one cause in the world

(b) ↑ incidence in women of childbearing age 2° to
menses

(c) **In the elderly, it is colon CA until proven otherwise**

(d) Dietary deficiency **virtually impossible in adults,
seen in children**

(3) Si/Sx = tachycardia, fatigue, pallor all from anemia,
smooth tongue, brittle nails, esophageal webs, and pica
all from iron deficiency

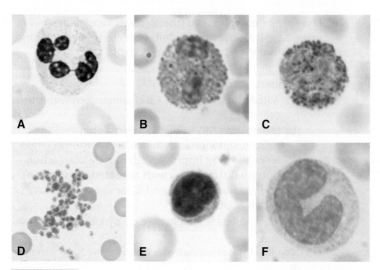

FIGURE 1.24

Nml blood cells. **A.** Neutrophil. **B.** Eosinophil. **C.** Basophil. **D.** Platelets. **E.** Lymphocyte. **F.** Monocyte. (From Cohen BJ, Wood DL. *Memmler's the human body in health and disease,* 9th Ed. Philadelphia, PA: Lippincott, Williams & Wilkins, 2000, with permission.)

     (4) Dx = ↓ **serum iron,** ↓ serum ferritin, ↑ **total iron-binding capacity (TIBC),** peripheral smear → target cells (Figure 1.25A)

     (5) Tx = iron sulfate; should achieve baseline hematocrit within 2 mos

  c. Sideroblastic anemia

     (1) Ineffective erythropoiesis because of disorder of porphyrin pathway

     (2) Etiologies = chronic alcoholism, drugs (commonly INH), genetic

FIGURE 1.25

A. Target cells on blood smear. (From Anderson SC. *Anderson's atlas of hematology.* Baltimore: Wolters Kluwer Health/Lippincott Williams & Wilkins, 2003.) **B.** Ringed sideroblasts on Prussian blue staining of iron in bone marrow. (McClatchey KD. *Clinical laboratory medicine,* 2nd Ed. Philadelphia, PA: Lippincott Williams & Wilkins, 2002.) **C.** Basophilic stippling of red cells on blood smear. (From Anderson SC. *Anderson's atlas of hematology.* Baltimore: Wolters Kluwer Health/Lippincott Williams & Wilkins, 2003.)

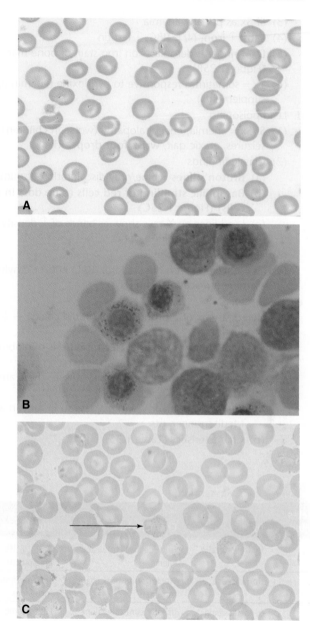

      (3) Si/Sx as per any anemia

      (4) Labs: ↑ **iron**, N/↑ TIBC, ↑ ferritin

      (5) Dx = ringed sideroblasts on iron stain of bone marrow (Figure 1.25B)

      (6) Tx = sometimes responsive to pyridoxine (vitamin B_6 supplements)

  d. Lead poisoning

      (1) Si/Sx = anemia, encephalopathy (worse in children), seizures, ataxic gait, **wrist/foot drops**, RTA

      (2) Classic findings

        (a) **Bruton's lines** = blue/gray discoloration at gumlines

        (b) **Basophilic stippling of red cells (blue dots in red cells)** (Figure 1.25C)

        (c) Lead lines on X-rays show as bands of ↑ density at metaphyses of long bones

      (3) Dx = serum lead level

      (4) Tx = chelation with dimercaprol (BAL) and/or ethylene-diaminetetraacetic acid (EDTA)

  e. Thalassemias

      (1) Hereditary dz of ↓ production of globin chains → ↓ Hb production

      (2) Differentiation through gel electrophoresis of globin proteins

      (3) α-Thalassemia (↓ α-globin chain synthesis; there are four α alleles)

        (a) Seen commonly in Asian pts, less so in African and Mediterranean pts

        (b) Characteristics (Table 1.35)

Table 1.35 α-Thalassemia

# Alleles Affected	Dz	Characteristic	Blood Smear
4	Hydrops fetalis	Fetal demise, total body edema	Bart's γ_4 Hb precipitations
3	HbH disease	Precipitation of β-chain tetramers	Intraerythrocytic inclusions
2	α-Thalassemia minor	Usually clinically silent	Mild microcytic anemia
1	Carrier state	No anemia, asymptomatic	No abnormalities

Table 1.36 β-Thalassemia

	Thalassemia Major (β–/β–)	Thalassemia Minor (β+/β–)
Si/Sx	Anemia develops at age 6 mos (due to switch from fetal γ Hb to adult β), splenomegaly, frontal bossing due to extramedullary hematopoiesis, iron overload (2° to transfusions)	Typically asymptomatic carriers
Dx	**Electrophoresis** ↓↓↓ HbA, ↑ HbA$_2$, ↑ HbF	**Electrophoresis** ↓ HbA, ↑ HbA$_2$ (γ), **N HbF**
Tx	Folate supplementation, splenectomy for hypersplenism, transfuse only for severe anemia	Avoid oxidative stress

    (4) β-Thalassemia (↓ β-globin chain synthesis; there are two β alleles)

        (a) Usually of Mediterranean or African descent

        (b) Characteristics (Table 1.36)

  f. Sickle cell anemia (Figure 1.26)

    (1) HbS tetramer polymerizes, causing sickling of deoxygenated RBCs

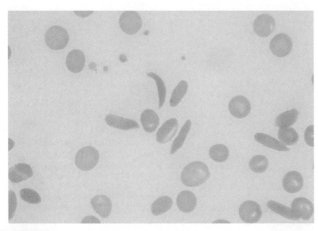

FIGURE 1.26

Sickle cell anemia on blood smear. (From Anderson SC. *Anderson's atlas of hematology.* Baltimore, MD: Wolters Kluwer Health/Lippincott Williams & Wilkins, 2003.)

(2) Si/Sx

    (a) Vaso-occlusion → pain crisis, myocardiopathy, infarcts of bone/CNS/lungs/kidneys, and autosplenectomy because of splenic infarct → ↑ susceptibility to encapsulated bacteria

    (b) **Intravascular hemolysis → gallstones in children or teens**

    (c) ↑ risk of aplastic anemia from parvovirus B19 infxns

(3) Dx = Hb electrophoresis → HbS phenotype

(4) Tx

    (a) O_2 (cells sickle when Hb desaturates), transfuse as needed

    (b) Hydroxyurea → ↓ incidence and severity of pain crises

    (c) Pneumococcal vaccination due to ↑ risk of infxn

2. **Megaloblastic Anemias (MCV >100)**

  a. **Results from ↓ DNA synthesis with nml RNA/protein synthesis**

  b. **Pathognomonic blood smear → hypersegmented neutrophils** (Figure 1.27)

  c. Vitamin B_{12} deficiency

    (1) Pernicious anemia is most common cause

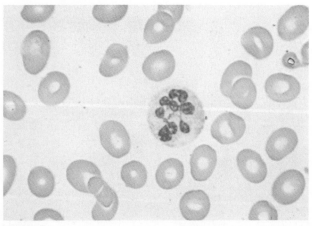

FIGURE 1.27

Hypersegmented neutrophil. (From Gold DH, Weingeist TA. *Color atlas of the eye in systemic disease.* Baltimore: Lippincott Williams & Wilkins, 2001.)

(a) Ab to gastric parietal cells $\rightarrow \downarrow$ production of intrinsic factor (necessary for uptake of B_{12} in the terminal ileum)

(b) Accompanied by achlorhydria and atrophic gastritis

(2) Other causes = malabsorption because of gastric resection, resection of terminal ileum, or intestinal infxn by *Diphyllobothrium latum*

(3) Si/Sx = megaloblastic anemia **with neurologic signs** = peripheral neuropathy, paresthesias, $\downarrow$ balance and position sense, **worse in legs**

(4) **Dx = $\uparrow$ serum methylmalonic acid and $\uparrow$ homocysteine levels**—more sensitive than B_{12} levels, which may or may not be $\downarrow$

(5) Tx = vitamin B_{12} high-dose oral Tx proven equivalent to parenteral

d. Folic acid deficiency

(1) Folic acid derived from green, leafy vegetables ("foliage")

(2) Causes = dietary deficiency (most common), pregnancy or hemolytic anemia ($\uparrow$ requirements), methotrexate or prolonged TMP-SMX Tx (inhibits reduction of folate into tetrahydrofolate)

(3) Si/Sx = megaloblastic anemia, no neurologic signs

(4) Dx = **nml serum methylmalonic acid but $\uparrow$ homocysteine levels**—more sensitive than folate levels, which may or may not be $\downarrow$

(5) Tx = oral folic acid supplementation

3. **Normocytic Anemias**

a. Hypoproliferative (Table 1.37)

b. Hemolytic (Table 1.38)

B. **Coagulation Disorders**

1. **Thrombocytopenia**

a. Caused by splenic sequestration, stem-cell failure, or $\uparrow$ destruction

b. Si/Sx = bleeding time $\uparrow$ at counts <50,000, clinically significant bleeds start at counts <20,000, CNS bleeds occur when counts <10,000

c. $\downarrow$ Production seen in leukemia, aplastic anemia, and alcohol (even minimal)

d. Causes (Table 1.39)

e. Lab values (Table 1.40)

Table 1.37 Hypoproliferative Anemias

Disease	Characteristics
Anemia of renal failure	• ↓ EPO production by kidney • Indicates chronic renal failure • Tx = EPO
Anemia of chronic dz	• Seen in chronic inflammation (e.g., cancer, TB or fungal infxn, collagen-vascular dz) • Caused by release of hepcidin from the liver as an acute phase reactant • Dx = ↓ serum iron, Nml/↑ ferritin, ↓ TIBC • Tx = for the underlying disease
Aplastic anemia	• Bone marrow failure, usually idiopathic, or due to parvovirus B19 (especially in sickle cell) hepatitis virus, radiation, drugs (e.g., chloramphenicol) • Dx = bone marrow Bx → hypocellular marrow • Tx = ATG, cyclosporine, marrow transplantation if refractory

ATG, antihymocyte globulin; BMT, bone marrow transplantation.

Table 1.38 Hemolytic Anemias

Disease	Characteristics
Spherocytosis	• Autosomal dominant defect of spectrin → spherical, stiff RBCs trapped in spleen • Si/Sx = childhood jaundice and gallstones, indirect hyperbilirubinemia, Coombs negative • Dx = clinical ⊕ peripheral smear → spherocytes • Tx = folic acid, splenectomy for severe dz
Autoimmune hemolysis (IgG-mediated)	• Etiologies = idiopathic (most common), lupus, drugs (e.g., penicillin), leukemia, lymphoma • Si/Sx = rapid-onset, spherocytes on blood smear, ↑ indirect bilirubin, jaundice, ↓ haptoglobin, ↑ urine hemosidern • Dx = ⊕ direct Coombs test • Tx = prednisone, if fails rituximab (anti-CD20 B cell MAb), if that fails, splenectomy
Cold-agglutinin disease (IgM-mediated)	• Most commonly idiopathic, can be due to *Mycoplasma pneumoniae* and mononucleosis (CMV, EBV infxns) • Si/Sx = anemia on exposure to cold or following URI • Dx = cold-agglutinin test and indirect Coombs test • Tx = prednisone, supportive
Mechanical destruction	• Causes = disseminated intravascular coagulation (DIC), thrombotic thrombocytopenic purpura (TTP), hemolytic-uremic syndrome (HUS), and artificial heart valve • Peripheral smear → schistocytes (see Figure 1.28) • Tx = underlying disease

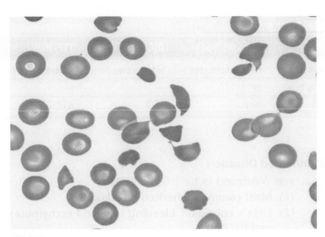

FIGURE 1.28

Schistocytes on blood smear. (From Anderson SC. *Anderson's atlas of hematology.* Baltimore, MD: Wolters Kluwer Health/Lippincott Williams & Wilkins, 2003.)

Table 1.39 Causes of Platelet Destruction (Thrombocytopenia)

Disease	Characteristics
Idiopathic thrombocytopenic purpura (ITP)	• Autoantibody-mediated platelet destruction • **In children, follows URI and is self-limiting, in adults it is chronic** • Tx = steroids, IVIG, splenectomy, rituximab (anti-CD20 MAb) for refractory dz
Thrombotic thrombocytopenic purpura (TTP)	• Idiopathic dz, often seen in HIV, can be fatal • **Pentad** = hemolytic anemia, thrombocytopenia, renal failure, fever, neurologic dz • Tx = plasma exchange
Hemolytic-uremic syndrome (HUS)	• Usually in kids, often due to *E. coli* 0157:H7 • Si/Sx = acute renal failure, bloody diarrhea, abdominal pain, seizures, **fulminant thrombocytopenia with hemolytic anemia** • Tx = dialysis
Disseminated intravascular coagulations	• Seen in adenocarcinoma, leukemia, sepsis, trauma • ↑ Fibrin split products, ↓ fibrinogen, ↑ PT/PTT • Tx = correct underlying cause
Drug-induced	• Causes = heparin, sulfonamides, valproic acid • Reverses within days of ceasing drug intake

Table 1.40 Labs in Platelet Destruction

Study	Autoantibody	DIC	TTP/HUS
Blood smear	Microspherocytes	Schistocytes (+)	**Schistocytes (+++)**
Coombs test	⊕	—	—
PT/PTT	Nml	↑↑↑	Nml/↑

2. **Inherited Disorders**
    a. von Willebrand factor (vWF) deficiency
        (1) **Most common inherited bleeding dz**
        (2) Si/Sx = **episodic ↑ bleeding time and ecchymoses, nml PT/PTT**
        (3) Dx = vWF levels and ristocetin–cofactor test
        (4) Tx = DDAVP (↑ vWF secretion) or cryoprecipitate for acute bleeding
    b. Hemophilia
        (1) X-linked deficiency of factor VIII (hemophilia A) or X-linked deficiency of factor IX (hemophilia B = Christmas dz)
        (2) Si/Sx = hemarthroses (bleeding into joint), ecchymoses with minor trauma, ↑ **PTT, nml PT, nml bleeding time**
        (3) Dx = ↓ factor levels
        (4) Tx = recombinant factor VIII or factor IX concentrate
3. **Hypercoagulable Dz** (Table 1.41)

Table 1.41 Hypercoagulable Diseases

Primary (Inherited)	Secondary (Acquired)	
Antithrombin III deficiency	Prolonged immobilization	L-Asparaginase
Protein C deficiency	Pregnancy	Hyperlipidemia
Protein S deficiency	Surgery/trauma	Anticariolipin Ab
Factor V Leiden deficiency	Oral contraceptives	Lupus anticoagulant
Dysfibrinogenemia	Homocystinuria	Disseminated
Plasminogen (activator)	Malignancy	intravascular
deficiency	(adenocarcinoma)	coagulation
Heparin cofactor II deficiency	Smoking	Vitamin K deficiency
Homocystinemia	Nephrotic syndrome	
Factor II (prothrombin) mutation		

Table 1.42 Myeloproliferative Diseases

Disease	Characteristics
Polycythemia vera	• Rare, peak onset at 50–60 yrs, male predominance • Si/Sx = headache, diplopia, retinal hemorrhages, stroke, angina, claudication (all due to vascular sludging), early satiety, splenomegaly, gout, **pruritus after showering, plethora, basophilia** • **5% progress to leukemia, 20% to myelofibrosis** • Tx = phlebotomy, hydroxyurea to keep blood counts low
Essential thrombocythemia	• Si/Sx = platelet count >1 × 10⁶ cells/ml, splenomegaly ecchymoses • Dx = rule out other causes (due to iron deficiency, malignancy, etc.) • 5% progress to myelofibrosis or acute leukemia • Tx = anagrelide, plateletpharesis
Idiopathic myelofibrosis	• Typically affects patients ≥50 yrs • Si/Sx = massive hepatosplenomegaly, blood smear → **teardrop cells** • Dx = hypercellular marrow on biopsy • Poor Px, median 5 yrs before marrow failure • Tx = supportive • Chronic myelogenous leukemia (see section D.3).

C. **Myeloproliferative Dz** (Table 1.42)

1. Caused by clonal proliferation of a myeloid stem cell → excessive production of mature, differentiated myeloid cell lines

2. All can transform into acute leukemias

3. Thrombocytosis

   a. 1° (bone marrow disorder) versus 2° (reactive)

   b. 1° can be essential thrombocythemia but also can see a thrombocytosis in polycythemia rubra vera or chronic myelogenous leukemia—typically count is >1 million

   c. 2° or reactive thrombocytosis can be seen in any chronic inflammatory disorder, serious infxn, acute bleed, iron-deficiency anemia (mechanism unclear), or following splenectomy—typically count is <1 million

D. **Leukemias**

1. **Acute Lymphoblastic Leukemia**

   a. **Peak age is 3–4 yrs;** most common neoplasm in children

   b. Si/Sx = fever, fatigue, anemia, pallor, petechiae, infxns

   c. Labs → leukocytosis, anemia, ↓ platelets, marrow bx → ↑ blasts, peripheral blood blasts are **PAS +, CALLA +, TdT +**

d. Tx = chemotherapy: induction, consolidation, maintenance intrathecal chemotherapy during consolidation

e. Px = 80% cure in children (much worse in adults)

2. **Acute Myelogenous Leukemia (AML)**

a. **Most common leukemia in adults**

b. Si/Sx = fever, fatigue, pallor, petechiae, infxns, lymphadenopathy

c. Labs → thrombocytopenia, peripheral blood, and marrow bx → myeloblasts that are **myeloperoxidase +, Sudan Black +, Auer Rods +**

d. Tx

(1) Chemotherapy → induction, consolidation (no maintenance)

(2) All-*trans* retinoic acid used for the M3 subtype of AML, causes differentiation of blasts—beware of onset of DIC in these pts

e. Px = overall 30% cure; BMT improves outcomes

3. **Chronic Myelogenous Leukemia**

a. Presents most commonly in the 50s but can be any age

b. Si/Sx = anorexia, early satiety, diaphoresis, arthritis, bone tenderness, leukostasis (WBC $\geq 1 \times 10^5$) → dyspnea, dizzy, slurred speech, diplopia

c. Labs → **Philadelphia (Ph) chromosome ⊕, peripheral blood → cells of all maturational stages,** ↓ leukocyte alkaline phosphatase

d. Ph chromosome is pathognomonic, seen in >90% of pts with CML, because of translocation of *abl* gene from chromosome 9 to *bcr* on 22

e. Tx = tyrosine kinase inhibitor (e.g., imatinib mesylate)—if fails, only BMT can be curative

f. **Blast crisis** = acute phase, invariably develops causing death in 3–6 mos; mean time to onset = **3–4 yrs**

4. **Chronic Lymphocytic Leukemia**

a. ↑ incidence with age, causes 30% of leukemias in the United States

b. Si/Sx = typically aSx for many yrs, and when it eventually does become Sx pts have organomegaly, hemolytic anemia, thrombocytopenia, blood smear and marrow → nml morphology lymphocytosis of blood and marrow

c. **Tx** = palliative, early Tx does NOT prolong life

d. Other presentations of similar leukemias

(1) Hairy cell leukemia (B-cell subtype)

(a) Si/Sx = characteristic hairy cell morphology (Figure 1.29A), pancytopenia

(b) Tx = IFN-α, splenectomy

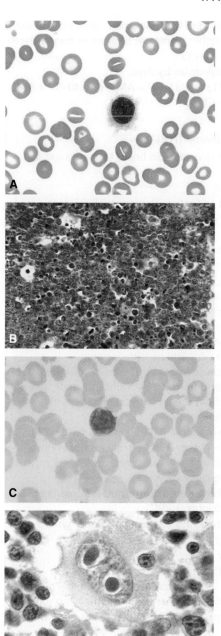

FIGURE 1.29

A. Hairy cell leukemic cell on blood smear. (From Anderson SC. *Anderson's atlas of hematology.* Baltimore: Wolters Kluwer Health/Lippincott Williams & Wilkins, 2003.) **B.** Starry sky pattern of Burkitt's lymphoma on bx. (Image from Rubin E, Farber JL. *Pathology,* 3rd Ed. Philadelphia, PA: Lippincott Williams & Wilkins, 1999.) **C.** Sézary cell of T-cell lymphoma. (From Anderson SC. *Anderson's atlas of hematology.* Baltimore: Wolters Kluwer Health/Lippincott Williams & Wilkins, 2003.) **D.** Reed–Sternberg cell in pt with Hodgkin's dz. Mirror-image, owl-eye nuclei contain large eosinophilic nucleoli. (Image from Rubin E, Farber JL. *Pathology,* 3rd Ed. Philadelphia, PA: Lippincott Williams & Wilkins, 1999.)

   (2) T-cell leukemias tend to involve skin, often present with erythematous rashes; some are because of human T-cell leukemia virus (HTLV)

   Most Common Leukemias by Age:

   Up to age 15 = ALL; age 15–39 = AML; age 40–59 ≥ AML & CML; ≥60 = CLL

E. **Lymphoma**

   1. **Non-Hodgkin's Lymphoma (NHL)**

      a. Commonly seen in HIV, often in brain, teenagers get in head and neck

      b. Burkitt's lymphoma

         (1) Closely related to Epstein–Barr virus (EBV) infxns

         (2) African Burkitt's involves jaw/neck; US Burkitt's involves abdomen

         (3) Burkitt's shows a classic "starry sky" pattern on histopathology, caused by spaces scattered within densely packed lymph tissue (Figure 1.29B)

      c. Non-Hodgkin's treatment

         (1) Chemotherapy with or without radiation

         (2) Typical chemotherapy is R-CHOP = Rituximab + Cyclophosphamide + Hydroxydaunarubicin (adriamycin) + Oncovin (vincristine) + Prednisone

         (3) Side effects include marrow suppression, hair loss, nausea, and vomiting from the cyclophosphamide, risk of cardiotoxicity from the adriamycin, and peripheral neuropathy from vincristine

      d. Cutaneous T-cell lymphoma (CTCL, mycosis fungoides)

         (1) Si/Sx = often in elderly, diffuse scaly rash or erythroderma (total body erythema), precedes clinically apparent malignancy by years

         (2) **Stained cells have cerebriform nuclei** (looks like cerebral gyri) (Figure 1.29C)

         (3) Leukemic phase of this dz is called "Sézary syndrome"

         (4) Tx = ultraviolet light Tx, consider systemic chemotherapy

      e. Angiocentric T-cell lymphoma

         (1) Two subtypes = nasal T-cell lymphoma (lethal midline granuloma) and pulmonary angiocentric lymphoma

         (2) Si/Sx = large mass, Bx often non-Dx because of diffuse necrosis

         (3) Tx = palliative radiation, Px very poor

2. **Hodgkin's Lymphoma**
   a. Occurs in a bimodal age distribution, young men and the elderly
   b. EBV infxn is present in up to 50% of cases
   c. Si/Sx = **Pel–Ebstein fevers** (fevers wax and wane over weeks), chills, night sweats, weight loss, pruritus; **Sx worsen with alcohol intake**
   d. Reed–Sternberg (RS) cells seen on Bx, **appear as binucleated giant cells ("owl eyes")** or **mononucleated giant cell (lacunar cell)** (Figure 1.29D)
   e. Tx depends on clinical staging
      (1) Stage I = 1 lymph node involved → radiation
      (2) Stage II = ≥2 lymph nodes on same side of diaphragm → radiation
      (3) Stage III = involvement on both sides of diaphragm → chemotherapy
      (4) Stage IV = disseminated to organs or extranodal tissue → chemotherapy
      (5) Chemotherapy regimens
         (a) MOPP = **m**echlorethamine, **O**ncovin (vincristine), **p**rocarbazine, **p**rednisone
         (b) ABVD = **A**driamycin (daunorubicin), **b**leomycin, **v**incristine, **d**acarbazine

VIII. Empiric Antibiotic Tx for Specific Infxns (Table 1.43)

Table 1.43 Empiric Antibiotic Treatment of Specific Infections

Disease	Microorganisms[a]	Empiric Antibiotics[a]
Abdominal infection	GNR, anaerobes	3rd gen ceph + metronidazole
Aspiration pneumonia	Mouth and throat anaerobes	3rd gen ceph + metronidazole OR clindamycin
Bites	GNR and anaerobes	Amoxicillin-clavulonic acid
Brain abscess	GPC, GNR, anaerobes	3rd gen ceph + metronidazole +/− vancomycin
Bronchitis	S. pneumoniae, H. influenzae, M. catarrhalis, viruses	None, or TMP-SMX or amoxicillin

(continued)

Table 1.43 *Continued*

Disease	Microorganisms[a]	Empiric Antibiotics[a]
CAP (community-acquired pneumonia)	*S. pneumoniae, H. influenzae, M. catarrhalis, Mycoplasma pneumoniae, Chlamydophila pneumoniae, Chlamydia psittaci, Legionella*	3rd gen ceph + macrolide OR fluoroquinolone
Cellulitis	*S. aureus,* Group A *Strep,* other *Strep*	Clindamycin, cefazolin + TMP-SMX, or vancomycin
Cholangitis	GNR, anaerobes	3rd gen ceph ⊕ metronidazole
Dental infection	Mouth anaerobes	Clindamycin
Diabetic foot	GNR, anaerobes, +/− *S. aureus*	(3rd gen ceph + metronidazole OR ampicillin-sulbactam) +/− vancomycin
Endocarditis	*S. aureus,* viridians *Strep,* HACEK, coag neg *Staph*	3rd gen ceph + vancomycin + oxacillin
Epididymitis and prostatitis	<35 yo → *N. gonorrhea* >35 yo → GNR	<35 yo → 3rd gen ceph >35 yo → 3rd gen ceph OR fluoroquinolone
Necrotizing fasciitis	Group A *Strep, Clostridium,* community MRSA	(PCN or 3rd gen ceph) + clindamycin + vancomycin
Gastroenteritis	GNR	Fluoroquinolone OR 3rd gen ceph
Urethritis	*N. gonorrhoeae, Chlamydia trachomatis*	3rd gen ceph + doxycycline
Liver abscess	GNR, anaerobes OR *Entamoeba histolytica*	3rd gen ceph + metronidazole OR metronidazole
Lung abscess	Mouth/throat anaerobes	3rd gen ceph + metronidazole OR clindamycin
Meningitis (adult)	*S. pneumoniae, N. meningitidis, H. influenzae, Listeria*	3rd gen ceph + vancomycin: add ampicillin if elderly, immune compromised or pregnant (for *Listeria*)
Meningitis (pediatric)	*E. coli, Listeria, S. pneumoniae, N. meningitidis*	3rd gen ceph + ampicillin + vancomycin
Neutropenic fever	GNR, GPC	(Ceftazidime OR cefepime OR imipenem OR piperacillin-tazobactam) ± gentamicin ± vancomycin

Table 1.43 *Continued*

Disease	Microorganisms[a]	Empiric Antibiotics[a]
Nosocomial pneumonia	GNR, *S. aureus*	(Ceftazidime OR cefepime OR imipenem OR piperacillin-tazobactam OR ciprofloxacin) + vancomycin
Osteomyelitis	GPC, GNR	3rd gen ceph + vancomycin
Pharyngitis	Group A Strep	PCN
PID	GNR, anaerobes, *Chlamydia/Neisseria*	Clindamycin + gentamicin + doxycycline
Pyelonephritis	GNR	3rd gen ceph or gentimicin
Spontaneous bacterial peritonitis	GNR, *S. pneumoniae*	3rd gen ceph
Septic arthritis	*S. aureus, Strep spp.*, GNR	Vancomycin + 3rd gen ceph
Septic shock	GPC, GNR	Vancomycin + (3rd gen ceph OR piperacillin-tazobactam OR imipenem) +/− fluoroquinolone +/− metronidazole
Bell's palsy	HSV, other	Valacyclovir/acyclovir
Herpes zoster	VZV	Valacyclovir/acyclovir
Retinitis in HIV	CMV	Valganciclovir/ganciclovir
Encephalitis	HSV, other	Acyclovir (iv)
Oral thrush	*Candida*	Nystatin swish and swallow if just oral, fluconazole if esophageal dz

[a]GNR, gram-negative rod, GPC, gram-positive cocci; 3rd gen ceph, third generation cephalosporin; for community acquired infections, pseudomonal coverage is not required, and ceftriaxone or cefotaxime are the preferred third generation cephalosporins; for nosocomial infections, pseudomonal coverage is required and ceftazidime or cefepime (actually a fourth generation cephalosporin) are the preferred agents.
After identification of the actual causative organism, the initial empiric treatment should always be narrowed as much as possible.

Algorithm 1.2

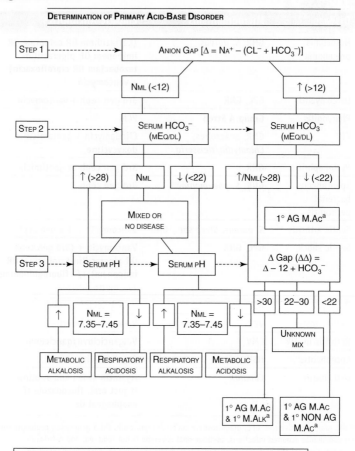

DETERMINATION OF PRIMARY ACID-BASE DISORDER

STEP 1 - - - - - - - - - → ANION GAP $[\Delta = Na^+ - (Cl^- + HCO_3^-)]$

NML (<12)   ↑ (>12)

STEP 2 - - - - - - - - - → SERUM HCO_3^- (MEQ/DL) - - - - - → SERUM HCO_3^- (MEQ/DL)

↑ (>28)   NML   ↓ (<22)   ↑/NML (>28)   ↓ (<22)

MIXED OR NO DISEASE

1° AG M.Ac[a]

STEP 3 - - - → SERUM pH - - - → SERUM pH - - - → Δ Gap ($\Delta\Delta$) = $\Delta - 12 + HCO_3^-$

↑   NML = 7.35–7.45   ↓   ↑   NML = 7.35–7.45   ↓   >30   22–30   <22

UNKNOWN MIX

METABOLIC ALKALOSIS   RESPIRATORY ACIDOSIS   RESPIRATORY ALKALOSIS   METABOLIC ACIDOSIS

1° AG M.Ac & 1° M.Alk[a]   1° AG M.Ac & 1° NON AG M.Ac[a]

[a]AG = anion gap. M.Alk = metabolic alkalosis. M.Ac = metabolic acidosis.

Algorithm 1.3

METABOLIC ACIDOSIS

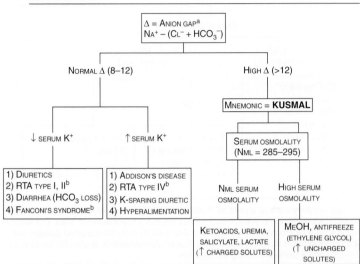

Check for compensation or the presence of a mixed disorder. Winter's formula predicts the CO_2 if there is compensation: $CO_2 = 1.5 * HCO_3^- + 8 \pm 2$. If the CO_2 is higher than expected, there is an additional acidotic process occurring. If the CO_2 is lower than expected, there is an additional alkalotic process occurring.

[a] Calculate Δ in *all* patients, regardless of pH or HCO_3^-. Mixed acidosis and alkalosis can cancel each other out, causing neutral pH. Perform the following steps to search for a mixed disorder.
1) Calculate Δ: if $\Delta \geq 12$, the disorder is a 1° anion gap acidosis
2) Calculate $\Delta\Delta = |\Delta - 12 + HCO_3^-|$: if $\Delta\Delta \geq 31$, there is also a 1° metabolic alkalosis
      if $\Delta\Delta \leq 21$, there is also a 1° nonanion gap acidosis
Example: A diabetic in ketoacidosis who is vomiting can have a 1° anion gap acidosis from the ketoacidosis and a 1° metabolic alkalosis from the vomiting. In this case, the $\Delta > 12$, the $\Delta\Delta \geq 31$. A diabetic with renal failure who presents with ketoacidosis can have a 1° anion gap and nonanion gap acidosis, with a $\Delta > 12$ and a $\Delta\Delta \leq 21$. Note that this patient may also be vomiting and either tachypneic or bradypneic from obtundation. Thus the patient may have three 1° metabolic acid-base disorders (1° AG acidosis, 1° nonAG acidosis, 1° metabolic alkaosis) and a respiratory disorder. In this case, the disorders must be discriminated clinically or by changes in status in response to therapy.
      Our thanks to Dr. Arian Torbati for his assistance with the $\Delta\Delta$ algorithm.
[b] See Section III.F for description of RTA and Fanconi's syndrome.

Algorithm 1.4

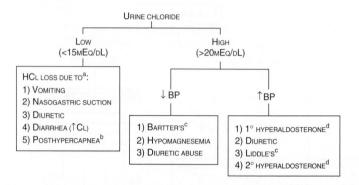

METABOLIC ALKALOSIS

URINE CHLORIDE

LOW (<15mEq/dL)

HIGH (>20mEq/dL)

HCL LOSS DUE TO[a]:
1) VOMITING
2) NASOGASTRIC SUCTION
3) DIURETIC
4) DIARRHEA (↑CL)
5) POSTHYPERCAPNEA[b]

↓ BP

1) BARTTER'S[c]
2) HYPOMAGNESEMIA
3) DIURETIC ABUSE

↑BP

1) 1° HYPERALDOSTERONE[d]
2) DIURETIC
3) LIDDLE'S[c]
4) 2° HYPERALDOSTERONE[d]

[a] These conditions are all known as "contraction alkaloses," or "chloride-responsive alkaloses." The contraction in extracellular volume creates a hypochloremic state. The kidney resorbs extra bicarbonate from the tubules due to the loss of chloride anion (tubules need a different anion to maintain electrical neutrality). Administration of chloride anion in the form of normal saline will correct the alkalosis.

[b] Patients who are hypercapnic undergo renal compensation, with resorption of extra bicard from the tubules to offset the respiratory acidosis. When the hypercapnia is corrected (e.g., via intubation) the kidneys must adjust and resorb less bicard. Until they adjust, the patient will have a posthypercapnic metabolic alkalosis.

[c] See Appendix B for Bartter's & Liddle's.

[d] 1° hyperaldosteronism is known as Conn's syndrome. See Endocrinology, Section III.D. 1.2° hyperaldosteronism can be caused by renal artery stenosis (see Nephrology, Section V), Cushing's syndrome (see Endocrine, Section III.B), congestive heart failure, and hepatic cirrhosis.

Algorithm 1.5

RESPIRATORY ACID-BASE DIFFERENTIAL

RESPIRATORY ALKALOSIS	RESPIRATORY ACIDOSIS
• CNS LESION	• MORPHINE/SEDATIVES
• PREGNANCY	• STROKE IN BULBAR AREA OF BRAIN STEM
• HIGH ALTITUDE	• ONDINE'S CURSE (CENTRAL SLEEP APNEA)
• SEPSIS/INFECTION	• COPD (EMPHYSEMA, ASTHMA, BRONCHITIS)
• SALICYLATE TOXICITY	• ADULT RESPIRATORY DISTRESS SYNDROME
• LIVER FAILURE	• CHEST WALL DISEASE (POLIO, KYPHOSCOLIOSIS,
• ANXIETY (HYPERVENTILATION)	MYASTHENIA GRAVIS, MUSCULAR DYSTROPHY)
• PAIN/FEAR (HYPERVENTILATION)	• OBESITY
• CONGESTIVE HEART FAILURE	• HYPOPHOSPHATEMIA (DIAPHRAGM REQUIRES
• PULMONARY EMBOLUS	LOTS OF ATP DUE TO HIGH ENERGY DEMAND)
• PNEUMONIA	• SUCCINYLCHOLINE (PARALYSIS FOR INTUBATION)
• HYPERTHYROIDISM	• PLEURAL EFFUSION
• COMPENSATION FOR A 1° ACIDOSIS	• PNEUMOTHORAX

Check for the presence of a mixed disorder by comparing the change in CO_2 and HCO_3 from normal (normal $CO_2 = 40$, normal $HCO_3 = 24$).

Acute respiratory acidosis:	HCO_3^- increases by 1 for every 10 the CO_2 increases.
Acute respiratory alkalosis:	HCO_3^- decreases by 2 for every 10 the CO_2 decreases.
Chronic respiratory acidosis:	HCO_3^- increases by 3.5 for every 10 the CO_2 increases.
Chronic respiratory alkalosis:	HCO_3^- decreases by 5 for every 10 the CO_2 decreases.

It's easy to remember the compensations by organizing them in the following table.

	ACIDOSIS	ALKALOSIS
Acute	1	2
Chronic	3–4 (3.5)	5

Change in HCO_3^- per 10 change in CO_2.
Just remember = 1 : 2 : 3–4 : 5!

As usual, if the CO_2 is higher than predicted, there is a mixed acidotic process. If the CO_2 is lower than predicted, there is a mixed alkalotic process.

Algorithm 1.6

EVALUATION OF HYPONATREMIA

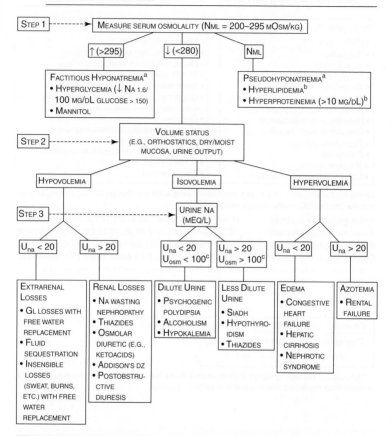

STEP 1 -----> MEASURE SERUM OSMOLALITY (NML = 200–295 MOSM/KG)

↑ (>295)   ↓ (<280)   NML

FACTITIOUS HYPONATREMIA[a]
• HYPERGLYCEMIA (↓ NA 1.6/ 100 MG/DL GLUCOSE > 150)
• MANNITOL

PSEUDOHYPONATREMIA[a]
• HYPERLIPIDEMIA[b]
• HYPERPROTEINEMIA (>10 MG/DL)[b]

STEP 2 ----- VOLUME STATUS (E.G., ORTHOSTATICS, DRY/MOIST MUCOSA, URINE OUTPUT)

HYPOVOLEMIA   ISOVOLEMIA   HYPERVOLEMIA

STEP 3 ----- URINE NA (MEQ/L)

$U_{na} < 20$ $U_{na} > 20$ $U_{na} < 20$ $U_{osm} < 100^c$ $U_{na} > 20$ $U_{osm} > 100^c$ $U_{na} < 20$ $U_{na} > 20$

EXTRARENAL LOSSES
• GI LOSSES WITH FREE WATER REPLACEMENT
• FLUID SEQUESTRATION
• INSENSIBLE LOSSES (SWEAT, BURNS, ETC.) WITH FREE WATER REPLACEMENT

RENAL LOSSES
• NA WASTING NEPHROPATHY
• THIAZIDES
• OSMOLAR DIURETIC (E.G., KETOACIDS)
• ADDISON'S DZ
• POSTOBSTRUCTIVE DIURESIS

DILUTE URINE
• PSYCHOGENIC POLYDIPSIA
• ALCOHOLISM
• HYPOKALEMIA

LESS DILUTE URINE
• SIADH
• HYPOTHYROIDISM
• THIAZIDES

EDEMA
• CONGESTIVE HEART FAILURE
• HEPATIC CIRRHOSIS
• NEPHROTIC SYNDROME

AZOTEMIA
• RENTAL FAILURE

[a] Pseudohyponatremia is a lab artifact due to serum volume occupation by lipid or protein, resulting in an apparent decrease in the amount of Na per given volume of serum. Factitious hyponatremia is a true decrease in serum Na concentration (but normal total body Na) caused by glucose or mannitol osmotically drawing water into the serum.
[b] These disorders are characterized by ≥ 10mOsm/kg gap between the calculated & and the measued serumosmolarity. Serum osmolality is calculated by $(2*Na) + (BUN/2.8) + (glucose/18)$. The gap is due to the presence of solutes detected by the lab but not accounted for in the osmolality calculation.
[c] U_{osm} = urine osmolality.

Algorithm 1.7

EVALUATION OF HYPERNATREMIA

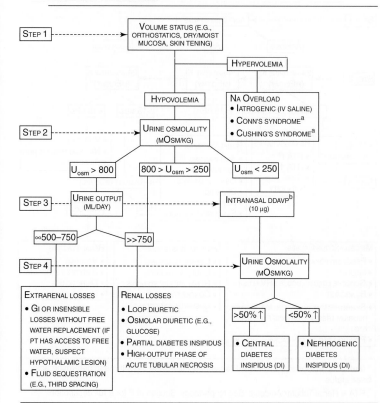

STEP 1 → VOLUME STATUS (E.G., ORTHOSTATICS, DRY/MOIST MUCOSA, SKIN TENING)

HYPERVOLEMIA

HYPOVOLEMIA

NA OVERLOAD
- IATROGENIC (IV SALINE)
- CONN'S SYNDROME[a]
- CUSHING'S SYNDROME[a]

STEP 2 → URINE OSMOLALITY (mOSM/KG)

$U_{osm} > 800$ | $800 > U_{osm} > 250$ | $U_{osm} < 250$

STEP 3 → URINE OUTPUT (ML/DAY)

INTRANASAL DDAVP[b] (10 μg)

∞500–750 | ≫750

STEP 4 → URINE OSMOLALITY (mOSM/KG)

EXTRARENAL LOSSES
- GI OR INSENSIBLE LOSSES WITHOUT FREE WATER REPLACEMENT (IF PT HAS ACCESS TO FREE WATER, SUSPECT HYPOTHALAMIC LESION)
- FLUID SEQUESTRATION (E.G., THIRD SPACING)

RENAL LOSSES
- LOOP DIURETIC
- OSMOLAR DIURETIC (E.G., GLUCOSE)
- PARTIAL DIABETES INSIPIDUS
- HIGH-OUTPUT PHASE OF ACUTE TUBULAR NECROSIS

>50% ↑ | <50% ↑

CENTRAL DIABETES INSIPIDUS (DI)

NEPHROGENIC DIABETES INSIPIDUS (DI)

[a] See Endocrinology, Section III.B.1 and III.D.1 for Cushing's syndrome and Conn's syndrome.
[b] DDAVP = long-acting antidiuretic hormone analogue. Patients with central DI respond by successfully increasing the concentration of their urine by 50%. Patients with nephrogenic DI are unable to concentrate their urine in the presence of DDAVP. Patients with DI tend to be only mildly hypernatremic.

Algorithm 1.8

EVALUATION OF HYPOKALEMIA

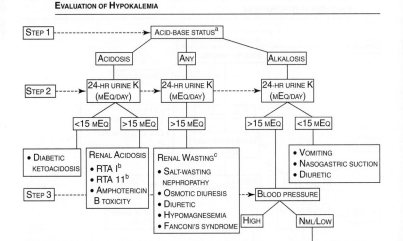

MISCELLANEOUS CAUSES:
- PSEUDOHYPOKALEMIA[d]
- INSULIN
- GLUCOSE LOAD (GLUCOSE IN IV FLUID)
- B[2] AGONIST
- SYMPATHETIC STIMULATION (M1, SEIZURE, DELIRIUM TREMENS, INTENSE EXERCISE, ETC.)
- POLYURIA DUE TO ANY CAUSE

HYPERALDOSTERONE[e]
- CONN'S SYNDROME
- LIDDLE'S SYNDROME
- RENAL ARTERY STENOSIS
- CONGESTIVE HEART FAILURE
- CUSHING'S SYNDROME

RENAL WASTING
- VOMITING
- BARTTER'S SYNOROME[e]
- DIURETIC USE
- HYPOMAGNESEMIA

[a] Metabolic acidosis or alkalosis. Please see Acid-Base algorithms to determine acid-base status.

[b] RTA = Renal Tubular Acidosis. See Nephrology, Section III.F for a full description.

[c] Salt wasting nephropathies are tubulointerstitial disorders (e.g., pyelonephritis, renal medullary dz, acute tubular necrosis & allergic interstitial nephritis). For Fanconi's syndrome, see Nephrology, Section III.F.2.

[d] Pseudohypokalemia is seen in conditions with very high white blood cell counts (e.g., leukernia). The while cells take up potassium while they are sitting in the blood draw tube, creating spurious results.

[e] See Endocrinology, Sections III.B & D for Cushing's & Conn's syndromes, IV.C for congenital adrenal hyperplasia, Nephrology, Section V for renal artery stenosis, and Appendix B for Liddle's & Bartter's syndromes.

IX. Electrolyte Disorders & Management

Table 1.44 Hypokalemia

1. For urgent K⁺ replacement give iv and oral K⁺ simultaneously
   - Give IV at 10 mEq/hr through peripheral line or 20 mEq/hr through central line (more rapid administration causes vessel necrosis).
   - Give oral K⁺ at up to 40 mEq/hr
   - Contrary to popular belief, oral K⁺ increases serum K⁺ much faster than IV (because you can't give IV quickly)
   - Each 10 mEq oral or IV should ↑ serum K⁺ by 0.1 mmol/L
2. If K⁺ repeatedly falls or remains low:
   - Check pt's meds for diuretics or toxins (e.g., amphotericin) that cause K⁺ wasting
   - Replete serum magnesium, normal Mg is required for maintenance of serum K⁺ levels
   - Start K⁺-sparing diuretic (e.g., spironolactone) or ACE inhibitor to help maintain K⁺ levels
   - Advise to eat high K⁺ food (e.g., banana)
3. Peri-MI, the K⁺ should be kept >4.0 to suppress arrhythmias—be aggressive!
4. In renal failure, small doses of oral or IV K⁺ will dramatically ↑ serum K⁺, so be careful!

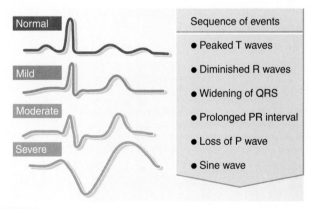

FIGURE 1.30

Hyperkalemia-related EKG changes.

Table 1.45 Hyperkalemia

Diagnosis

Plasma potassium >6.5 mmol/L
Dangerous level of K^+ depends on if acute ($\approx$ 5 mmol/L) or chronic ($\approx$6.5 mmol/L)
May be associated with muscle weakness and EKG abnormalities (e.g., widening of QRS complexes, peaked T waves, loss of the P wave)
Predominantly occurs in patients with renal failure or muscle breakdown

Emergency Treatment: Hyperkalemia Associated with EKG Abnormalities

Give:
10 mL of 10% calcium gluconate bolus IV, repeated if necessary (up to 100 mL/24 hrs) to stabilize myocardial cell membranes
It does not lower potassium
Then:
Glucose + insulin: give 50 mL of dextrose 50% with 10 units of short-acting insulin. This will lower plasma potassium for several hours (4–6 hrs)
±05 mL 8.4% sodium bicarbonate if pH <7.4
±Kayexalate oral or per rectum ($\downarrow K^+$ for 24 hrs)

Longer-Term Treatment

Remove the cause
Diet ($\leq$60 mmol K^+/day)
Regular dialysis in renal failure

Algorithm 1.9

EVALUATION OF HYPERKALEMIA

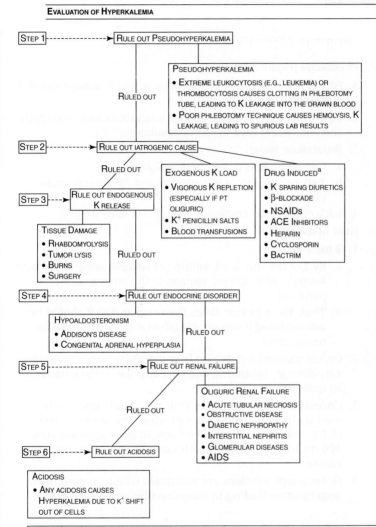

STEP 1 - - - - - - - - - - - - - ▶ RULE OUT PSEUDOHYPERKALEMIA

PSEUDOHYPERKALEMIA
- EXTREME LEUKOCYTOSIS (E.G., LEUKEMIA) OR THROMBOCYTOSIS CAUSES CLOTTING IN PHLEBOTOMY TUBE, LEADING TO K LEAKAGE INTO THE DRAWN BLOOD
- POOR PHLEBOTOMY TECHNIQUE CAUSES HEMOLYSIS, K LEAKAGE, LEADING TO SPURIOUS LAB RESULTS

RULED OUT

STEP 2 - - - - - - - - - ▶ RULE OUT IATROGENIC CAUSE

RULED OUT

EXOGENOUS K LOAD
- VIGOROUS K REPLETION (ESPECIALLY IF PT OLIGURIC)
- K^+ PENICILLIN SALTS
- BLOOD TRANSFUSIONS

DRUG INDUCED[a]
- K SPARING DIURETICS
- β-BLOCKADE
- NSAIDs
- ACE INHIBITORS
- HEPARIN
- CYCLOSPORIN
- BACTRIM

STEP 3 - - - ▶ RULE OUT ENDOGENOUS K RELEASE

TISSUE DAMAGE
- RHABDOMYOLYSIS
- TUMOR LYSIS
- BURNS
- SURGERY

RULED OUT

STEP 4 - - - - - - - - - - - - - ▶ RULE OUT ENDOCRINE DISORDER

HYPOALDOSTERONISM
- ADDISON'S DISEASE
- CONGENITAL ADRENAL HYPERPLASIA

RULED OUT

STEP 5 - - - - - - - - - - - - - ▶ RULE OUT RENAL FAILURE

RULED OUT

OLIGURIC RENAL FAILURE
- ACUTE TUBULAR NECROSIS
- OBSTRUCTIVE DISEASE
- DIABETIC NEPHROPATHY
- INTERSTITIAL NEPHRITIS
- GLOMERULAR DISEASES
- AIDS

STEP 6 - - - - - - - - ▶ RULE OUT ACIDOSIS

ACIDOSIS
- ANY ACIDOSIS CAUSES HYPERKALEMIA DUE TO K^+ SHIFT OUT OF CELLS

---

[a] NSAIDs = nonsteroidal anti-inflammatories, inhibit prostaglandins → ↓ renal perfusion → ↓ K delivery to nephron. ACE inhibitors block efferent arteriole constriction → ↓ CFR → ↓ K delivery to the nephron. Heparin blocks aldosterone production, while cyclosporine blocks aldosterone activity. Bactrim (trimethoprim) has K-sparing diuretic effect on tubules.

2. SURGERY

I. Fluid and Electrolytes

A. **Physiology** (Figure 2.1)

1. Fifty to seventy percent of lean body weight is water; most of it is in skeletal muscle

2. Total body water (TBW) is divided into extracellular (one-third) and intracellular (two-thirds) compartments

3. Extracellular water

   a. Comprises 20% of lean body weight

   b. Twenty-five percent intravascular and 75% extravascular (interstitial)

4. Intracellular water comprises 40% of lean body weight

B. **Fluid Management**

1. **3 for 1 Rule**

   a. By 1–2 hrs after a 1-L infusion of isotonic saline or lactated Ringer's, only 300 mL remains in the intravascular compartment

   b. **Thus, three to four times the vascular deficit should be administered** if isotonic crystalloid solutions are used for resuscitation

2. Colloid solutions (containing high-molecular-weight molecules; e.g., albumin, hetastarch, and dextrans) stay in the intravascular space longer

3. Colloids are more expensive than crystalloids and may be most useful in the edematous pt where, for instance, 100 mL of 1% albumin solution will be able to draw approximately 400 mL from the extravascular compartment, thus decreasing edema

4. **Note: Starch solutions are associated with increased tissue accumulation leading to coagulopathy and renal failure.**

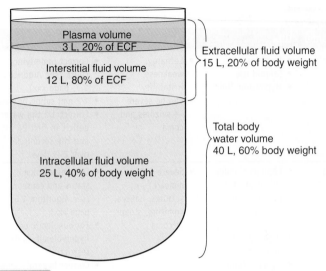

FIGURE 2.1

Distribution of fluid within the body. (From Premkumar K. *The massage connection anatomy and physiology.* Baltimore, MD: Lippincott Williams & Wilkins, 2004.)

C. **Hydration of Surgical Pts**
  1. Pts are commonly NPO (nothing by mouth) and require IV fluid hydration
  2. An uncomplicated pt without oral intake loses ≥1 L of fluid per day from sweat, urine, feces, and respiration
  3. Adequate fluid hydration is indicated by **urine output ≥0.5 cc/kg/hr (for typical pt ≥30 cc/hr)** and by measuring daily weight changes
  4. Electrolytes should be replaced as necessary
     a. Salivary and colon secretions are high in potassium (K+)
     b. Stomach, ileum, and bile secretions are high in Cl⁻
     c. Salivary, ileum, pancreas, and bile secretions are high in HCO_3^-

D. **Common Electrolyte Disorders** (Table 2.1)

Text continues on page 142

Table 2.1 Common Electrolyte Disorders

Disorder	DDx	Si/Sx	Tx
↑ Na⁺	• Fluid loss • Steroid use • Hypertonic fluids	• Lethargy, weakness, irritability • Can be severe → seizures and coma	• Correct underlying cause (see Algorithm 1.7, page xxx) • 1/2 nml saline or water • Correct 1/2 the water deficit in first 24 hrs and the second 1/2 over 2–3 days
↓ Na⁺	• Copious bladder irrigation status post transurethral resection of the prostate (TURP) • High-output ileostomy • Hyperglycemia • Adrenal insufficiency	• Severe (<115 mmol/L) → seizures, nausea, vomiting, stupor, or coma	• Determine volume status and cause (see Algorithm 1.6, page xxx) • For euvolemic or hypervolemic, water restrict • Correct hyperglycemia • Refractory dz → hypertonic saline
↑ K⁺	• Acidosis • ↓ Insulin • Leukocytosis • Burns • Crush injury	• Neuromuscular and cardiac sequelae (heart block, ventricular fibrillation, asystole) • EKG → peaked T waves, flattened P waves, wide QRS, eventually a sinusoidal pattern	• Stabilize cardiac membranes with IV calcium gluconate • Glucose and insulin infusion • Albuterol and loop diuretics • Binding resins (Kayexalate) and dialysis longer term • Reverse cause (see Algorithm 1.9, page xxx)
↓ K⁺	• Diarrhea, nasogastric suction, vomiting • Diuretics, metabolic alkalosis • Cushing's, burns, β-agonists, ↓ Mg²¹	• Ectopy, T-wave depression, prominent U waves • Also ventricular tachycardia and ↑ sensitivity to digoxin	• See Table 1.41 • Reverse cause (see Algorithm 1.8, page xxx)

Table 2.1 *Continued*

Disorder	DDx	Si/Sx	Tx
↑Ca²⁺	• Malignancy (number one cause in inpatients) • Disorders involving bone, parathyroid, or kidneys • Acute pancreatitis	• Altered mental status, muscle weakness, ileus, constipation, nausea, vomiting • Nephrolithiasis • QT-interval shortening	• Hydration and loop diuretics • Bisphosphonates • Calcitonin
↓ Ca²⁺	• Blood transfusion • Parathyroid resection • ↓ Mg⁺⁺ • Renal failure	• Chvostek's and Trousseau's signs • Paresthesias, tetany, seizures, weakness, mental status changes • QT interval prolonged	• Calcium gluconate • Vitamin D supplement
↑ Mg²⁺	• Overzealous Mg²⁺ supplements in patients with renal failure	• Lethargy, weakness, ↓ deep tendon reflexes • Paralysis, ↓ BP and heart rate (HR) • Prolonged PR and QT intervals	• Calcium gluconate • Nml saline infusion with a loop diuretic • Dialysis
↓ Mg²⁺	• Diarrhea, malabsorption • Vomiting • Aggressive diuresis, alcoholism, chemoTx	• T wave and QRS widening, PR and QT intervals prolonged	• MgSO₄
↑ Phos	• Usually iatrogenic • Rhabdomyolysis • Hypoparathyroid • Hypocalcemia • Villous adenoma	• Can cause soft-tissue calcification • Heart block	• ↓ Dietary phosphorus • Aluminum hydroxide • Hydration and acetazolamide • Dialysis
↓ Phos	• Excessive IV glucose • Hyperpara thyroidism • Osmotic diuresis • Refeeding syndrome	• Diffuse weakness and flaccid paralysis (all because of ↓ adenosine triphosphate (ATP) production)	• Potassium phosphate or sodium phosphate

Note: Refeeding syndrome caused by a large glucose load too soon after prolonged NPO status; see ↓ in Mg²⁺, K⁺, and Phos.

II. Blood Product Replacement

A. **Nml Hemostasis**

1. Coagulation involves endothelium, platelets, and coagulation factors

2. Endothelial damage allows platelets to bind to the **subendo-thelium through interaction with von Willebrand factor (vWF),** inducing platelet release of adenosine diphosphate (ADP), (5-HT) and platelet-derived growth factor (PDGF), which promote platelet aggregation.

3. **Platelet–platelet interactions occur via GPIIB-IIIA to form thrombus**

4. Coagulation Cascades
   a. Two coagulation pathways share factors I, II, V, and X
   b. Extrinsic pathway
      (1) Tissue thromboplastin (tissue factor) activates factor VII, which then activates factor X
      (2) Measured in vitro by prothrombin time (PT)
   c. Intrinsic pathway
      (1) Factors XII → XI → IX → VIII, activated factor VIII causes activation of the common factor X
      (2) Measured in vitro by partial thromboplastin time (PTT)
   d. Factor I = fibrin, which cross-links platelets to provide the tensile strength needed to stabilize the **thrombus mediated by GPIIB-IIIA.**

5. Vitamin K is fat soluble, derived from leafy vegetables and colonic flora
   a. Cofactors for γ-carboxylation of factors II, VII, IX, and X and the anticoagulation factors proteins C and S enable them to interact with Ca^{2+}
   b. Deficiency caused by malabsorption, prolonged parenteral feeding, prolonged oral antibiotics, or ingestion of oral anti-coagulants **(warfarin)**
   c. First sign is prolonged PT, because of the short half-life of factor VII (3–6 hrs)

B. **Preoperative Evaluation of Bleeding Disorders**

1. Si/Sx = Hx or FHx of ↑ bleeding following minor cuts, dental procedures, menses, or past surgeries, ecchymoses, or sequelae of liver dz

2. Ask about nonsteroidal anti-inflammatory drugs (NSAID) or herbal medicine intake during the week of surgery

3. Bleeding Time
   a. Evaluates platelet function
   b. ↑ bleeding time indicates quantitative or qualitative platelet dz
   c. Also ↑ in von Willebrand's dz and vasculitis
4. Thrombin Time (TT)
   a. Measures the time to clot after the addition of thrombin, which is responsible for conversion of fibrinogen to fibrin
   b. ↑ TT may be due to ↑ fibrin, dysfibrinogenemia, disseminated intravascular coagulation (DIC), or heparin
5. **Routine preoperative lab screening is not warranted without Si/Sx suggestive of underlying disorder**

C. **Transfusions**
   1. Packed Red Blood Cells (pRBCs)
      a. Type and screen = pt's RBCs tested for A, B, and Rh antigens and donor's serum screened for antibodies to common RBC antigens
      b. Cross-match = pt's serum checked for preformed antibodies against the donor's RBCs
      c. In trauma situations, type O negative blood is given while additional units are being typed and crossed (O positive blood can be given to male pts and postmenopausal women if no O negative is available)
      d. **1 unit pRBCs should ↑ hemoglobin by 1 g/dL and ↑ hematocrit 3%**
      e. Complications
         (1) Acute rejection
            (a) Because of preformed antibodies against the donor RBCs
            (b) Si/Sx = anxiety, flushing, tachycardia, renal failure, shock
            (c) **Most common cause is clerical error**
            (d) Recheck all paperwork and repeat cross-match
            (e) Tx = stop transfusion, IV fluids to maintain urine output
         (2) Infectious diseases
            (a) Hepatitis C virus (HCV) is by far the most common cause of hepatitis in pts who received prior transfusions, although risk of new HCV infxn now is lower with blood bank screening
            (b) Current risks (Table 2.2)

Table 2.2 Risk of Viral Infection from Blood Transfusions

Disease	Estimated Risk[a]
Hepatitis B	1 case per 220,000 units transfused
Hepatitis C	1 case per 230,000 units transfused
HIV	1 per 1.2 million units transfused

[a]Mean estimates from Jackson BR, Busch MP, Stramer SL, et al. The cost-effectiveness of NAT for HIV, HCV, and HBV in whole blood donations. *Transfusion* 2003;43:721–729.

2. Platelet Transfusions
   a. Pts do not bleed significantly until platelets <50,000/μL, so transfusion should be given only to maintain this level
   b. If pt is anticipated to experience severe blood loss intraoperatively or the pt is actively bleeding, transfuse to maintain even higher
   c. Most common complication is alloimmunization
      (1) Platelet counts fail to rise despite continued transfusion
      (2) Caused by induction of antibodies against the donor's major histocompatibility complex (MHC) type
      (3) Single-donor, human leukocyte antigen (HLA)-matched platelets may overcome problem

3. Plasma Component Transfusion
   a. Plasma products do not require cross-matching, but donor and recipient should be ABO compatible
   b. Fresh-frozen plasma (FFP)
      (1) Contains all the coagulation factors
      (2) Used to correct all clotting factor deficiencies
   c. Cryoprecipitate is rich in factor VIII, fibrinogen, and fibronectin
   d. **Note: Uremic patients may have severe bleeding secondary to platelet dysfunction, treatment with DDAVP or cryoprecipitate. Do not transfuse platelets because new platelets will become dysfunctional.**

4. Other Products
   a. Factor VIII concentrate—useful in hemophilia A patients
   b. Factor IX or prothrombin complex concentrate (PCC)—contains II, VII, IX, X. Can be used to reverse warfarin overdose
   c. Activated Factor VIIa—initiates coagulation in areas where tissue factor is located, developed for patients with rare factor VII deficiency or inhibitors against coagulation factor, and has had limited use in uncontrolled hemorrhage.

III. Perioperative Care

A. Preoperative Care

1. All pts require detailed H&P
2. Laboratory Tests
   a. CBC for pts undergoing procedure that may incur large blood loss
   b. Electrolytes, blood urea nitrogen (BUN), and creatinine in pts >60 yrs or who have illnesses (e.g., diarrhea, liver, and renal dz) or take medications (e.g., diuretics) that predispose them to electrolyte disorders
   c. Urinalysis (UA) in pts with urologic Sx or those having urologic procedures
   d. PT and PTT in pts with bleeding diathesis or liver disease or who are undergoing neurosurgery or cardiac surgery
   e. Liver function tests (LFTs) in pts with liver disease
   f. CXR in pts with ↑ risk of pulmonary complications (e.g., obesity or thoracic procedures) and those with preexisting pulmonary problems
   g. EKG in men >40, women >50, or young pts with preexisting cardiac dz

B. Perioperative Review of Systems

1. Neurologic—Cerebrovascular Disease
   a. Strokes usually occur postoperatively and are caused by hypotension or emboli from atrial fibrillation
   b. Pts with a recent history of strokes should have their surgical procedure delayed at least 6 wks
   c. Aspirin should be discontinued 2 wks prior to surgery.
2. Cardiovascular
   a. Atrial fibrillation most common postoperative cardiac event
   b. Goldman cardiac risk index stratifies the operative risk of noncardiac surgery pts and helps in the decision of pursuing further Dx testing
   c. See Table 2.3
3. Pulmonary
   a. Pulmonary complications rarely occur in healthy pts
   b. Chronic obstructive pulmonary disease (COPD) is the most important and significant risk factor to consider
   c. Obesity, abd, and intrathoracic procedures predispose pts to pulmonary complications in the postoperative period

Table 2.3 Goldman Cardiac Risk Index

Condition	Points	Concern
S_3 gallop, jugular venous distention (JVD)	11	Congestive heart failure
MI within 6 mos	10	Cardiac injury
Abnormal EKG rhythm	7	Diseased cardiac conduction
>5 premature ventricular contractions/min	7	Cardiac excitability/arrhythmia
Age >70	5	↑ comorbidity
General poor health	3	↑ morbidity
Aortic stenosis	3	Left ventricular outflow obstruction
Peritoneal/thoracic/aortic surgery	3	Major surgery
Emergency	3	Emergency surgery

Note: 26 points warrants life-saving procedures only, because of ↓ risk of cardiac-related death.

    d. Smoking Hx, independent of COPD, is also an important risk factor

4. Renal
   a. Postoperative acute renal failure → ≥50% mortality despite hemodialysis
   b. Chronic renal failure is a significant risk factor not only because of the ↑ risk of developing acute failure but also because of the associated metabolic disturbances and underlying medical conditions
   c. Azotemia, sepsis, intraoperative hypotension, nephrotoxic drugs, and radiocontrast agents are risk factors for postoperative renal failure
   d. Expanding the intravascular volume with IV fluids and using **N-acetylcysteine** or sodium bicarbonate prior to administration of radiocontrast dye will help prevent contrast associated nephropathy (CAN)

5. Infxn/Immunity
   a. Infxn risk depends upon pt characteristics and surgery
   b. Advanced age, diabetes, immunosuppression, obesity, preexisting infxn, and preexisting illness all ↑ risk
   c. Surgical risk factors include GI surgery, prosthetic implantation, preoperative wound contamination, and duration of the operation

d. Prophylaxis
   (1) To prevent surgical wound infxns, antibiotics should be administered within 1 hour, before the skin incision is made—stop prophylactic antibiotics within 24 hrs postoperatively
   (2) Appropriate choice of the antibiotics depends on the procedure
   (3) Give all pts with prosthetic heart valves antibiotic prophylaxis to prevent bacterial endocarditis

6. Hematologic
   a. Deep venous thrombosis (DVT) prevented by early ambulation and mechanical compression stockings
   b. Subcutaneous heparin may be substituted for compression stockings
   c. Pulmonary embolus should always be considered as a cause of postoperative acute-onset dyspnea

7. Endocrinology
   a. Adrenal insufficiency
      (1) Surgery creates stress for the body; normally the body reacts to stress by secreting more corticosteroids
      (2) Response may be diminished in pts taking corticosteroids for ≥1 wk preoperatively and pts with primary adrenal insufficiency
      (3) Hence, for these pts, steroid replacement is needed, and **hydrocortisone is given before, during, and after surgery to approximate the response of the nml adrenal gland.** If these measures are not taken, then adrenal crisis may occur.
      (4) Adrenal crisis
         (a) Life-threatening complication of adrenal insufficiency
         (b) **Si/Sx = unexplained hypotension and tachycardia despite fluid and vasopressor administration**
         (c) Tx = corticosteroids dramatically improve BP

C. **Fever**
   1. Intraoperative Fever
      a. DDx = transfusion reaction, malignant hyperthermia, or prior infxn
      b. Malignant hyperthermia
         (1) Triggered by several anesthetic agents, for example, halothane, isoflurane, and succinylcholine
         (2) Tx = dantrolene, cooling measures, ICU monitoring

2. Postoperative Fever
   a. **Mnemonic for causes: the 5Ws**
      (1) **W**ind (lungs)
      (2) **W**ater (urinary tract)
      (3) **W**ound
      (4) **W**alking (DVT)
      (5) **W**onder drug (drug reaction)
   b. Immediate postoperative fever includes atelectasis, *Streptococcus* and *Clostridium* wound infxns, and aspiration pneumonia
   c. One to two days postoperatively look for indwelling vascular line infxn, aspiration pneumonia, and infectious pneumonia
   d. Tx = encourage early postoperative ambulation, incentive spirometry use postoperatively, treat infxns with appropriate antibiotics

IV. Trauma

A. **General**
   1. Trauma is the major cause of death in those <40 yrs
   2. Management broken into 1° and 2° surveys

B. **Primary Survey = ABCDE**
   1. **A** = **A**irway
      a. All pts immobilized due to ↑ risk of spinal injury
      b. Maintain airway with jaw thrust or mandible/tongue traction, protecting cervical spine
      c. If pt is likely to vomit, position them in a slightly lateral and head-down position to prevent aspiration
      d. If airway cannot be established, a large-bore (14-gauge) needle can be inserted into the cricothyroid membrane
      e. Do not perform tracheotomy in the field or ambulance
      f. Unconscious pts need endotracheal (ET) tube (Glasgow Coma Scale <8 intubate)
   2. **B** = **B**reathing
      a. Assess chest expansion, breath sounds, respiratory rate, rib fractures, subQ emphysema, and penetrating wounds
      b. Life-threatening injuries to the lungs or thoracic cavity are
         (1) Tension pneumothorax
            (a) Causes contralateral mediastinal shift, distended neck veins (↑ central venous pressure [CVP]),

hypotension, absent breath sounds, and hyperresonance to percussion on the affected side

    (b) Tx = immediate chest tube or 14-gauge needle puncture of affected side

(2) Open pneumothorax → Tx = immediate closure of the wound with dressings and placement of a chest tube

(3) Flail chest

    (a) Caused by multiple rib fractures that form a free-floating segment of chest wall that moves paradoxically to the rest of the chest wall, resulting in an inability to generate sufficient inspiratory or expiratory pressure to drive ventilation

    (b) Tx = intubation with mechanical ventilation

(4) Massive hemothorax

    (a) Injury to the great vessels with subsequent hemorrhage into the thoracic cavity

    (b) Tx = chest tube, surgical control of the bleeding site

    (c) **Surgical indications—Approximately 90% of penetrating thoracic injuries can be treated with tube thoracostomy alone, indications for thoracotomy include (1) 1,500-cc initial output from chest tube or (2) 250 cc/hr for 4 hrs**

c. Neck injuries can be life-threatening (Figure 2.2)

  (1) Neck trauma: three zones

    (a) Zone I: clavicle to cricoid cartilage. Structures at greatest risk in this zone are the great vessels, aortic arch, trachea, esophagus, lung apices, cervical spine, spinal cord, and cervical nerve roots

    (b) Zone II: cricoid cartilage to the angle of the mandible. Important structures in this region include the carotid and vertebral arteries, jugular veins, pharynx, larynx, trachea, esophagus, cervical spine, and spinal cord

    (c) Zone III: angle of the mandible to the base of the skull. Salivary and parotid glands, esophagus, trachea, cervical spine, carotid arteries, jugular veins, and major cranial nerves

  (2) Assessment: four-vessel angiography is routinely used to evaluate stable pts sustaining penetrating wounds to Zones I and III that pierce the platysma

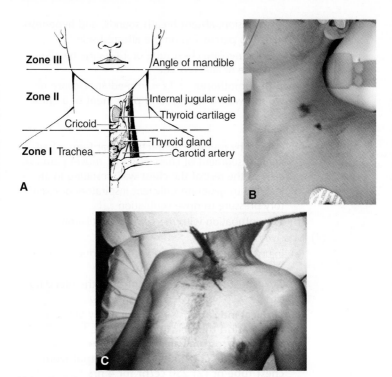

FIGURE 2.2

A. Anterior view of the neck. Significant structures and the zones of the neck are illustrated. (From Harwood-Nuss A, Wolfson AB, Londen CD, et al., eds. *The clinical practice of emergency medicine,* 3rd Ed. Philadelphia, MD: Lippincott Williams & Wilkins, 2001, with permission.) **B.** Gunshot wound in Zone 1 of neck. (Courtesy of Mark Silverberg, MD.) **C.** Stab wound in Zone 1 of neck. (Courtesy of Lewis J. Kaplan, MD.) (B,C from Greenberg MI, Hendrickson RG, Silverberg M, et al. *Greenberg's text-atlas of emergency medicine.* Philadelphia, PA: Lippincott Williams & Wilkins, 2004, with permission.)

      (3) Tx
         (a) Zone II injuries are routinely explored especially if platysma is pierced or if pt is unstable
         (b) Never send an unstable pt to a radiographic suite
         (c) If surgical exposure and access to bleeding vessels proves impractical, such as in Zone III, then therapeutic embolization or occlusion of damaged vessels may be warranted

d. For esophageal injury, conduct gastrografin swallow or direct visualization

e. Thoracic surgery consult

(1) Follow Advanced Trauma Life Support (ATLS) guidelines for pt stabilization and surgical exploration.

3. **C = C**irculation

a. Two large-bore IVs placed in upper extremities (if possible)

b. For severe shock, place a central venous line

c. O-negative blood on standby for any suspected significant hemorrhage

d. Consider **a Focused Assessment with Sonography for Trauma (FAST)**

(1) **A rapid, bedside, ultrasound examination performed to identify intraperitoneal hemorrhage or pericardial tamponade**

(2) **FAST assessment is indicated in trauma patients who give a history of abdominal trauma, are hypotensive, or are unable to provide a reliable history because of impaired consciousness due to head injury or drugs**

(3) **FAST is an adjunct to the ATLS primary survey and therefore follows the performance of the ABCs**

(4) **Four areas assessed are**

(a) **Perihepatic (hepatorenal space)**

(b) **Perisplenic**

(c) **Pelvis**

(d) **Pericardium**

4. **D = D**isability

a. Neurologic disability assessed by history, careful neurologic examination (Glasgow coma scale), laboratory tests (blood alcohol level, blood cultures, blood glucose, ammonia, electrolytes, UA), and skull X-rays

b. Loss of consciousness

(1) DDx = **AEIOU TIPS** = **A**lcohol, **E**pilepsy, **E**nvironment (temp), **I**nsulin (+/−), **O**verdose, **U**remia (electrolytes), **T**rauma, **I**nfection, **P**sychogenic, **S**troke

(2) Tx = Coma cocktail = dextrose, thiamine, naloxone, and O_2

c. ↑ Intracranial pressure (ICP) → HTN, bradycardia, and bradypnea = Cushing's triad

d. Tx = ventilation to keep $PaCO_2$ at 30–40 mm Hg, controlling fever, administration of osmotic diuretics (mannitol), corticosteroids, and even bony decompression (burr hole)

Table 2.4 Glasgow Coma Scale

Finding		Finding	
Eye Opening	**Points**	**Motor Response**	**Points**
Spontaneous	4	To command	6
To voice	3	Localizes	5
To stimulation (pain)	2	Withdraws	4
No response	1	Abnormal flexion	3
Verbal Response		Extension	2
Oriented	5	No response	1
Confused	4		
Incoherent	3		
Incomprehensible	2		
No response	1		

Note: Glasgow coma scale score <8 indicates severe neurologic injury; intubation must be performed to secure airway.

5. **E = E**xposure
   a. Remove all clothes without moving pt (cut off if necessary)
   b. Examine all skin surfaces and back for possible exit wounds
   c. Ensure pt not at risk for hypothermia (small children)

C. **Secondary Survey**
   1. Identify all injuries, examine all body orifices
   2. Periorbital and mastoid hematomas ("raccoon eyes" and Battle's sign), hemotympanum, and cerebrospinal fluid (CSF) otorrhea/rhinorrhea → basilar skull fractures
   3. Glasgow coma scale should be performed (Table 2.4)
   4. Deaths from abd trauma usually result from sepsis because of hollow viscus perforation or hemorrhage if major vessels are penetrated
   5. Dx
      a. If pt stable, diagnostic peritoneal lavage, abd Utz, or CT scan
      b. If pt unstable, surgical laparotomy
      c. If blood noted at urethra, perform retrograde urethrogram before placement of a bladder catheter; hematuria suggests significant retroperitoneal injury and requires CT

Table 2.5 Differential Diagnosis of Shock

Type	Cardiac Output	Pulmonary Capillary Wedge Pressure	Peripheral Vascular Resistance
Hypovolemic	↓	↓	↑
Cardiogenic	↓	↑	↑
Septic	↑	↓	↓

scan for evaluation; take pt to OR for surgical exploration if unstable

    d. Check for compartment syndrome of extremities; Si/Sx = tense, pale, paralyzed, paresthetic, and painful extremity; Tx = fasciotomy

  6. Tx = Surgical hemostasis

D. **Shock**

  1. Most commonly hypovolemic DDx (Table 2.5)

  2. Correction of defect (Table 2.6)

  3. Shock in trauma can also be neurogenic or cardiogenic

  4. Neurogenic because of blood pooling in splenic bed and muscle from loss of autonomic innervation

  5. Tx = usually self-limiting; can be managed by placing pt in supine or Trendelenburg position, **will need volume resuscitation and vasoactive medication (e.g., dopamine) for a short time until neurogenic tone returns.**

Table 2.6 Correction of Defect in Shock

Type	Defect	First-Line Treatment
Hypovolemic	↓ Preload	Two large-bore IVs, crystalloid or colloid infusions (see Section I), replace blood losses with the **3 for 1** rule = give 3 L of fluid per liter of blood loss
Cardiogenic	Myocardial failure	Pressors—dobutamine first line, can add dopamine and/or norepinephrine, supplemental oxygen
Septic	↓ Peripheral vascular resistance	Norepinephrine to vasoconstrict peripheral arterioles, prevent vascular progression to multiple organ dysfunction syndrome (MODS), give resistance IV antibiotics as indicated, supplemental oxygen

SURGERY

V. Burns

A. Partial Thickness

1. 1° and 2° burns are limited to epidermis and superficial dermis
2. Si/Sx = skin is red, blistered, edematous, skin underneath blister is pink or white in appearance, very painful
3. Infxn may convert to full-thickness burns

B. Full Thickness

1. 3° and 4° burns affect all layers of skin and subcutaneous tissues
2. Si/Sx = skin initially is painless, dry, white, charred, cracked, insensate
3. 4° burns also involve muscle and bone
4. All full-thickness burns require surgical excision and skin grafting.
5. Percentage of body surface area (BSA) affected (Figure 2.3 and Table 2.7)
6. Tx = Resuscitation, monitor fluid status, transfer to burn center.
   a. Consider any facial burns or burning of nasal hairs as a potential candidate for acute respiratory distress syndrome (ARDS) and airway compromise
   b. Fluid resuscitation
      (1) Parkland formula = % BSA × weight (kg) × 4, formula used to calculate volume of crystalloid needed
      (2) Give half of fluid in first 8 hrs; remainder given over next 16 hrs
   c. CXR to rule out inhalation injury
   d. Labs → PT/PTT, CBC, type and cross, arterial blood gas (ABGs), electrolytes, UA
   e. Irrigate and débride wound, topical antibiotics (silver sulfadiazine, mafenide, Polysporin), tetanus prophylaxis, and stress ulcer prophylaxis
   f. Transfer to burn center if pt is very young <10 yrs old or >50 yrs old. Burns >20% BSA, full-thickness burns >5% BSA, coexisting chemical or electrical injury, facial burns, genitalia, perineum, hands, feet, or preexisting medical problems
   g. Make pt NPO until bowel function returns; pt will have extremely ↑ protein and caloric requirements with vitamin supplementation

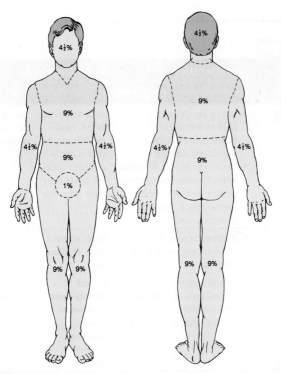

Rule of nines for calculating body surface area. (From Nettina SM. *The Lippincott manual of nursing practice,* 7th Ed. Philadelphia: Lippincott Williams & Wilkins, 2001.)

    h. Excision of eschar to level of bleeding capillaries and split-thickness skin grafts

    i. **Marjolin's ulcer = squamous cell carcinoma arising in an ulcer or burn**

    j. **Curling's ulcer =** acute duodenal ulcer seen in burn patients

Table 2.7 Body Surface Area in Burns

Palm of hand	1%	Upper extremities[a]	9%
Head and neck[a]	9%	Lower extremities[a]	18%
Anterior trunk[a]	18%	Genital area[a]	1%
Posterior trunk[a]	18%		

[a]In adults.

Text continues on page 158

VI. Neck Mass Differential (Table 2.8)

Table 2.8 Neck Mass Differential Diagnosis

Disease	Characteristics	Dx Findings	Tx
Congenital			
Torticollis	• Lateral deviation of head because of hypertrophy of unilateral sternocleidomastoid • Can be congenital, neoplasm, infxn, trauma, degenerative disease, or drug toxicity (particularly D_2 blockers → phenothiazines)	Rock hard knot in the sterno-cleidomastoid that is easily confused with the hyoid bone upon palpation	Muscle relaxants and/or surgical repair
Thyroglossal duct cyst	• **Midline** congenital cysts, which usually presents in childhood	**Cysts elevate upon swallowing**	Surgical removal
Branchial cleft cyst	• **Lateral** congenital cysts, which usually do not present until adulthood, when they become infected or inflamed	**Do not elevate upon swallowing,** aspirate contains cholesterol crystals	Surgical excision
Cystic hygroma	• Occluded lymphatics, which usually present within first 2 yrs of life • **Lateral or midline**	Translucent, benign mass painless, soft and compressible	Surgical excision
Dermoid cyst	• **Lateral or midline** • Solid mass composed of an overgrowth of epithelium	**No elevation with swallowing**	Surgical excision
Carotid body tumor → paraganglioma	• Palpable mass at bifurcation of common carotid artery • Not a vascular tumor, but originate from neural crest cells in the carotid body within the carotid sheath • Rule of 10: 10% malignant, 10% familial, 10% secrete catecholamines	**Pressure on tumor can cause bradycardia and dizziness, will move in horizontal direction but not in vertical direction**	Surgical excision with prior emobolization of feeding vessels

Table 2.8 *Continued*

Disease	Characteristics	Dx Findings	Tx
Acquired-Inflammatory			
Cervical lymphadenitis	• Bilateral lymphadenopathy is usually viral, caused by Epstein–Barr virus, cytomegalovirus, or HIV • Unilateral is usually bacterial, caused by *Staphylococcus. aureus,* group A and B Strep • Cat scratch fever (*Bartonella henselae*), transmitted via scratch of young cats • Scrofula because of tuberculosis • *Actinomyces israelii* → sinuses drain pus containing "sulfur granules" • Kawasaki's syndrome • Lymphoma	Fine-needle aspirate and culture	Per cause: Viral → supportive; bacteria → antibiotics; Kawasaki's → IVIG; Lymphoma→ chemotherapy
Thyroid			
Goiter	• Enlargement of thyroid gland • Usually 2° to ↓ iodine intake, inflammation or use of goitrogens	Fine-needle aspirate, thyroid-stimulating hormone, levels	Treat underlying condition
Malignancy	• See Internal Medicine, Section V.F	Fine-needle aspirate	Surgical excision, followed by radioactive iodine as indicated

SURGERY

VII. Surgical Abdomen (Figures 2.4–2.6)

A. **Right Upper Quadrant (RUQ)** (Table 2.9A)

B. **Right Lower Quadrant (RLQ)** (Table 2.9B)

C. **Left Upper Quadrant (LUQ)** (Table 2.9C)

D. **Left Lower Quadrant (LLQ)** (Table 2.9D)

E. **Midline** (Table 2.9E)

F. **Tx**

 1. Generally all above surgical conditions will require **NPO, naso-gastric (NG) tube, IV fluids, and cardiac monitoring**

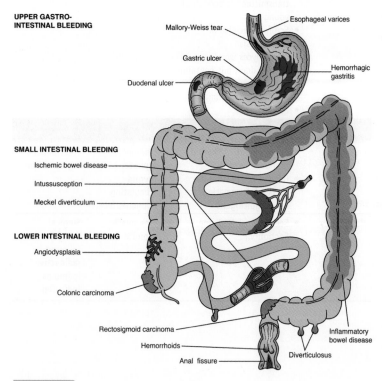

UPPER GASTRO-INTESTINAL BLEEDING

Mallory-Weiss tear

Esophageal varices

Gastric ulcer

Hemorrhagic gastritis

Duodenal ulcer

SMALL INTESTINAL BLEEDING

Ischemic bowel disease

Intussusception

Meckel diverticulum

LOWER INTESTINAL BLEEDING

Angiodysplasia

Colonic carcinoma

Rectosigmoid carcinoma

Hemorrhoids

Anal fissure

Inflammatory bowel disease

Diverticulosus

FIGURE 2.4

Common causes of GI bleeding. (Image from Rubin E, Farber JL. *Pathology*, 3rd Ed. Philadelphia: Lippincott Williams & Wilkins, 1999.)

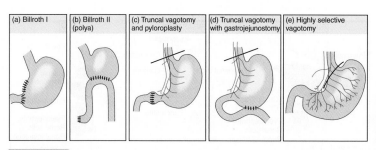

FIGURE 2.5

Operations for peptic ulceration. **A.** Partial gastrectomy with Billroth I anastomosis. The ulcer and the ulcer-bearing portion of the stomach are resected. **B.** Partial gastrectomy with creation of a duodenal loop (Billroth II, Polya). **C.** Truncal vagotomy and pyloroplasty. The main nerves are divided to eliminate nervous stimulation of the stomach, reducing the acid secretory capacity, and gastric emptying is maintained with pyloroplasty. **D.** Truncal vagotomy with gastrojejunostomy. The main nerves are divided and gastric emptying maintained with gastrojejunostomy. **E.** Highly selective vagotomy. Innervation of the acid-producing area of the stomach is interrupted, leaving the nerve supply to the antrum and pylorus intact. This does not affect gastric emptying, so a drainage procedure is not required. (Adapted from Axford JS. *Medicine.* Oxford: Blackwell Science, 1996, with permission.)

2. IV antibiotics as needed
3. Surgery for hemostasis and life-threatening conditions, consult appropriate surgical service (obstetric, pediatric surgery, etc.) as indicated

VIII. Esophagus

A. **Hiatal Hernia**
   1. Majority of pts with reflux have hiatal hernia (80%)
   2. Si/Sx = gastroesophageal reflux disease (GERD) and chest pain
   3. Dx = barium swallow to identify anatomic variations
   4. Two Types of Hiatal Hernias
      a. Type I
         (1) Sliding hiatal hernia, most common.
         (2) Consists of movement of the gastroesophageal junction and stomach up into the mediastinum
         (3) Tx = antacids as per GERD

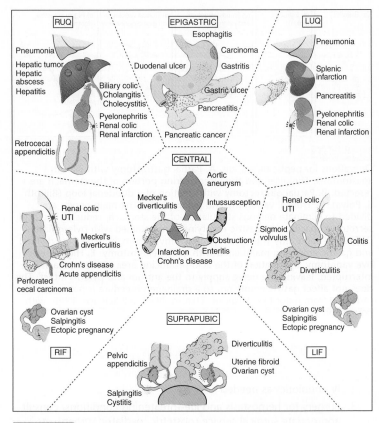

FIGURE 2.6 Acute abd pain.

 b. Type II
  (1) Herniation of the stomach fundus through the diaphragm parallel to the esophagus
  (2) Tx = mandatory surgical repair due to ↑ risk of strangu-
   lation
 c. **Type III**
  (1) **Herniation of the stomach fundus as well as sliding
   of the gastroesophageal junction above the diaphragm**
  (2) **Tx = surgical reduction and repair**

Text continues on page 165

Table 2.9A Right Upper Quadrant Differential Diagnosis

Disease	Characteristics
Biliary colic	• Si/Sx = constant right upper quadrant (RUQ) to epigastric pain • Utz → gallstones but no gallbladder wall thickening or pericholecystic fluid
Cholecystitis	• Si/Sx = fever, RUQ tenderness, **Murphy's sign** (inspiratory arrest upon deep palpation of RUQ) • Labs → moderate to severe leukocytosis, ↑ LFTs, ↑ bilirubin • Utz → gallstones, **pericholecystic fluid,** thickened gallbladder wall
Choledocholithiasis	• Si/Sx = RUQ pain worse with fatty meals, jaundice • Utz → CBD dilatation • Labs → ↑ LFTs, ↑ bilirubin
Pneumonia[a]	• Si/Sx = pleuritic chest pain and fever • CXR → infiltrate, labs → leukocytosis
Fitz-Hugh–Curtis syndrome[a]	• Syndrome of perihepatitis caused by ascending *Chlamydia* or *N. gonorrhoeae* salpingitis • Si/Sx = RUQ pain, fever, Hx or Si/Sx of salpingitis • Labs → leukocytosis but nml bilirubin and LFTs • Utz → nml gallbladder and biliary tree but fluid around the liver and gallbladder

Cholangitis	• Life threatening
	• Si/S
	   ◊ **Charcot's triad** = fever, jaundice, and RUQ pain
	   ◊ **Reynolds' pentad:** add hypotension and mental status change
	• Labs → leukocytosis, blood Cx → enteric organisms, ↑ LFTs, ↑ bilirubin
	• Utz and CT → biliary duct dilatation from obstructing gallstones
	• Dx with endoscopic retrograde cholangiopancreatography (ERCP) or percutaneous transhepatic cholangiography (PTC)

Hepatitis[a]	• Si/Sx = RUQ pain/tenderness, jaundice, fever • Labs → ↑ LFTs, ↑ bilirubin, leukocytosis, ⊕ hepatitis virus serologies • Utz rules out other causes of RUQ pain

[a]Medical treatment indicated unless patient absolutely requires surgery for cure.

Table 2.9B Right Lower Quadrant Differential Diagnosis

Disease	Characteristics
Appendicitis	• Si/Sx = right lower quadrant (RLQ) pain/tenderness originally diffuse and then migrating to **McBurney's point** (1/3 the distance from the anterior superior iliac spine to the umbilicus), fever, diarrhea • Perform rectal exam to rule out retroperitoneal appendicitis • Labs → leukocytosis, fecalith on plain film or abd CT • Decision to take to OR based mostly on clinical picture
Yersinia enterocolitis[a]	• Si/Sx = fever, diarrhea, severe RLQ pain make it hard to distinguish from appendicitis • Labs → fecal culture
Ectopic pregnancy	• Si/Sx = crampy to constant lower abd pain, vaginal bleeding, tender adnexal mass, menstrual irregularity • Labs → anemia, ↑ human chorionic gonadotropin (hCG), culdocentesis reveals blood
Salpingitis/ tubo-ovarian abscess (TOA)	• Si/Sx = lower abd/pelvic pain (constant to crampy, sharp to dull), purulent vaginal discharge, cervical motion tenderness, adnexal mass • Wet mount → white blood cells (WBC), endocervical Cx ⊕ for *N. gonorrhoeae* or *Chlamydia* • Utz → TOA, CT scan can help rule out appendicitis
Meckel's diverticulum	• **1–10–100 rule: 1%–2%** prevalence, **1–10** cm in length, **50–100** cm proximal to ileocecal valve, or rule of 2s: **2% of the population, 2% are symptomatic (usually before age 2), remnants are roughly 2 in, found 2 ft from ileocecal valve and found 2× as common in males** • Si/Sx = GI bleed (melena, hematochezia), small bowel obstruction (intussusception, Littre's hernia), Meckel's diverticulitis (similar presentation to appendicitis) • Nuclear medicine gastric scan to detect gastric mucosa present in 50% of Meckel's diverticula or tagged red blood cell (RBC) scan to detect bleeding source
Ovarian torsion	• Si/Sx = acute onset, sharp unilateral lower abd/pelvic pain, pain may be intermittent because of incomplete torsion, pain related to change in position, nausea and fever present, tender adnexal mass • Utz and laparoscopy confirm Dx
Intussus- ception	• Most common in infants 5–10 mos • SiSx = infant crying with pulling legs up to abdomen, dark, red stool (**currant jelly**), vomiting, shock • Barium or air contrast enema → diagnostic "coiled spring" sign

[a]Medical treatment indicated unless patient absolutely requires surgery for cure.

Table 2.9C Left Upper Quadrant Differential Diagnosis

Disease	Characteristics
Peptic ulcer[a]	• Si/Sx = epigastric pain relieved by food or antacids • Perforated ulcers present with sudden upper abd pain, shoulder pain, GI bleed • Labs → endoscopy or upper GI series
Myocardial infarction[a]	• Si/Sx = chest pain, dyspnea, diaphoresis, nausea • Labs → EKG, troponins, creatine kinase–MB
Splenic rupture	• Si/Sx = tachycardia, broken ribs, Hx of trauma, hypotension • **Kehr's sign** = left upper quadrant pain and referred left shoulder pain • Labs → leukocytosis • X-ray → fractured ribs, medially displaced gastric bubble • CT scan of abdomen preferred method of Dx

[a]Medical treatment indicated unless patient absolutely requires surgery for cure.

Table 2.9D Left Lower Quadrant Differential Diagnosis

Disease	Characteristics
Diverticulitis[a]	• Si/Sx = left lower quadrant (LLQ) pain and mass, fever, urinary urgency • Labs → leukocytosis • CT scan and Utz → thickened bowel wall, abscess—do not use contrast enema
Sigmoid volvulus	• Si/Sx = elderly, chronically constipated patient, abd pain, distention, obstipation • X-ray → **inverted U**, contrast enema → **bird's beak deformity**
Pyelonephritis[a]	• Si/Sx = high fever, rigors, costovertebral angle tenderness, Hx of UTI • Labs → pyuria, ≈ urine culture
Ovarian torsion	• See RLQ (Table 2.9B)
Ectopic pregnancy	• See RLQ (Table 2.9B)
Salpingitis	• See RLQ (Table 2.9B)

[a]Medical treatment indicated unless patient absolutely requires surgery for cure.

SURGERY

Table 2.9E Midline Differential Diagnosis

Disease	Characteristics
Pancreatitis	• Si/Sx = severe epigastric pain radiating to the back, nausea/vomiting, signs of hypovolemia because of "third spacing," ↓ bowel sounds • In hemorrhagic pancreatitis, there are ecchymotic appearing skin findings in the flank (**Grey Turner's sign**) or periumbilical area (**Cullen's sign**) • Labs → leukocytosis, ↑ serum and urine amylase, ↑ lipase • X-ray → dilated small bowel or transverse colon adjacent to the pancreas, called **"sentinel loop"** • CT → phlegmon, pseudocyst, necrosis, abscess
Pancreatic pseudocyst	• Si/Sx = sequelae of pancreatitis, if pancreatitis Sx do not improve, check for pseudocyst; may cause fever or shock in infected or hemorrhagic cases • CT and Utz → fluid-filled cystic mass
Abd aortic aneurysm (AAA)	• Si/Sx = usually aSx, rupture presents with back or abd pain and shock, compression on duodenum or ureters can cause obstructive Sx, palpable pulsatile periumbilical mass • X-ray (cross-table lateral films), Utz, CT, aortography reveal aneurysm
Gastroesophageal reflux disease[a]	• Si/Sx = position-dependent (supine worse) substernal or epigastric burning pain, regurgitation, dysphagia, hoarse voice • Dx by barium swallow, manometric or pH testing, esophagoscopy
Myocardial infarction[a]	• See LUQ (Table 2.9C)
Peptic ulcer[a]	• See LUQ (Table 2.9C)
Gastroenteritis[a]	• Si/Sx = diarrhea, vomiting, abd pain, fever, malaise, headache • Labs → stool studies not usually indicated except in severe cases

[a]Medical treatment indicated unless patient absolutely requires surgery for cure.

    d. **Type IV**

      (1) **Herniation of abdominal organs (e.g., spleen, intestines, liver, pancreas) above the diaphragm**

      (2) **Tx = surgical reduction and repair**

B. **Achalasia**

  1. Most common motility disorder.

  2. Loss of esophageal motility and failure of lower esophageal sphincter (LES) relaxation; may be caused by ganglionic degeneration or Chagas disease; results in the dilatation of the proximal esophagus

  3. Si/Sx = dysphagia of both solids and liquids, weight loss, and repulsion of undigested foodstuffs that may produce a foul odor

  4. May ↑ risk of esophageal CA because stasis promotes development of Barrett esophagus

  5. Dx

    a. Barium swallow → dilatation of the proximal esophagus with subsequent narrowing of the distal esophagus; studies may also reveal esophageal diverticula

    b. Manometry → ↑ LES pressure and failure to relax

  6. Tx

    a. Endoscopic dilation of LES with balloon cures 80% of pts

    b. Alternative is a myotomy with a modified fundoplication

    c. Surgical Tx or Botox injection of LES may be considered.

C. **Esophageal Diverticula (Zenker's Diverticulum)**

  1. Proximal diverticula are usually Zenker's

  2. Pulsion diverticula involving only the mucosa, located between the thyropharyngeal and cricopharyngeus muscle fibers (condition associated with muscle dysfunction/spasms)

  3. Si/Sx = dysphagia, regurgitation of solid foods, choking, left-sided neck mass, and bad breath

  4. Dx = clinically + barium swallow

  5. Tx = myotomy of cricopharyngeus muscle and removal of diverticulum

D. **Esophageal Tumors**

  1. Squamous Cell CA

    a. Most common esophageal CA, alcohol and tobacco synergistically ↑ risk of development

    b. Most commonly seen in men in the sixth decade of life

SURGERY

2. AdenoCA
   a. Seen in pts with chronic reflux → Barrett's esophagus = squamous to columnar metaplasia
   b. Ten percent of pts with Barrett's esophagus will develop adenoCA
3. Si/Sx for both = **dysphagia**, weight loss, hoarseness, tracheo-esophageal fistula, recurrent aspiration, and possibly symptoms of metastatic disease
4. Dx = barium study demonstrates **classic apple-core lesion;** Dx confirmed with endoscopy with biopsy, CT of abdomen and chest is also performed to determine extent of spread
5. Tx = esophagectomy with gastric pull-up or colonic interposition with or without chemotherapy/radiation
6. Px poor unless resected prior to spread (very rare); however, palliation should be attempted to restore effective swallowing

IX. Gastric Tumors

A. Benign tumors comprise <10% of all gastric tumors; most commonly polyps and leiomyoma
B. Stomach CA most common after 50 yrs, ↑ incidence in men
C. Linked to blood group A (suggesting genetic predisposition), immunosuppression, and environmental factors
D. Nitrosamines, excess salt intake, low fiber intake, *Helicobacter pylori,* achlorhydria, chronic gastritis are all risk factors
E. Almost always adenocarcinoma; usually involves antrum, rarely fundus; aggressive spread to nodes/liver
F. Rarer Gastric Tumors
   1. Lymphoma
      a. Causes 4% of gastric CA, better Px than adenoCA
      b. Associated with *H. pylori* infxn
   2. Linitis Plastica
      a. Infiltrating, diffuse adenoCA, invariably fatal within months
      b. **This is the deadliest form of gastric CA**
G. Several classic physical findings in metastatic gastric CA
   1. **Virchow's node = large rock-hard supraclavicular node**
   2. **Krukenberg tumor = mucinous, signet-ring cells that metastasize from gastric CA to bilateral ovaries, so palpate for ovarian masses in women**

3. **Sister Mary Joseph sign** = metastasis to umbilicus, feel for hard nodule there, associated with poor Px
4. **Blumer's shelf** = palpable nodule superiorly on rectal exam, caused by metastasis of GI CA

H. Si/Sx for all = weight loss, anemia, anorexia, GI upset

I. Dx = biopsy

J. Tx = mostly palliative; combination surgery and chemotherapy when tolerated

K. Px = approximately 5% survival at 5 yrs

X. Hernia (Table 2.10)

A. **Inguinal Hernias (Figure 2.7)**
   1. Most common hernia; more common in men
   2. Direct type = viscera protrudes directly through abd wall at Hesselbach's triangle (inferior epigastric artery, rectus sheath, and inguinal ligament), medial to inferior epigastric artery
   3. Indirect type is more common (two-thirds are indirect), pass lateral to inferior epigastric artery into spermatic cord covered by cremasteric muscle
   4. Si/Sx = intermittent groin mass with bowel sounds that appear during Valsalva maneuvers
   5. DDx = femoral hernias, which protrude below the inguinal ligament

Table 2.10 Hernia Definitions

Combined (pantaloon)	Concurrent direct and indirect hernias
Sliding	Part of the hernia sac wall is formed by a visceral organ
Richter	Part of the bowel is trapped in the hernia sac
Littre	Meckel's diverticulum contained inside hernia
Reducible	Able to replace herniated tissue to its usual anatomic location
Incarcerated	Hernias that are not reducible
Strangulated	Incarcerated hernia with vascular compromise → ischemia
Incisional	Herniation through surgical incision, commonly 2° to wound infxn

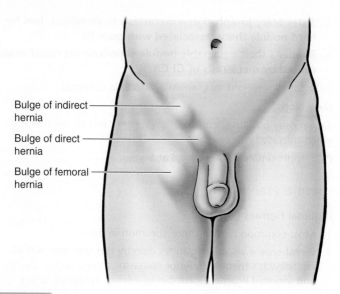

Bulge of indirect hernia

Bulge of direct hernia

Bulge of femoral hernia

FIGURE 2.7

Inguinal and femoral hernias. (From Moore KL, Dalley AF. *Clinical oriented anatomy,* 4th Ed. Baltimore, MD: Lippincott Williams & Wilkins, 1999.)

6. Dx = physical exam some unable to completely differentiate until surgery

7. Tx = surgical repair with mesh placement

B. **Femoral Hernias** (Figure 2.7)

1. More common in women

2. Si/Sx = bulge above or below the inguinal ligament, ↑ risk of incarceration

3. Dx = clinical and/or surgical

4. Tx = surgical repair should not be delayed

C. **Visceral Hernias**

1. Cause intestinal obstruction

2. Si/Sx = as per bowel obstruction (e.g., obstipation, abd pain, etc.)

3. X-ray → no gas in rectum, distended bowel, air–fluid levels

4. DDx = other causes of bowel obstruction such as adhesions, external hernia, malignancy, etc.

5. Dx = clinical or surgical

6. Tx = surgical repair if hernia is not reducible

XI. Hepatic Tumors

A. **Benign Tumors**

1. Hemangioma is most common benign tumor of the liver
2. Hepatic adenoma incidence related to oral contraceptives
3. Adenomas may rupture → severe intraperitoneal bleed
4. Dx = Utz, CT scan
5. Tx = surgery only indicated if danger of rupture, pt symptomatic, or large amount of liver involved

B. **Malignant Tumors**

1. Metastases are the most common malignant hepatic tumors
2. Hepatocellular CA is the most common 1° hepatic malignancy
   a. Note also called "hepatoma," incorrectly implying benign tumor (historical misnomer)
   b. Most common malignancy in the world, endemic in Southeast Asia and sub-Saharan Africa because of vertical transmission of hepatitis B virus (HBV)
   c. Associated with cirrhosis, HBV and HCV infxn, alcoholism, hemochromatosis, Wilson's disease
   d. Si/Sx = weight loss, jaundice, weakness, dull and constant RUQ or epigastric pain, hepatomegaly; palpable mass or bloody ascites may also be present
   e. Labs → ↑ bilirubin, ⊕ HBV or HCV serologies, **very high** α-fetoprotein (AFP) level
   f. Dx = Utz or CT scan
   g. Tx = (1) surgical resection, (2) liver transplant, (3) chemo-Sorafenib
3. Hemangiosarcoma
   a. Associated with toxic exposure to polyvinyl chloride, Thorotrast, and arsenic
   b. Dx = Utz or CT scan
   c. Tx = surgical resection, may be curative if liver function is nml; in presence of cirrhosis, usually not effective

XII. Gallbladder

A. **Cholelithiasis = Gallstones**

1. Higher incidence in women, multiple pregnancies, obesity (**the four Fs = female, forty, fertile, fat**)
2. Ten percent of U.S. population has gallstones; complications of the disorder are what necessitate intervention

3. Pts ≤20 yrs with gallstones should undergo workup for congenital spherocytosis or hemoglobinopathy

4. Si/Sx = aSx by definition

5. Dx = Utz, often incidental finding that does not require therapy

6. Tx

   a. aSx pts with gallstones do not require cholecystectomy unless there is ↑ risk for developing CA

   b. Pts with a porcelain gallbladder (calcified gallbladder walls) and those of Native American descent with gallstones are at ↑ risk of developing gallbladder CA and should receive a cholecystectomy

B. **Biliary Colic**

1. Because of gallstone impaction in cystic or common bile duct (CBD)

2. **The vast majority of people who have aSx gallstones WILL NEVER progress to biliary colic** (2%–3% progress per year; lifelong risk = 20%)

3. Sx = sharp colicky pain made worse by eating, particularly fats

4. May have multiple episodes that resolve, but eventually this condition leads to further complications, so surgical resection of the gallbladder is required

5. Dx = Ultrasound; hepatobiliary iminodiacetic acid **(HIDA) scan may help with the diagnosis in the absence of stones. An ejection fraction of <20% is highly suggestive of acalculous cholecystitis**

6. Tx = cholecystectomy to prevent future complications

C. **Cholecystitis**

1. Cholecystitis is due to 2° infxn of obstructed gallbladder

   a. The EEEK! bugs: *Escherichia coli, Enterobacter, Enterococcus, Klebsiella* spp.

   b. Si/Sx = sudden onset, severe, steady pain in RUQ/epigastrium; muscle guarding/rebound; ⊕ **Murphy's sign** (RUQ palpation during inspiration causes sharp pain and sudden cessation of inspiration)

   c. Labs → leukocytosis (may be >20,000 in emphysematous cholecystitis = presence of gas in gallbladder wall), ↑ aspartate aminotransferase/alanine aminotransferase (AST/ALT), ↑ bilirubin

   d. Dx = Utz → gallstones, pericholecystic fluid, and thickened gallbladder wall; if results equivocal can confirm with radionuclide cholescintigraphy (e.g., HIDA scan)—CT scan usually is not the test of choice to diagnose cholecystitis

  e. Tx

    (1) NPO, IV hydration, and antibiotics to cover Gram-negative rods and anaerobes

    (2) Demerol better for pain as morphine causes spasm of the sphincter of Oddi

    (3) Surgical resection if unresponsive or worsening

D. **Choledocholithiasis**

  1. Passage of stone through the cystic duct, can obstruct CBD

  2. Si/Sx = obstructive jaundice, ↑ conjugated bilirubin, hypercholesterolemia, ↑ alkaline phosphatase

  3. Dx = Utz → CBD >9-mm diameter (Utz first line for Dx)

  4. Surgical Pearl—**Normal CBD 3–4 mm, increases by 1 mm per 10 years over the age of 50. For example, 5 mm at 50, 6 mm at 60.**

  5. **Passage of stone to CBD can cause acute pancreatitis if the ampulla of Vater is obstructed by the stone**

  6. Tx = laparoscopic cholecystectomy, or ERCP

E. **Ascending Cholangitis**

  1. Results from 2° bacterial infxn of obstructed CBD, facilitated by obstructed bile flow

  2. Obstruction usually because of choledocholithiasis but can be 2° to strictures, foreign bodies (e.g., surgical clips from prior abd surgery), and parasites

  3. **Charcot's triad = jaundice, RUQ pain, fever (85% sensitive for cholangitis)—for Reynolds' pentad add altered mental status and hypotension**

  4. Dx = Utz or CT → CBD dilation.

  5. This is a life-threatening emergency!

  6. Tx

    a. NPO, IV hydration, and antibiotics to cover Gram-negative rods and anaerobes

    b. ERCP or PTC to decompress the biliary tree and remove obstructing stones followed by cholecystectomy once clinically improved

F. **CA**

  1. Very rare, usually occurs in seventh decade of life

  2. More commonly seen in females; gallstones are risk factors for developing CA

3. Most common 1° tumor of gallbladder is adenoCA

4. Frequently seen in Far East, associated with *Clonorchis sinensis* (liver fluke) infestation

5. When the tumor occurs at the confluence of the hepatic ducts forming the common duct, the tumor is called **"Klatskin's tumor"**

6. **Courvoisier's law** = gallbladder enlarges when CBD is obstructed by pancreatic CA but not enlarged when CBD is obstructed by stone

7. Courvoisier's sign is a palpable gallbladder

8. Si/Sx = as for biliary colic but persistent

9. Dx = Utz or CT to show tumor, but preoperative Dx of gallbladder CA is often incorrect

10. Tx = palliative stenting of bile ducts; can consider surgical resection for palliation only

11. Px = terminal, almost all pts die within 1 yr of Dx

XIII. Exocrine Pancreas

A. Acute Pancreatitis

1. Pancreatic enzymes autodigest pancreas → hemorrhagic fat necrosis, calcium deposition, and sometimes formation of pseudocysts (cysts not lined with ductal epithelium)

2. Most common causes in US = gallstones and alcohol

3. Other causes include infxn, trauma, radiation, drug (thiazides, azidothymidine [AZT], protease inhibitors), hyperlipidemia, hypercalcemia, vascular events, tumors, scorpion sting

4. Si/Sx = severe abd pain, prostration (fetal position opens up retroperitoneal space and allows more room for swollen pancreas), hypotension (because of retroperitoneal fluid sequestration), tachycardia, fever, ↑ serum amylase (90% sensitive)/lipase, hyperglycemia, hypocalcemia

5. Dx = clinically and/or abd CT, **classic x-ray finding = sentinel loop or colon cutoff sign** (loop of distended bowel adjacent to pancreas)

6. **Classic physical findings = Grey Turner's sign (discoloration of flank) and Cullen's sign (periumbilical discoloration)**

7. Tx is aimed at decreasing stress to pancreas

   a. NPO until symptoms/amylase subside; total parenteral nutrition (TPN) if NPO for >7–10 days

Table 2.11 Ranson's Criteria	
On Admission	**Within 24–48 hrs**
Age >55, WBCs >16,000/mL, aspartate aminotransferase >250 IU/dL, lactate dehydrogenase >350, blood glucose >200, base deficit >4 mEq/L	↓ hematocrit >10%, blood urea nitrogen rise >5 mg/dL, serum calcium <8 mg/dL, arterial pO_2<60 mmHg, fluid sequestration >6 L
• 0–2 of these → minimal mortality	
• 3–5 → 10%–20% mortality	
• >5 → ≥50% mortality	

SURGERY

    b. Demerol to control pain

    c. IV fluid resuscitation

    d. Alcohol withdrawal prophylaxis

    e. May require ICU admission if severe

  8. Complications = abscess, pseudocysts, duodenal obstruction, shock lung, and acute renal failure

  9. Repeated bouts of pancreatitis cause chronic pancreatitis, resulting in fibrosis and atrophy of the organ with early exocrine and later endocrine insufficiency

  10. Px of acute pancreatitis determined by **Ranson's criteria** (Table 2.11)

B. **Pancreatic Pseudocyst**

  1. Collection of fluid in pancreas surrounded by a fibrous capsule, no communication with fibrous ducts

  2. **Suspect anytime a pt is readmitted with pancreatitis for complaints within several weeks of being discharged after a bout of pancreatitis**

  3. 2° to pancreatitis or trauma, as in steering wheel injury

  4. Dx = Abd Utz/CT (Figure 2.8A)

  5. Tx = percutaneous surgical drainage or pancreaticogastrostomy or **pancreaticojejunostomy** (creation of surgical fistula to drain cyst into the stomach or jejunum), but small cysts will resorb on their own

  6. New cysts contain blood, necrotic debris, leukocytes; old cysts contain straw-colored fluid

  7. Can become infected with purulent contents, causing peritonitis after rupture

FIGURE 2.8

A. CT scan showing a well-defined, low-density pancreatic pseudocyst (*arrows*). (From Patel PR. *Lecture notes on radiology.* Oxford: Blackwell Science, 1998, with permission.) **B.** Pancreatic tumors.

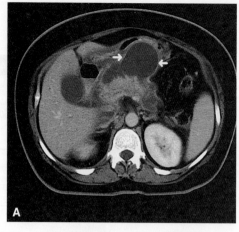

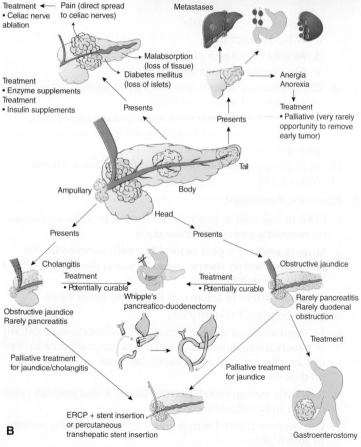

C. **Pancreatic CA**

1. Epidemiology = 90% are adenoCA, with 60% of these arising in the head of pancreas

2. More common in African-Americans, cigarette smokers, and males; linked to chronic pancreatitis and diabetes mellitus

3. Si/Sx = painless jaundice, weight loss, abd pain; **classic sign is Trousseau's syndrome = migratory thrombophlebitis, which occurs in 10% of pts**

4. Frequently invades duodenum, ampulla of Vater, and CBD; can also cause biliary obstruction

5. Dx = Labs: ↑ bilirubin, ↑ alkaline phosphatase, ↑ CA 19–9 (not diagnostic), **CT scan** (Figure 2.8B)

6. Tx = Whipple's procedure, resection of pancreas, part of small bowel, stomach, gallbladder

7. Site of CA and extent of disease at time of Dx determines Px: usually very poor; 5-yr survival rate after palliative resection is 5%

D. **Endocrine Pancreatic Neoplasm**

1. Insulinoma **(Most common pancreatic islet cell tumor)** because hyperplasia of insulin-producing β-cells

2. Glucagonoma = α-cell tumor → hyperglycemia and exfoliative dermatitis. Note: Most malignant tumor, 70% metastasis rate.

3. Somatostatinoma = delta cell tumor → produces somatostatin, develop diabetes mellitus

4. VIPoma = secretes vasoactive intestinal peptide (VIP), prolonged watery diarrhea with severe electrolyte imbalances

5. Zollinger–Ellison syndrome (Gastrinoma)

   a. Dx = clinically, elevated serum levels of insulin, glucagon, or gastrin + secretin test.

   b. Tx = surgical resection of the tumor and aggressive PPI therapy.

   c. **Surgical Pearl—Associated with MEN 1, sporadic tumors (66%) often located in the gastrinoma triangle (confluence of the cystic and CBD superiorly, the second and third portions of the duodenum inferiorly, and the neck and body of the pancreas medially)**

XIV. Small Intestine

A. **Small Bowel Obstruction (SBO)**

1. Most common surgical condition of the small bowel

2. Causes = peritoneal adhesions from prior surgery, hernias, and neoplasms in order of occurrence in the adult population

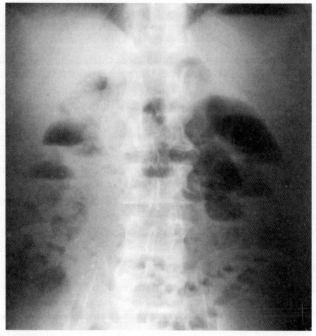

FIGURE 2.9

"Stepladder" pattern of air–fluid levels on upright view in patient with small bowel obstruction. (From Harwood-Nuss A, Wolfson AB, Linden CH, et al. *The clinical practice of emergency medicine*, 3rd Ed. Philadelphia, PA: Lippincott Williams & Wilkins, 2001.)

3. Other causes include Crohn's disease, Meckel's diverticulum, radiation enteritis, gallstone ileus, hypokalemia, narcotics, anticholinergics, acute pancreatitis, gastroenteritis, and cholecystitis

4. Si/Sx = crampy abd pain, nausea, vomiting, lack of flatus, abd tenderness, abd distention, and hyperactive, high-pitched bowel sounds

5. DDx = paralytic ileus (similar Si/Sx)

6. Dx = abd series → distended loops of small bowel proximal to the obstruction, upright film → air–fluid levels or free air beneath the diaphragm (if accompanied by bowel perforation) on a posterior/anterior (PA) chest film (Figure 2.9)

7. Tx

   a. Conservative Tx = IV fluids, NG tube decompression, and Foley catheter; partial obstructions may be successfully treated with conservative therapy

    b. Surgical candidates receive antibiotics to include both anaerobic and Gram-negative coverage

    c. Objective of surgery is to remove obstruction and resect nonviable bowel

    d. **Surgical Pearl—90% of early postoperative SBO (within 30 days) are due to adhesions, 80% will resolve without surgery, 95% within 2 wks of starting conservative treatment.**

B. **Small Bowel Neoplasms**

1. Leiomyoma is most common benign tumor of the small bowel

2. Si/Sx = pain, anemia, weight loss, nausea, and vomiting; common complication is obstruction that is caused primarily by leiomyomas

3. Carcinoid tumors (small bowel is the second most common location, appendix is first) → cutaneous flushing, diarrhea, and respiratory distress

4. Malignant neoplasms in order of decreasing incidence: **adeno-CA, carcinoid, lymphoma, and sarcomas**

5. Dx = biopsy, not necessarily reliable

6. Tx = surgical resection of primary tumor along with lymph nodes and liver metastases, if possible

XV. Colon

A. **Colonic Polyps: neoplastic, hamartoma, inflammatory, hyperplastic**

1. Neoplastic Polyps

    a. Most commonly adenomas and can be classified as tubular adenoma (smallest malignant potential), tubulovillous adenoma, or villous adenoma (greatest malignant potential)

    b. Mean age of pts with polyps is 55; incidence ↑ with age

    c. Fifty percent of polyps occur in the sigmoid or rectum

    d. Si/Sx = intermittent rectal **bleeding** is most common presenting complaint

    e. Dx = colonoscopy, sigmoidoscopy, always consider family Hx

    f. Tx

        (1) Colonoscopic polypectomy or laparotomy

        (2) If invasive adenoCA is found, a colectomy is not mandatory if gross and microscopic margins are clear, if tissue

is well differentiated without lymphatic or venous drainage, and polyp stalk does not invade

2. Hyperplastic Polyps
   a. Common in distal colon; comprise 90% of all polyps
   b. Most commonly benign, but can be associated with malignancy in hyperplastic polyposis syndrome
   c. Patients with multiple or large hyperplastic polyps are at ↑ risk for malignancy

3. Familial Polyposis Syndromes
   a. Familial adenomatous polyposis (FAP) has autosomal dominant inheritance of *APC* gene; abundant polyps throughout the colon and rectum beginning at puberty
   b. Gardner's syndrome consists of polyposis, desmoid tumors, osteomas of mandible or skull, and sebaceous cysts
   c. Turcot's syndrome is polyposis with medulloblastoma or glioma
   d. Dx = family Hx, colonoscopy; presence of congenital hypertrophy of retinal pigment epithelium predicts FAP with 97% sensitivity
   e. Tx = colectomy and upper GI endoscopy to rule out gastroduodenal lesions—a favored operation is an abd colectomy, mucosal proctectomy, and ileoanal anastomosis

4. Peutz–Jeghers Syndrome (Figure 2.10)
   a. Si/Sx = autosomal dominant inheritance, nonneoplastic hamartomatous polyps in stomach, small intestine, and colon, skin, and mucous membrane hyperpigmentation, **particularly freckles on lips**
   b. ↑ **Risk of developing CA in other tissues** (e.g., breast, pancreas)
   c. Dx = clinical and family Hx
   d. Tx = careful, regular monitoring for malignancy

5. Juvenile Polyposis Syndromes
   a. Examples include juvenile polyposis coli, generalized juvenile GI polyposis, and Cronkhite–Canada syndrome
   b. Si/Sx = hamartomatous polyps and thus carry ↓ malignant potential, similar to Peutz–Jeghers; pts with familial juvenile polyposis carry ↑ risk for GI CA
   c. Dx = clinical and family Hx
   d. Tx = polypectomy is generally reserved for symptomatic polyps

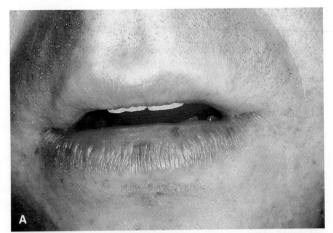

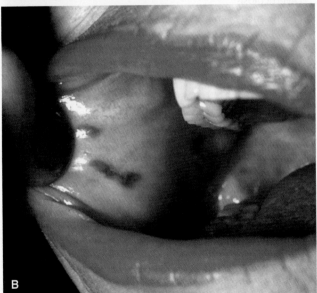

FIGURE 2.10

Peutz–Jeghers syndrome. **A.** Pigmented macules on the lips that cross the vermilion border. (Courtesy of Jeffrey P. Callen, MD.) **B.** Buccal and perioral pigment spots are characteristic of this syndrome. (From Yamada T, Alpers DH, Kaplowitz N, et al., eds. *Atlas of gastroenterology,* 3rd Ed. Philadelphia, PA: Lippincott Williams & Wilkins, 2003, with permission.)

B. **Diverticular Disease**
1. General Characteristics
    a. Approximately 50% of people have diverticula, ↑ incidence between fifth and eighth decade of life in Western countries, but **only 10%–20% cause Sx**
    b. True diverticula = herniations involving the full bowel wall thickness
    c. True diverticula are rare, often found in cecum and ascending colon
    d. False diverticula = only mucosal herniations through muscular wall
    e. False diverticula are common, >90% found in sigmoid colon
    f. It is believed that ↑ intraluminal pressure (perhaps promoted by ↓ fiber diet) causes herniation
2. Diverticulosis
    a. Presence of multiple false (acquired) diverticula
    b. Si/Sx = 80% are aSx and are found incidentally; can cause recurrent abd pain in LLQ and changes in bowel habits; 5%–10% of pts present with lower GI hemorrhage that can be massive
    c. Dx = colonoscopy or barium enema to reveal herniations
    d. Tx
        (1) aSx pts should ↑ fiber content of diet, ↓ fatty food intake, and avoid foods that exacerbate diverticular obstruction (e.g., seeds)
        (2) Surgical therapy for uncomplicated diverticulosis is **rare**
        (3) See Section C for management of GI hemorrhage
3. Diverticulitis
    a. Diverticular infxn and macroperforation resulting in inflammation
    b. Inflammation may be limited to the bowel, extend to pericolic tissues, form an abscess, or result in peritonitis
    c. Si/Sx
        (1) LLQ pain, diarrhea or constipation, fever, anorexia, and leukocytosis—**bleeding is more consistent with diverticulosis, not diverticulitis**
        (2) **Life-threatening complications from diverticulitis include large perforations, abscess or fistula formation, and obstruction**
        (3) Most common fistula associated with diverticular dz is **colovesicular** (presenting with recurrent UTIs, **and/or pneumaturia**)

d. Dx
  (1) CT scan may demonstrate edema of the bowel wall and the presence/location of formed abscesses
  (2) Barium enema and colonoscopy are generally contra-indicated for the acute pt, but if the pt's Sx point to obstruction or to presence of a fistula, a contrast enema is warranted
  (3) **Colonoscopy 4–6 wks after resolution of symptoms to exclude underlying neoplasm.**

e. Tx
  (1) Majority of pts respond to conservative Tx with IV hydration, antibiotics with coverage for Gram-negative rods and anaerobes, and NPO orders
  (2) Abscess requires CT- or Utz-guided percutaneous drainage
  (3) If pt experiences recurrent bouts after acute resolution, a sigmoid colectomy is usually considered on an elective basis
  (4) Perforation or obstruction → resection of affected bowel and construction of a temporary diverting colostomy and a Hartman pouch—reanastomosis performed 2–3 mos postoperatively. Alternatively, **sigmoid colectomy with colocolonic anastamosis with proximal loop ileostomy can be done.**

C. GI Hemorrhage

1. **Bright-red blood per rectum** (BRBPR) usually points to bleeding in the **distal small bowel or colon,** although a proximal bleeding site must be considered
2. Massive lower GI hemorrhage usually is caused by diverticular disease, angiodysplasia, ulcerative colitis, ischemic colitis, or solitary ulcer (Figure 2.11)
3. Chronic rectal bleed usually is because of hemorrhoids, fissures, CA, or polyps
4. Dx
   a. Digital rectal exam (DRE) and visualization with an anoscope and sigmoidoscope to locate and Tx obvious bleeding site
   b. Endoscopy to evaluate for an upper GI bleed
   c. Angiography if pt continues to bleed despite rule out upper GI source
   d. If bleeding is minimal/stopped or angiography is indeterminate and the pt is stable, the bowel should be prepped and colonoscopy performed
   e. Tagged RBC scan or barium enema if colonoscopy is non-Dx

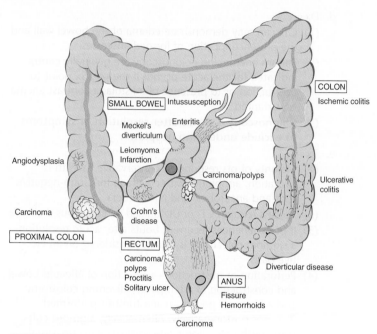

FIGURE 2.11

Lower GI bleeding.

5. Tx

    a. IV fluids and transfusions as needed to maintain hemodynamic stability

    b. Surgery is rarely required and should be considered only if bleeding persists (>90% of bleeding ceases spontaneously) despite intervention

D. **Large Intestine Obstruction**

    1. Accounts for 15% of obstructions—most common site is sigmoid colon

    2. Three most common causes are **adenoCA, scarring 2° to diverticulitis, and volvulus—consider adhesions if pt had previous abd surgery**

    3. Other causes are fecal impaction, inflammatory disorders, foreign bodies, and other benign tumors

    4. Si/Sx = abd distention, crampy abd pain, nausea/vomiting

    5. **X-ray → distended proximal colon, air–fluid levels, no gas in rectum**

6. Dx = clinical + X-ray, consider barium enema if X-rays are equivocal—**DO NOT GIVE BARIUM ORALLY WITH SUSPECTED OBSTRUCTION**

7. Tx = emergency laparotomy if cecal diameter >12 cm or for severe tenderness, peritonitis, sepsis, free air

8. Pseudo-obstruction (**Ogilvie's Syndrome**)

   a. Presence of massive right-sided colon dilatation with no evidence of obstruction

   b. Tx = colonoscopy and rectal tube for decompression

   c. **Consider Neostigmine (acetylcholinesterase inhibitor) to cause rapid bowel evacuation once a distal obstruction is ruled out and the patient has no hx of cardiac disease, will cause bradycardia so patient needs to be monitored when administered.**

E. **Volvulus**

   1. Rotation of the large intestine along its mesenteric axis—twisting can promote ischemic bowel, gangrene, and subsequent perforation

   2. Most common site is **sigmoid** (70%) followed by **cecum** (30%)

   3. **Commonly occurs in elderly individuals**

   4. Si/Sx = obstructive symptoms, including distention, tympany, rushes, and high-pitched bowel sounds

   5. Dx = clinical, confirmed by radiographic studies

      a. X-ray → dilated loops of bowel with loss of haustra with **a kidney bean appearance**

      b. Barium enema → a narrowing mimicking a **"bird's beak"** or **"ace of spades"** picture, with point of beak pointing to site of bowel rotation

   6. Tx

      a. Sigmoidoscopy or colonoscopy for decompression

      b. If not successful, laparotomy with a two-stage resection and anastomosis is necessary

      c. Cecal volvulus is treated with right hemicolectomy. Cecopexy (attachment of mobile cecum to peritoneal membrane) can be done but increased risk of recurrence

F. **Colon CA**

   1. Epidemiology

      a. Second leading cause of CA deaths

      b. Genetic influences include tumor suppressor and proto-oncogenes

c. **Obtain preoperative carcinoembryonic antigen (CEA) levels to follow disease, if the CEA is elevated, it should be negligible after resection allowing it to be followed postoperatively for recurrence of disease.**

d. Lynch syndromes I and II or hereditary nonpolyposis colorectal CA (HNPCC)

   (1) **Lynch syndrome I** is an autosomal dominant predisposition to colorectal CA with right-sided predominance (70% proximal to the splenic flexure)

   (2) **Lynch syndrome II** shows all of the features of Lynch syndrome I and also causes extracolonic CA, particularly endometrial CA, CA of the ovary, small bowel, stomach, and pancreas, and transitional cell CA of the ureter and renal pelvis

2. Screening

a. **Age >50 yrs without risk factors (strong family Hx, ulcerative colitis, etc.) → yearly stool occult blood tests, flexible sigmoidoscopy q3–5 yrs or colonoscopy q10 yrs or barium enema q5–10 yrs**

b. Colonoscopy/barium enema if polyps found

c. Pts with risk factors require more frequent and full colonoscopies

3. Dx

a. Endoscopy or barium enema—biopsy not essential

b. Obtain preoperative CEA to follow disease; these levels will be elevated before any physical evidence of disease

4. Surgical = resection and regional lymph node dissection

5. Adjuvant Tx for metastatic dz = **FOLFOX (5-fluorouracil + leucovorin or levamisole and oxaliplatin)—30% improvement in survival, bevacizumab (Avastin) can be added for distant disease**

6. Follow-Up

a. Hx, physical, and CEA level q3 mos for 3 yrs, then follow-up every 6 mos for 2 yrs

b. Colonoscopy at 6 mos, 12 mos, 3 yrs, and 5 yrs

c. CT and MRI for suspected recurrences

XVI. Rectum and Anus (Figure 2.11)

A. Hemorrhoids

1. Varicosity in the lower rectum or anus caused by congestion in the veins of the hemorrhoidal plexus

2. Si/Sx = anal mass, bleeding, itching, discomfort
3. Presence or absence of pain depends on the location of the hemorrhoid: internal hemorrhoid is generally not painful, whereas an external hemorrhoid can be extremely painful
4. **Thrombosed External Hemorrhoid**
   a. Not a true hemorrhoid, but subcutaneous external hemorrhoidal veins of the anal canal
   b. It is classically **painful**, tense, bluish elevation beneath the skin or anoderm
5. Hemorrhoids are classified by degrees
   a. 1° = no prolapse
   b. 2° = prolapse with defecation, but returns on its own
   c. 3° = prolapse with defecation or straining, require manual reduction
   d. 4° = not capable of being reduced
6. Dx = H&P inspection of the perianal area, DRE, anoscopy, and sigmoidoscopy
7. Tx = conservative therapy consists of a high-fiber diet, Sitz baths, stool-bulking agents, stool softeners, cortisone cream, astringent medicated pads
8. Definitive Tx = sclerotherapy, cryosurgery, rubber band ligation, and surgical hemorrhoidectomy

B. **Fistula-in-Ano**
1. Communication between the rectum to the perianal skin, usually 2° to anal crypt infxn
2. Infxn in the crypt forms abscess then ruptures and a fistulous tract is formed; can be seen in Crohn's disease
3. Si/Sx = intermittent or constant discharge, may exude pus, incontinence
4. Dx = physical exam
5. Tx = fistulotomy
6. Factors that predispose to maintenance of fistula patency = **FRIEND = F**oreign body, **R**adiation, **I**nfection, **E**pithelialization, **N**eoplasm, **D**istal obstruction

C. **Anal Fissure**
1. Epithelium in the anal canal denuded 2° to passage of irritating diarrhea and a tightening of the anal canal related to nervous tension
2. Si/Sx = **classic** presentation, a severely painful bowel movement associated with bright red bleeding

3. Dx = anoscopy under anesthesia.

4. **Surgical Pearl—90% of fissures are located in the posterior midline**

5. Tx = stool softeners, dietary modifications, and bulking agents, Botox type A, or nitroglycerin ointment

6. Surgical Tx = lateral internal sphincterotomy if pain is unbearable and fissure persists

D. Rectal CA

1. More common in males

2. Si/Sx = **rectal bleeding,** obstruction, altered bowel habits, and tenesmus

3. Dx = colonoscopy, sigmoidoscopy, biopsy, barium enema

4. Tx

   a. sphincter preserving surgery, neoadjuvant therapy has been shown to decrease the local recurrence rate and increase the number of tumors amenable to sphincter preserving surgery

   b. Neoadjuvant is appropriate for nodal positive or transmural involvement

   c. 5-Fluorouracil used to presensitize tumor cells before radiation administered

   d. Local recurrence rate for those treated with surgery alone is 30%–50%.

E. Anal CA

1. Most commonly squamous cell CA, others include transitional cell, adenoCA, melanoma, and mucoepidermal

2. Risk factors include fistulas, abscess, infxns, and Crohn's disease

3. Si/Sx = **anal bleeding,** pain, and mucus evacuation

4. Dx = biopsy

5. Tx = Nigro Protocol (5-fluorouracil, mitomycin, and radiation)— first-line therapy for all anal cancers except melanoma

XVII. Bariatric Surgery

1. Indications: National Institutes of Health (NIH)-recommended criteria for bariatric surgery:

   a. People who have a body mass index (BMI) of 40 or higher, or

   b. People with a BMI of 35 or higher with one or more related comorbid conditions.

2. Patients must undergo a 6-mo supervised medical weight loss program before consideration of surgery.

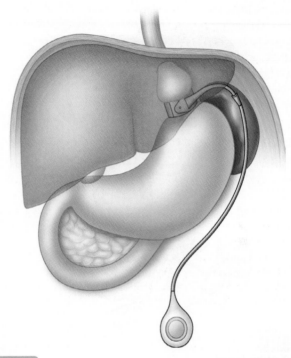

FIGURE 2.12

Lap band.

3. Types
   a. Lap Band (Figure 2.12)
      (1) Restrictive procedure, adjustable
      (2) Sixty percent excess weight loss at 10 years
      (3) Most serious complication associated with slippage or band erosion which needs surgical correction
   b. Roux-en-Y gastric bypass (Figure 2.13)
      (1) Restrictive and malabsorption
      (2) Seventy percent excess weight loss at 10 yrs
      (3) Associated with "dumping syndrome"
      (4) More vitamin and protein deficiency
      (5) Most serious short-term complication associated with leak (1%–2%), long-term stomal narrowing, gastrogastric fistula (1%–2%), and marginal ulcer (3%–10%)

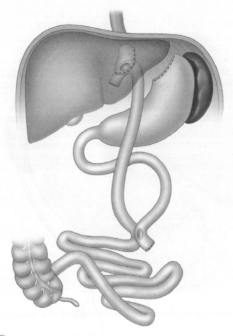

FIGURE 2.13
Roux-en-Y gastric bypass.

    c. Vertical Sleeve Gastrectomy (Figure 2.14)
      (1) Restrictive
      (2) Sixty to seventy percent excess weight loss at 2 yrs (long-term results pending)
      (3) Not associated with "dumping syndrome"
      (4) Often utilized for high risk or high BMI patients (BMI >60)
4. Potential Complications
    a. Pulmonary embolism is the leading cause of perioperative death (1%–2% of patients with up to 30% mortality)
    b. Nutritional Deficiencies
      (1) **Hyperparathyroidism**—due to hypocalcemia from bypass of the duodenum in gastric bypass patients (GBP). Need supplementation with calcium citrate and vitamin D.

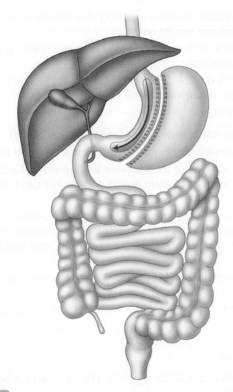

FIGURE 2.14

Vertical sleeve gastrectomy.

(2) **Iron**—also absorbed in the duodenum. Should be monitored and supplemented. Especially a problem in menstruating females.

(3) **Vitamin B12**—needs intrinsic factor from the gastric mucosa to be absorbed. The remaining gastric pouch may be too small for absorption. These patients may need parenteral administration of B12.

(4) **Zinc**—leads to acne, eczema, memory loss, lethargy, and hair loss.

XVIII. Breast

A. Mastalgia

1. Cyclical or noncyclical breast pain NOT because of lumps

2. Tx = danazol, works by inducing amenorrhea (side effects are hirsutism and weight gain)

3. Pain worse with respiration may be due to Tietze syndrome (costochondritis)

4. Mondor's disease = thoracoepigastric vein phlebitis → skin retraction along vein course

B. **Gynecomastia**

1. Enlargement of male breast (unilateral or bilateral)

2. Lobules not found in male breast as in the female breast

3. Occurs as result of an imbalance in estrogen and androgen hormones usually occurring during puberty but can occur in old age

4. Can also be seen in hyperestrogen states, such as liver cirrhosis or drug use that inhibits liver breakdown of estrogen, for example, alcohol, marijuana, heroin, and psychoactive drugs

5. Medication induced-cimetidine, spironolactone, antipsychotics, isoniazid, and digitalis

6. Seen in Klinefelter's syndrome and pts with a testicular neoplasm

C. **CA Risks**

1. Risk ↑ by

    a. Number one factor is gender (1% of breast CA occur in men)

    b. Age (number one factor in women)

    c. Young first menarche (<11 yrs)

    d. Old at first pregnancy (>30 yrs)

    e. Late menopause (>50 yrs)

    f. FHx

       (1) Ninety-five percent of CA are not familial

       (2) ↑ incidence in pt having a first-degree relative with history of breast CA

       (3) Autosomal dominant (not 100% penetrance) conditions with ↑ risk: breast cancer (BRCA)-1, BRCA-2, Li–Fraumeni syndrome, Cowden's disease, and Peutz–Jeghers

    g. Prior breast CA in opposite breast

2. Risk NOT ↑ by caffeine, sexual orientation

3. Risk NOT ↑ by fibroadenoma (FA) or fibrocystic disease

4. CA occurs most frequently in upper outer quadrant (tail of Spencer)

D. **Breast Tumors**

1. **FA** (Figure 2.15)

a. Most common tumor in teens and young women (peak in 20s)

b. Histology = myxoid stroma and curvilinear, slit ducts

c. FAs grow rapidly, no ↑ risk for developing CA

d. Tx NOT required, often will resorb within several weeks; reevaluation after 1 mo is standard

Algorithm 2.1

WORKUP OF A BREAST MASS

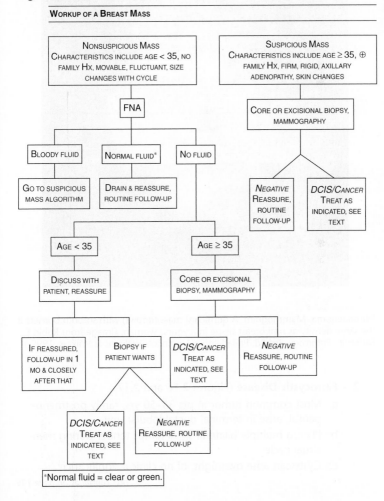

*Normal fluid = clear or green.

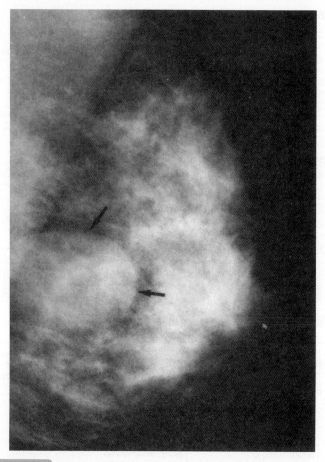

FIGURE 2.15

Fibroadenoma. Mammogram. A dominant mass (*arrows*) with smooth borders is the same density as nml breast tissue in a young woman. (Image from Rubin E, Farber JL. *Pathology,* 3rd Ed. Philadelphia: Lippincott Williams & Wilkins, 1999.)

2. **Fibrocystic Disease** (Figures 2.16 and 2.17)
   a. Most common tumor in pts 35–50 yrs, rarely postmenopausal, arise in terminal ductal lobular unit
   b. Pts c/o multiple bilateral small lumps tender during menstrual cycle
   c. Cysts can arise overnight, of no clinical significance

Text continues on page 195

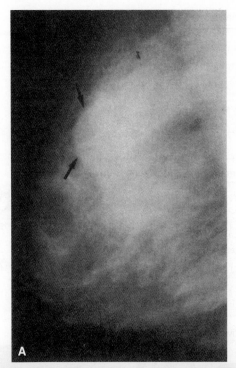

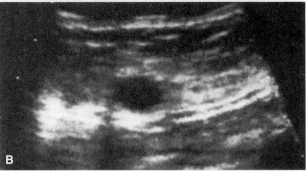

FIGURE 2.16

Fibrocystic breast disease. **A.** Mammogram showing oval, very well-defined mass without calcifications (*arrows*). **B.** The mass was shown to be cystic on Utz. (Both images from Rubin E, Farber JL. *Pathology,* 3rd Ed. Philadelphia: Lippincott Williams & Wilkins, 1999.)

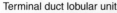
Terminal duct lobular unit

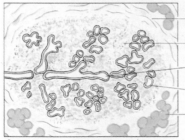

- Interlobular stroma
- Intralobular stroma
- Intralobular duct
- Terminal duct or acinus
- Fat

A Nonproliferative fibrocystic change

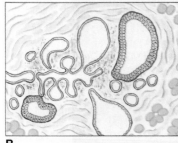

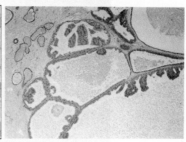

B Proliferative fibrocystic change

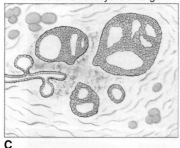

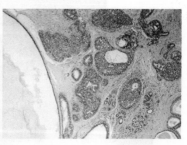

C

FIGURE 2.17

Histology of fibrocystic change. **A.** Nml terminal lobular unit. **B.** Nonproliferative fibrocystic change. This lesion combines cystic dilation of the terminal ducts with varying degrees of apocrine metaplasia of the epithelium and ↑ fibrous stroma. **C.** Proliferative fibrocystic change. Terminal duct dilation and intraductal epithelial hyperplasia are present. (From Rubin E, Gorstein F, Rubin R, et al. *Rubin's pathology: clinicopathologic foundations of medicine,* 4th Ed. Baltimore, MD: Lippincott Williams & Wilkins, 2005, with permission.)

d. Not associated with ↑ risk for CA, **unless biopsy specimen reveals epithelial (ductal or lobular) hyperplasia with atypia then a 4–5x increased risk of CA.**

e. Dx/Tx = fine-needle aspiration (FNA), drainage of fluid—if aspirated fluid is bloody, send for cytology to rule out cystic malignancy

3. **Fibrous Pseudo-Lump**

   a. Parenchymal atrophy in premenopausal breast

   b. Multiple nodules will be present

4. **Intraductal Papilloma**

   a. Often presents with serous/**bloody nipple discharge (guaiac-positive)**

   b. Will be solitary growth in perimenopause but can have multiple nodules if younger

   c. **Solitary papillomas do not ↑ CA risk, but multiple papillomas DO**

5. **Intraductal Hyperplasia**

   a. Dx by biopsy, >two-cell layers in ductal epithelium, either with or without atypia

   b. If atypia is present, ↑ risk for CA later developing in EITHER breast

   c. It is NOT premalignant, it is a MARKER for future malignancy, which will not be in the same place

6. **Ductal CA In Situ (DCIS)** (Figure 2.18)

   a. Usually nonpalpable, seen as irregularly shaped ductal calcifications on mammography

   b. Unless comedonecrosis is present, not be visibly detectable

   c. Comedonecrosis common in *her2/neu* + (*c-erbB-2*+) disease

   d. This is a true premalignancy; will lead to invasive ductal CA (IDC)

   e. Histology = haphazard cells along papillae (in contrast to hyperplasia, which is orderly), punched-out areas in ducts with "Roman bridge" pattern because of cells infiltrating open spaces

   f. Tx = excision of mass, ensure clean margins on excision (if not excise again with wider margins), and add postoperative radiation to reduce rate of recurrence

   g. **Hormonal therapy—In estrogen receptor positive patients, tamoxifen therapy for 5 years decreased the risk of recurrence of invasive or DCIS by half compared to women not treated with tamoxifen.**

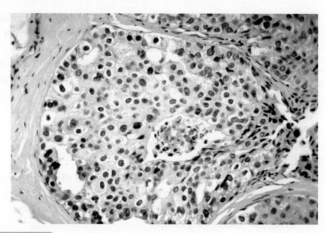

FIGURE 2.18

Ductal CA in situ, comedo-type. The terminal ducts are distended by CA in situ (intraductal CA). The centers of the tumor masses are necrotic and display dystrophic calcification. (From Rubin E, Gorstein F, Rubin R, et al. *Rubin's pathology: clinicopathologic foundations of medicine,* 4th Ed. Baltimore, MD: Lippincott Williams & Wilkins, 2005, with permission.)

7. **Lobular Carcinoma In Situ (LCIS)**

   a. Cannot be detected clinically or by gross examination; mammography is also a poor tool for diagnosing this disease

   b. It is NOT precancerous like DCIS is, but it IS a marker for future IDC risk in both breasts.

   c. Histology shows mucinous cells almost always present; "sawtooth" and clover-leaf configurations occur in the ducts

8. **IDC** (Figure 2.19)

   a. Most common breast CA, occurs commonly in mid-30s to late 50s, forms solid tumors

   b. Tumor size is the most important Px factor; node involvement is also an important Px factor

   c. Moderately differentiated IDC comes from cribriform or papillary intraductal originators

   d. Poorly differentiated IDC comes from intraductal comedo originator

   e. Forms solid tumor; many subtypes of this tumor exist (e.g., mucinous, medullary)

9. **Invasive Lobular CA**

   a. Only 3%–5% of invasive CA is lobular, present at age 45–56 yrs, vague appearance on mammogram

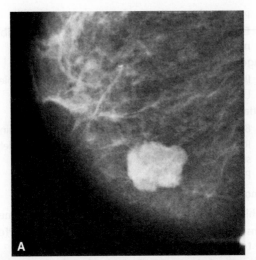

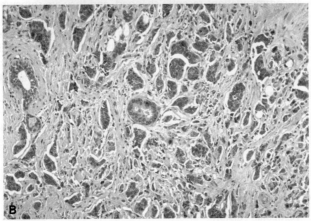

FIGURE 2.19

A. Mammogram of breast CA (note the irregular shape and borders of the growth). (Reprinted with permission from Mitchell GW. *The female breast and its disorders,* 1st Ed. Baltimore, MD: Williams & Wilkins, 1990.) **B.** Ductal CA. Invasive ductal CA. Irregular cords and nests of tumor cells, derived from the same cells that compose the intraductal component **(A)**, invade the stroma. Many of the cells form ductlike structures. (Image from Rubin E, Farber JL. *Pathology,* 3rd Ed. Philadelphia. PA: Lippincott Williams & Wilkins, 1999.)

   b. Pts have ↑ frequency of bilateral CA
   c. **Exhibits single file growth pattern within a fibrous stroma** (Figure 2.20)
10. **Paget Breast Disease (NOT BONE DISEASE!)**
    a. Presents with dermatitis/macular rash over nipple or areola
    b. Underlying ductal CA almost always present
11. **Inflammatory CA**
    a. Breast has classic Sx of inflammation: redness, pain, and heat
    b. Rapidly progressive breast CA, almost always widely metastatic at presentation
    c. Px poor

E. **Mammography**
   1. Highly effective screening tool in all but young women
   2. **Dense breast tissue found in young women interferes with the test's sensitivity and specificity**
   3. Recommendations recently changed, and they are somewhat controversial, with some organizations recommending annual screening and some recommending NO routine screening every 2 years screening between ages 40–49, and instead discussing risks and benefits with individual patients. American Cancer Society recommends yearly mammograms starting at age 40.
   4. Recommendations for age 50 and above vary from annual to every 2nd year mammograms.
   5. Additionally, high-risk women (family history, or genetic tendency) should be screened with an MRI in addition to mammogram.

XIX. Urology

A. **Scrotal Emergencies**
   1. Testicular Torsion
      a. Usually peripubertal pt
      b. Si/Sx = acute onset testicular pain and edema, nausea and vomiting, tender, swollen testicle with transverse lie, **absent cremasteric reflex on affected side**
      c. Dx = Doppler Utz to assess testicular artery flow
      d. Tx = emergent surgical decompression, with excision of testicle if it infarcts
   2. Epididymitis
      a. Si/Sx = unilateral testicular pain, dysuria, occasional urethral discharge, fever, leukocytosis in severe cases, painful and swollen epididymis

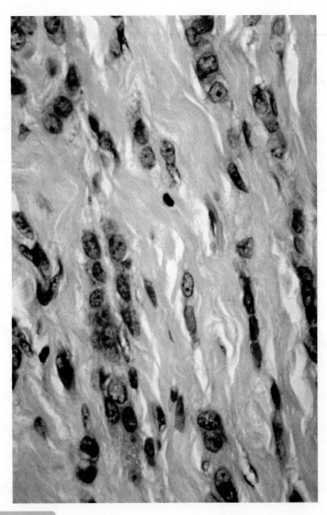

FIGURE 2.20

Invasive lobular CA. In contrast to invasive ductal CA, the cells of lobular CA tend to form single strands that invade between collagen fibers in a single pattern. The tumor cells are similar to those seen in lobular CA in situ. (From Rubin E, Gorstein F, Rubin R, et al. *Rubin's pathology: clinicopathologic foundations of medicine,* 4th Ed. Baltimore, MD: Lippincott Williams & Wilkins, 2005, with permission.)

    b. Dx = history and physical, labs → UA can be negative or show pyuria, urine Cx should be obtained, swab for *Neisseria gonorrhoeae* and *Chlamydia*

    c. Tx = antibiotics and NSAIDs

  3. Appendix Testis Torsion of Testicular Appendage

    a. Si/Sx = similar to testicular torsion, severe tenderness over superior pole of testicle, **"blue dot" sign** of ischemic appendage, nml position and lie, **cremasteric reflex present,** testicle and epididymis not tender

    b. Dx = Utz, perfusion confirmed with nuclear medicine scan

    c. Tx = supportive, should resolve in 2 wks

  4. Fournier's Gangrene

    a. Necrotizing fasciitis of the genital area

    b. Si/Sx = acute pruritus, rapidly progressing edema, erythema, tenderness, fever, chills, malaise, necrosis of skin and subcutaneous tissues, crepitus caused by gas-forming organisms

    c. Dx = history of diabetes mellitus, or immunocompromise, physical exam, labs → leukocytosis, positive blood and wound cultures (polymicrobial), X-ray → subcutaneous gas

    d. Tx emergently with wide surgical débridement and antibiotics

B. **Prostate CA**

  1. Si/Sx = advanced dz causes obstructive Sx, UTI, urinary retention; pts may also present with Sx due to metastases (bone pain, weight loss, and anemia), rock-hard nodule in prostate

  2. Dx = labs → anemia, azotemia, elevated serum acid phosphatase, and prostate-specific antigen (PSA)—note that use of these tests for screening is controversial because of relatively low sensitivity and specificity

  3. Transrectal Utz, CT scan, MRI, plain films for metastatic workup, biopsy to confirm Dx

  4. Bone scan helpful to detect bony metastases (Figure 2.21)

  5. Tx

    a. May not require Tx, most are indolent CA, but note that some are very aggressive and may warrant Tx depending on pt's wishes

    b. Modalities include finasteride, local irradiation, nerve sparing, or radical prostatectomy—risks of surgery include impotence and incontinence

    c. Aggressiveness of Tx depends on extent of disease and pt's age

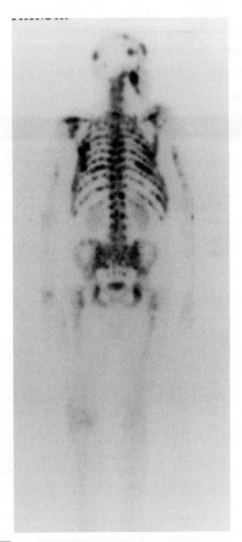

FIGURE 2.21

Bone scan showing multiple metastases secondary to prostatic CA. (From Crushieri A, Hennessy TPJ, Greenhalgh RM, et al. *Clinical surgery.* Oxford: Blackwell Science, 1996, with permission.)

XX. Neurosurgery

A. Head Injury

1. Intracranial Hemorrhage (Table 2.12; Figures 2.22 and 2.23)

Table 2.12	Intracranial Hemorrhage		
Type	**Bleeding Site**	**Characteristics**	**Treatment**
Epidural (Figure 2.22)	Middle meningeal artery	• **Dx = CT → biconcave disk not crossing sutures** • This is a medical emergency!	Evacuate hematoma via burr holes
Subdural (Figure 2.22)	Cortical bridging veins	• Causes = trauma, coagulopathy, common in elderly • Sx may start 1–2 wks after trauma • **Dx = CT → crescentic pattern extends across suture lines** • Px worse than epidural due to ↑ risk of concurrent brain injury	Evacuate hematoma via burr holes
Subarachnoid (Figure 2.23)	Circle of Willis, often at middle cerebral artery (MCA) branch	• Causes = arteriovenous malformation, berry aneurysm, trauma • Berry aneurysms → severe sudden headache, **CN III palsy**	Berry aneurysm = surgical excision or fill with metal coil
		• Cerebrospinal fluid (CSF) xanthochromia (also seen any time CSF protein>150 mg/dL or serum bilirubin >6 mg/dL) • Dx berry aneurysm with cerebral angiogram	Nimodipine to prevent vasospasm and result ant 2° infarcts
Parenchymal	Basal ganglia, internal capsule, thalamus	• Causes = hypertension, trauma, arteriovenous malformation, coagulopathy • CT/MRI → focal edema, hypodensity	↑ ICP → mannitol, hyperventilate, steroids and/ or ventricular shunt

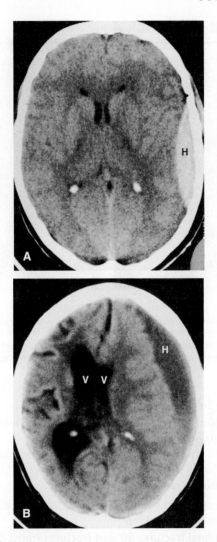

FIGURE 2.22

Extracerebral hematoma. **A.** CT scan showing a high-density lentiform area typical of an acute epidural hematoma (*H*). **B.** CT scan in another pt taken 1 mo after injury showing a subdural hematoma (*H*) as a low-density area. Note the substantial ventricular displacement. *V,* ventricle. (From Berg D. *Advanced clinical skills and physical diagnosis.* Oxford: Blackwell Science, 1999; Armstrong P, Wastie M. *Diagnostic imaging,* 4th Ed. Oxford: Blackwell Science, 1998, with permission.)

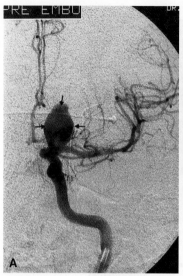 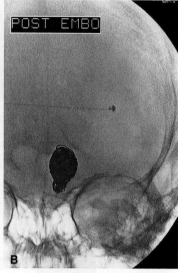

FIGURE 2.23

Aneurysm occlusion. **A.** Carotid angiogram showing a large aneurysm (*arrows*) arising at the termination of the internal carotid artery. **B.** Plain film after embolization of the aneurysm that is occluded with metal coils. (From Armstrong P, Wastie M. *Diagnostic imaging,* 4th Ed. Oxford: Blackwell Science, 1998, with permission.)

    2. General Treatment

        a. Establish ABCs, intubate, and ventilate unconscious pts

        b. Maintain cervical spine precautions

        c. ↑ ICP → mannitol, hyperventilate, steroids, and/or ventricular shunt

B. **Temporal Bone Fractures**

    1. Transverse fractures 20% of fractures, facial nerve injury, and loss of hearing more likely

    2. **Longitudinal fractures 80% of fractures (most common)**

    3. Dx by fine cut CT of temporal bone and audiogram

    4. IV antibiotics and ear drops if CSF leak noted

    5. Facial nerve decompression may be needed if facial nerve affected

C. **Basilar Skull Fractures**

    1. **Present with four classic physical findings: "raccoon eyes" and Battle's sign, hemotympanum, CSF rhinorrhea, and otorrhea**

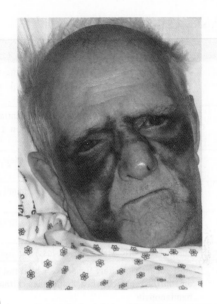

FIGURE 2.24

Raccoon eyes in basilar skull fracture.

2. "Raccoon eyes" are dark circles (bruising) about the eyes, signi-fying orbital fractures (Figure 2.24)
3. Battle's sign is ecchymoses over the mastoid process, indicating a fracture there
4. Dx = clinical + CT
5. Tx = supportive-HOB elevated, monitor ICP

D. **Tumors**

1. Si/Sx

   a. Headache awakening pt at night or is worse in morning after waking
   b. ↑ ICP → nausea/vomiting, **bradycardia with hypertension, Cheyne–Stokes respirations (Cushing's triad),** and papill-edema
   c. ⊕ Focal deficits, frequently of CN III → fixed, dilated pupil

2. DDx (Table 2.13)

3. Dx

   a. Bx → definitive Dx

Table 2.13 CNS Malignancy

Type	Characteristics
Metastatic	Small circular lesion, often multiple, at gray–white junction—**most common CNS neoplasm:** 1° = lung, breast, melanoma, renal cell, colon, thyroid
Glioblastoma multiforme	Large, irregular, ring enhancing due to central infarction (outgrows blood supply)—**most common 1° CNS neoplasm**
Meningioma	Second most common 1° CNS neoplasm, slow growing and benign
Retinoblastoma	Occurs in children, 60% sporadic, 40% familial (often bilateral)
Medulloblastoma	Found in cerebellum in floor of fourth ventricle, common in children
Craniopharyngioma	Compresses optic chiasm (visual loss) and hypothalamus
Prolactinoma	Most common pituitary tumor; Sx = **bilateral gynecomastia, amenorrhea, galactorrhea, impotence, bitemporal hemianopsia**
Lymphoma	Most common CNS tumor in AIDS pts (100× ↑ incidence), **MRI ring-enhancing lesion difficult to distinguish from toxoplasmosis**
Schwannoma	Usually affects CN VIII (acoustic neuroma) → tinnitus, deafness, ↑ ICP

b. Clinical suspicion + CT/MRI can diagnose lymphoma, pro-lactinoma, meningioma

c. Demographics important for retinoblastoma

4. Tx = excision for all 1° tumors except prolactinoma and lym-phoma

a. First-line Tx for prolactinoma = bromocriptine (D_2 agonist inhibits prolactin secretion); second line = surgery

b. Tx for lymphoma is radiation therapy, poor Px

c. Tx for metastases is generally radiation therapy and support

E. **Hydrocephalus**

1. Definition = ↑ CSF → enlarged ventricles

2. Si/Sx = ↑ ICP, ↓ cognition, headache, focal findings; in children, separation of cranial bones leads to grossly enlarged calvaria

3. **Dx made by finding dilated ventricles on CT/MRI** (Figure 2.25)

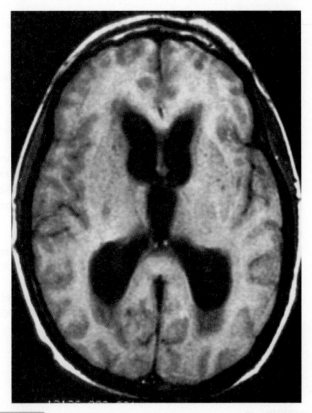

FIGURE 2.25

CT scan showing hydrocephalus. (From Cuschieri A, Thomas PJ, Henness RM, et al. *Clinical surgery.* Oxford: Blackwell Science, 1996, with permission.)

4. Lumbar puncture opening pressure and CT appearance are crucial to determine type of hydrocephalus

5. Nml ICP is always communicating

   a. Hydrocephalus ex vacuo

      (1) Ventricle dilation after neuron loss (e.g., stroke, CNS dz)

      (2) Sx due to neuron loss, not ventricular dilation in this case

      (3) Tx = none indicated

   b. Nml pressure hydrocephalus

      (1) **Si/Sx** = classic triad: bladder incontinence, dementia, ataxia ("wet, wacky, wobbly")

(2) Causes: 50% idiopathic, also meningitis, cerebral hemorrhage, trauma, atherosclerosis

(3) Because of ↓ CSF resorption across arachnoid villi

(4) Dx = clinically, or radionucleotide CSF studies

(5) Tx = diuretic therapy, repeated spinal taps, consider shunt placement

6. ↑ ICP can be communicating or noncommunicating

  a. Pseudotumor cerebri

   (1) Communicating spontaneous ↑ ICP

   (2) **Commonly seen in obese, young females;** can be idiopathic; massive quantities of vitamin A can cause it

   (3) **CT → no ventricle dilation (may even be shrunken)**

   (4) Tx = symptomatic (acetazolamide or surgical lumboperitoneal shunt); dz is typically self-limiting

  b. Noncommunicating

   (1) Because of block between ventricles and subarachnoid space → CSF outflow obstruction at fourth ventricle, foramina of Luschka/Magendie/Munro/Magnum

   (2) Causes = congenital (e.g., Arnold–Chiari syndrome), tumor effacing outflow path, or scarring 2° meningitis or subarachnoid hemorrhage

   (3) Dx = CT

   (4) Tx = treat underlying cause if possible

XXI. Vascular Diseases

A. Aneurysms

1. Abnormal dilation of an artery to **more than twice** its nml diameter

2. Most common cause is atherosclerosis

3. Common sites include abd aorta aneurysms (AAAs) and peripheral vessels including femoral and popliteal arteries

4. True aneurysms involve all three layers of the vessel wall— caused by atherosclerosis and congenital defects such as Marfan's syndrome

5. False aneurysms are "pulsatile hematomas" covered only by a thickened fibrous capsule (adventitia)—usually caused by traumatic disruption of the vessel wall or at an anastomotic site

6. Si/Sx = mostly aSx; however, pts can present with rupture, thrombosis, and embolization; some pts complain of referred back pain and/or epigastric discomfort

7. Rupture of AAA

   a. **Ruptured AAA is a surgical emergency,** and pt may present with **classic** abd pain, pulsatile abd mass, and hypotension

   b. The rate of rupture for a 5-cm diameter AAA is 6% per year; rate for 6-cm diameter AAA is 10% per year

   c. Pt's risk for rupture is ↑ by large diameter (Laplace's law), recent expansion, hypertension, and COPD; as a result, regular follow-up and control of hypertension are critical

8. Dx

   a. Palpation of a pulsatile mass in the abdomen on physical exam, confirmed with abd Utz or CT (Figures 2.26 and 2.27)

   b. CT or MRA are the best modalities to determine the size of the aneurysm in a stable pt

   c. Plain film of the abdomen may demonstrate a calcified wall

   d. Aortogram most definitive Dx, also reveals size and extent

9. Tx

   a. BP control, beta-blockade, and ↓ risk factors, or surgical intervention

   b. Surgical intervention usually involves placement of a synthetic graft within the dilated wall of the AAA; surgery is recommended for infrarenal or juxtarenal **aneurysms >5.5 cm** or growth spurt in diameter in a good surgical candidate

10. Complications

    a. Myocardial infarction (MI), renal failure (because of proximity of renal vasculature off of aorta), colonic ischemia (AAAs usually involve the inferior mesenteric artery [IMA])

    b. Be aware of formation of **aortoduodenal fistula** in pts who have had a synthetic graft placed for AAA disease and present with GI bleeding

11. **Peripheral aneurysms**

    a. Most commonly in the popliteal artery

    b. Dx-Duplex ultrasound, perform CTA or MRA to r/o contralateral aneurysm or AAA

    c. Fifty percent of popliteal aneurysms are bilateral, and 33% of pts with a popliteal aneurysm have an AAA.

    d. Si/Sx = rupture is rare, and pts usually present with thrombosis, embolization, or claudication

    e. Tx = surgical if pt is symptomatic or if >2 cm

B. **Aortic Dissection**

   1. Intimal tear through which blood can flow, creating a plane between the intima and remainder of vessel wall

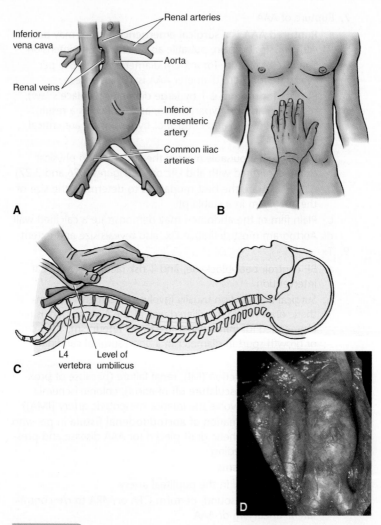

FIGURE 2.26

Pulsations of the aorta and AAA. (From Moore KL, Dalley AF II. *Clinical oriented anatomy,* 4th Ed. Baltimore, MD: Lippincott Williams & Wilkins, 1999.)

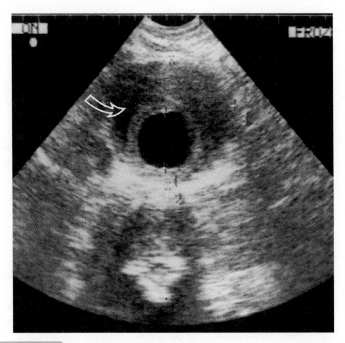

FIGURE 2.27

Abd aortic aneurysm. This is a transverse image of a large AAA with mural thrombus (*arrow*). The spine is well outlined posteriorly. (From Harwood-Nuss A, Wolfson AB, Linden CH, et al. *The clinical practice of emergency medicine,* 3rd Ed. Philadelphia, PA: Lippincott Williams & Wilkins, 2001.)

2. Usually confined to thoracic aorta (e.g., syphilis)

3. These planes can progress proximally and distally to disrupt blood supply to intestines, spinal cord, kidneys, and even the coronary vessels

4. In general, type A affects ascending aorta only; type B can affect both ascending and descending aorta

5. Si/Sx = **classic severe tearing (ripping) chest pain in hypertensive pts that radiates toward the back**

6. Dx = clinical, confirm with CT or aortogram, but if pt unstable take immediately to
OR

7. Tx

   a. Descending aortic dissection is usually medical (e.g., control of HTN and heart rate) unless life-threatening complications arise

b. In contrast, ascending dissection → immediate surgical intervention with graft placement

C. **Peripheral Vascular Disease (PVD)**

1. Caused by atherosclerotic dz in the lower extremities
2. Associated with cigarette smoking, diabetes mellitus, lipid abnormalities, hypertension, elevated levels of homocysteine, and elevated levels of C-reactive protein
3. Si/Sx = intermittent claudication, rest pain, ulceration, gangrene, reduced femoral, popliteal, and pedal pulses, dependent rubor, muscular atrophy, trophic changes, and skin blanching on foot elevation
4. Dry gangrene is the result of a chronic ischemic state and necrosis of tissue without signs of active infxn (Figure 2.28)
5. Wet gangrene is the superimposition of cellulitis and active infxn to necrotic tissue
6. Leriche Syndrome
   a. Aortoiliac disease → claudication in hip and gluteal muscles, impotence
   b. Five percent have limb loss at 5 yrs with rest pain (represents more severe ischemia); if not treated, almost 50% of pts will need amputation 2° to gangrene

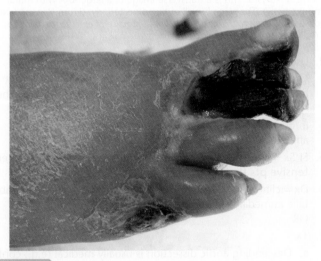

FIGURE 2.28

Dry gangrene of the toes. Image provided by Stedman's.

7. Dx
   a. Complete H&P, important to assess risk factors for athero-sclerosis and limitations of lifestyle from PVD
   b. Noninvasive testing includes but is not limited to measurement of the ankle–brachial index (ABI) and duplex examination
      (1) ABI is the ratio of BP in the ankle to the BP in the arm
      (2) Pts without disease have ABIs >1.0 given the higher absolute pressure in the ankle
      (3) Pts with severe occlusive disease (e.g., rest pain) gener-ally have indices <0.4; pts with claudication generally have indices <0.7
      (4) Exercise ABI most useful diagnostically; ABI may drop with exercise in a pt with PVD
      (5) Duplex (Utz) examination combines Utz and Doppler instruments, can provide information regarding blood flow velocity (related to stenosis), and display blood flow as a waveform: **nml waveform is triphasic, moderate occlusive disease waveform is biphasic, and severe disease waveform is monophasic**
      (6) Preoperative angiograms are classically done to confirm Dx and establish distal vessel runoff, or "road-map," vessels for the surgeon
      7. MRA and CTA may be used to supplement anatomic and physiologic data
8. Tx
   a. Lifestyle modifications include smoking cessation and increasing moderate exercise
   b. Pharmacotherapy is Cilostazol (vasodilator and platelet inhibitory properties) or second-line pentoxifylline
   c. Minimally invasive therapy includes percutaneous balloon angioplasty (PTA) and/or atherectomy—best results for iso-lated lesions of high-grade stenosis in the iliac and superior femoral arteries (SFA) vessels
   d. Treatment of iliac disease now involves PTA plus the place-ment of endoluminal stents
   e. Indications for surgical intervention are severe **rest pain, tissue necrosis, nonhealing infxn, and intractable claudication**
   f. Surgical treatment includes local endarterectomy with or without patch angioplasty and bypass procedures
   g. Results are better with autologous vein grafts; common operation for aortoiliac disease is the aortobifemoral bypass graft, whereas disease of the SFA is commonly treated with a femoral–popliteal bypass graft

9. Potential complication = **thrombosis,** must be addressed with thrombolytic agents, balloon thrombectomy, or graft revision

D. **Vessel Disease**

1. Varicose Veins

   a. Dilated, prominent tortuous superficial veins in the lower limbs

   b. Commonly seen in pregnancy (progesterone causes dilation of veins) and prolonged standing professions; may have an inherited predisposition

   c. Si/Sx = may be aSx or cause itching; may have dull aching and heaviness in legs, especially at day's end

   d. Dx = clinically

   e. Tx = support hose, elevate limbs, avoid prolonged standing; sclerotherapy or surgical ablation may be indicated

2. Venous Ulcers

   a. 2° to venous hypertension, DVT, or varicose veins; usually located on the medial ankle and calf

   b. Si/Sx = **painless ulcers,** large and shallow, contain bleeding granulation tissue (Figure 2.29)

   c. Phlegmasia alba dolens (milk leg)

      (1) Venous thrombosis usually occurring in postpartum women

      (2) Si/Sx = cool, pale, swollen leg with impalpable pulses

      (3) Tx = heparin and elevation

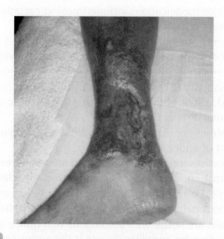

FIGURE 2.29

Venous stasis ulcer of the leg. (From Nettina SM. *The Lippincott manual of nursing practice,* 7th Ed. Philadelphia, PA: Lippincott Williams & Wilkins, 2001.)

   d. Phlegmasia cerulea dolens (venous gangrene)
      (1) Venous thrombosis with complete obstruction of arterial inflow
      (2) Si/Sx = sudden intense pain, massive edema, and cyanosis
      (3) Tx = heparin, elevation, venous thrombectomy if unresolved
   e. Dx = clinical, Doppler studies of extremities
   f. Tx = reduction of swelling by elevation, compression stockings, and Unna's boots (zinc oxide paste impregnated bandage); skin grafting is rarely indicated
3. Arterial Ulcers
   a. 2° to occlusive arterial disease
   b. Si/Sx = **painful in contrast to venous ulcers**, usually found on lower leg and lateral ankle, particularly on dorsum of the foot, toes, and heel, absent pulses, pallor, claudication, and may have "blue toes" (Figure 2.30)
   c. Dx = clinical, workup of PVD
   d. Tx = conservative management or bypass surgery

E. **Carotid Vascular Disease**
   1. Atherosclerotic plaques in carotid arteries (most commonly at carotid bifurcation)
   2. DDx of carotid insufficiency = trauma, anatomic kinking, fibromuscular dysplasia, and Takayasu's arteritis

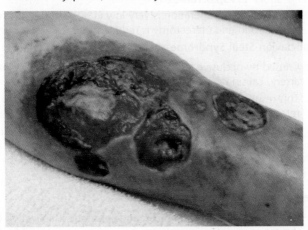

FIGURE 2.30

Arterial ulcer of the leg. (From Nettina SM. *The Lippincott manual of nursing practice,* 7th Ed. Philadelphia, PA: Lippincott Williams & Wilkins, 2001.)

3. Si/Sx = carotid bruit, transient ischemic attacks (TIAs; neurologic changes that reverse in <24 hrs), amaurosis fugax (transient monocular blindness), reversible ischemic neurologic deficits (lasting up to 3 days with no permanent changes), and cerebrovascular accidents (CVAs) that result in permanent neurologic changes

4. Dx = angiography; however, duplex scanning is noninvasive, can determine location and percent stenosis, and assess plaque characteristics (e.g., soft versus calcified)

5. Tx = modification of risk factors important, anticoagulation, and use of antiplatelet agents (aspirin, dipyridamole) intended to prevent thrombosis

6. Surgical therapy is carotid endarterectomy; pts usually placed on postoperative aspirin therapy

7. **Surgical Indications**
   a. **Symptomatic pt**
      (1) Carotid stenosis >70%
      (2) Multiple TIAs (risk of stroke 10% per year)
      (3) Pts who have experienced a CVA and have lesion amenable to surgery (stroke recurrence as high as 50% without surgery)
   b. In an **aSx pt** endarterectomy is controversial, but stenosis >75% is an accepted indication (AHA Consensus Statement, *Stroke* 1995;26:188–201)

8. Mortality rate of operation is very low (1%), and risk of stroke after carotid endarterectomy is reduced to 0.5%–2%

F. **Subclavian Steal Syndrome**

1. Caused by occlusive lesion in subclavian artery or innominate artery, causing ↓ blood flow distal to the obstruction

2. This results in the "stealing" of blood from vertebral artery via retrograde flow

3. Si/Sx = arm claudication, syncope, vertigo, nausea, confusion, and supraclavicular bruits

4. Dx = angiogram, Doppler, MRI

5. Tx = **carotid–subclavian bypass**

G. **Renovascular Hypertension**

1. Caused by renal artery stenosis and subsequent activation of the renin–angiotensin pathway

2. Commonly because of atherosclerotic lesions

3. Can also be 2° to fibromuscular dysplasia, subintimal dissections, and hypoplasia of renal artery

4. Si/Sx = most pts are aSx; some present with headache, abd bruits, or cardiac, cerebrovascular, or renal dysfunction related to hypertension; sudden onset of hypertension is more consistent with a dysplastic process when compared with the slower evolving atherosclerosis

5. Surgically correctable HTN = **renal artery stenosis (most common),** pheochromocytoma, unilateral renal parenchymal disease, Cushing's syndrome, primary hyperaldosteronism, hyperthyroidism, hyperparathyroidism, coarctation of the aorta, CA, and ↑ ICP

6. Dx = CTA, or MRA, definitive Dx (gold standard) obtained by **angiography (string of beads appearance);** others include IV pyelogram (IVP), renal duplex ultrasonography, and renal/vein renin ratio (Captopril test).

7. Tx = BP control and consider balloon catheter dilation of stenosis—results better with fibromuscular dysplasia versus atherosclerotic lesions; surgical correction involves endarterectomy, bypass, or resection

H. **Mesenteric Ischemia**

1. **Chronic Intestinal Ischemia**

   a. 2° to atherosclerotic lesions of at least two of the three major vessels supplying the bowel

   b. Si/Sx = **weight loss, postprandial pain, and abd bruit**

   c. Dx = definitive diagnosis is made with aortogram CTA or MRA are also useful.

   d. Tx = Percutaneous endovascular treatment (angioplasty or stenting) may be considered, surgical intervention (endarterectomy, bypass from aorta to involved graft) is **indicated** in absence of malignancy (particularly pancreatic CA must be ruled out)

2. **Acute Intestinal Ischemia**

   a. Acute thrombosis of a mesenteric vessel secondary to atherosclerotic changes or emboli from the heart

   b. Si/Sx = rapid onset of pain that is out of proportion to exam, vomiting, diarrhea, and history of heart condition predisposing to emboli formation (e.g., atrial fibrillation)

   c. Dx = angiogram should be performed immediately to confirm or rule out diagnosis

   d. Tx = surgical treatment of acute obstructive intestinal ischemia includes revascularization, resection of necrotic bowel, and when appropriate a "second look" operation 24–48 hrs after revascularization

3. OBSTETRICS AND GYNECOLOGY

I. Obstetrics

A. Terminology

1. Gravidity—total number of pregnancies
2. Parity—number of pregnancies carried to viability—can also express parity as four numbers: term pregnancies, preterm, abortions, and living children (TPAL)
3. Term delivery—delivery of infant after 37 wks of gestation
4. Premature delivery—delivery of infant weighing between 500 and 2,500 g and delivery between 20 and 37 wks

B. Prenatal Care

1. The First Visit

    a. Pregnancy Dx

    (1) Si/Sx = amenorrhea, ↑ urinary frequency, breast engorgement and tenderness, nausea, fatigue, bluish discoloration of vagina due to vascular congestion (Chadwick's sign), and softening of cervix (Hegar's sign)

    (2) Pregnancy test

        (a) Detects human chorionic gonadotropin (hCG) or its β-subunit

        (b) Rapidly dividing fertilized egg produces hCG even before implantation occurs

        (c) Commercial kits detect pregnancy 12–15 days after conception

        (d) Home tests have low false-positive rate but high false-negative rate

    (3) Utz

        (a) Gestational sac identified at 5 wk, fetal image detected by 6–7 wks, cardiac activity first noted at 8 wk

        (b) In first trimester, Utz is most accurate method to determine gestational age

    b. Obstetrical Hx

    (1) Duration of previous gestations and mode of delivery (e.g., nml spontaneous vaginal delivery versus cesarean section [C-section] versus vacuum assisted)

(2) Duration of labor, maternal, postpartum, and neonatal complications, newborn weight, newborn sex

c. Menstrual Hx including last menstrual period (LMP), regularity of cycles, age at menarche

d. Contraceptive Hx (important for risk assessment, oral contraceptive pills [OCPs] have been associated with birth defects)

e. Medical Hx

   (1) Medicines; consider potential teratogens (Tables 3.1 and 3.2)

   (2) FHx, social Hx including tobacco, ethanol, drug use, type of work, exposure to animals

   (3) Diabetes and HTN

f. Estimated date of confinement (EDC)

   (1) **Nägele's rule = LMP + 7 days − 3 mo + 1 yr,** e.g., if LMP began 05/20/2007, delivery due 02/27/2008

   (2) This calculation depends on regular 28-day cycles (only 20%–25% of women), adjustments must be made for longer or shorter cycles

g. Complete physical exam with pelvic examination including Papanicolaou (Pap) smear, cultures for *Neisseria gonorrhea* and *Chlamydia,* and estimation of uterine size

h. Labs include CBC, blood type with Rh status, urinalysis with culture, RPR test for syphilis, rubella titer, tuberculosis (TB) skin testing, can offer HIV antibody test

Table 3.1 Teratogens

Drug	Birth Defect
Lithium	Ebstein's anomaly (single-chambered right side of heart)
Carbamazepine, valproate	Neural tube defects
Retinoic acid	CNS defects, craniofacial defects, cardiovascular effects
Angiotensin-converting enzyme inhibitor	Renal failure in neonates, renal tubule dysgenesis, ↓ skull ossification
Oral hypoglycemic	Neonatal hypoglycemia
Warfarin (Coumadin)	Skeletal and CNS defects
NSAIDs	Constriction of ductus arteriosus, necrotizing enterocolitis
Thalidomide	Phocomelia—underdevelopment of limbs, face, ears, and vessels

Table 3.2 US Food and Drug Administration Drug Categories

Category	Description
A	Medication has not shown ↑ risk for birth defects in human studies.
B	Animal studies have not demonstrated a risk, and there are no adequate studies in humans, OR animal studies have shown a risk, but the risk has not been seen in humans
C	Animal studies have shown adverse effects, but no studies are available in humans, OR studies in humans and animals are not available
D	Medications are associated with birth defects in humans; however, potential benefits in rare cases may outweigh their known risks
X	Medications are contraindicated (should not be used) in human pregnancy because of known fetal abnormalities that have been demonstrated in both human and animal studies

    i. If pt is not already immune to rubella, do NOT vaccinate, as the vaccine is live virus

    j. Genetic testing as indicated by Hx (e.g., hemoglobin electrophoresis in African-American pt to determine sickle cell anemia likelihood)

    k. Recommend 25- to 35-lb weight gain during pregnancy

    l. Consider folate, iron, and multivitamin supplements

2. First-Trimester Visits (1–12 wks)

    a. Visit every 4 wks

    b. Assess weight gain/loss, BP, pedal edema, fundal height, urine dip for glucosuria and proteinuria (**trace glucosuria is nml because of ↑ glomerular filtration rate (GFR), but anything more than trace protein should be evaluated**)

    c. Estimation of gestational age by uterine size (Table 3.3)

       (1) Nml uterus is $3 \times 4 \times 7$ cm

       (2) Gravid uterus begins to enlarge and soften by 5–6 wks

Table 3.3 Height of Uterus by Gestational Week

12 wk	16 wk	20 wk	20–36 wk
At pubic symphysis	Midway from symphysis to umbilicus	At umbilicus	Height (cm) correlates with weeks of gestation[a]

[a]If uterine size (cm) > gestational age (wk) by >3 wks, consider multiple gestations, molar pregnancy, or MOST COMMONLY inaccurate dating.

    d. All pregnant women, regardless of age, should undergo first-trimester screening for Down's syndrome

       (1) Screen with combination of Utz and blood tests

       (2) Utz test is for nuchal translucency (NT), which measures the thickness at the back of the neck of the fetus

       (3) Blood tests include the standard triple-marker screen, including alpha-fetoprotein (AFP), βhCG, and estriol

          (a) AFP is ↓ in Down's syndrome, and ↑ in multiple gestational pregnancies and neural tube defects

          (b) Estriol is also ↓ in Down's syndrome

          (c) βHCG is ↑ in Down's syndrome

          (d) The triple-marker test detects ~70% of cases of Down's syndrome, with a ~5% false positive rate

       (4) Newer test, inhibin, is also ↑ in Down's syndrome, and adding it to the triple-marker test ↑ detection of Down's syndrome to 80% (*Obstetrics & Gynecology* 2005;106:260–67)

       (5) Adding the PAPP-A blood test ↑ detection to >85% (*NEJM* 2005;353:2001–2011)

3. Second-Trimester Visits (13–28 wks)

    a. Continue every 4 wks

    b. After 12 wks, use Doppler Utz to evaluate fetal heartbeat at each visit

    c. At 17–19 wks (quickening) and beyond, document fetal movement

    d. Amniocentesis for higher-risk mothers >35 yrs old or if Hx indicates (e.g., recurrent miscarriages, previous child with chromosomal or single gene defect, abnormal triple-marker or quadruple-marker screening test)

    e. Glucose screening at 24 wk (1-hr Glucola)

    f. Repeat hematocrit at 25–28 wk

4. Third-Trimester Visits (29–40 wks)

    a. Every 4 wks until wk 32, every 2 wks from wks 32–36, every wk until delivery

    b. Inquire about preterm labor (PTL) Sx: **vaginal bleeding, contractions, rupture of membranes (ROM)**

    c. Inquire about pregnancy-induced hypertension (PIH) (discussed further in Section I.D.3)

    d. Screen for *Streptococcus agalactiae* (**Group B *Streptococcus* [GBS]**) at 35–37 wks

    e. RhoGAM at 28–30 wks if indicated (discussed further in Section I.E.5.h)

OBSTETRICS AND GYNECOLOGY

C. Physiologic Changes in Pregnancy
   1. Hematologic
      a. Pregnancy is a **hypercoagulable** state
         (1) ↑ Clotting factor levels
         (2) Venous stasis due to uterine pressure on lower-extremity great veins
      b. Anemia of pregnancy
         (1) Plasma volume ↑ approximately 50% from wk 6 to wks 30–34
         (2) Red cell mass ↑ later and to a smaller degree, causing a relative anemia of approximately 15% due to dilution
      c. Slight leukocytosis due to granulocyte demargination
      d. Platelets ↓ slightly but remain within nml limits
   2. Cardiac
      a. Cardiac output ↑ 50% (↑ in both heart rate and stroke volume)
      b. Because of ↑ flow, ↑ S_2 split with inspiration, distended neck veins, systolic ejection murmur, and S_3 gallop are nml findings
      c. **Diastolic murmurs are not nml findings in pregnancy**
      d. ↓ Peripheral vascular resistance due to progesterone-mediated smooth muscle relaxation
      e. BP ↓ during first 24 wks of pregnancy with gradual return to nonpregnant levels by term
   3. Pulmonary
      a. Nasal stuffiness and ↑ nasal secretions due to mucosal hyperemia
      b. 4-cm elevation of diaphragm due to expanding uterus
      c. Tidal volume and minute ventilation ↑ 30%–40% (progesterone mediated)
      d. Functional residual capacity and residual volume ↓ 20%
      e. Hyperventilation →↑ PO_2, ↓ PCO_2—this allows the fetal PCO_2 to remain near 40 and still be able to give off CO_2 to maternal blood (sets up a CO_2 concentration gradient across maternal–fetal circulation and PO_2 gradient allowing maternal to fetal O_2 transfer)
      f. Respiratory rate, vital capacity, and inspiratory reserve do not change, total lung capacity ↓ approximately 5%
   4. GI
      a. ↓ GI motility due to progesterone
      b. ↓ Esophageal sphincter tone → gastric reflux also due to progesterone

    c. ↑ Alkaline phosphatase

    d. Hemorrhoids due to constipation and ↑ venous pressure due to enlarging uterus compressing inferior vena cava

5. Renal

    a. ↓ Bladder tone due to progesterone predisposes pregnant women to urinary stasis and urinary tract infxns (UTIs)/pyelonephritis

    b. GFR ↑ 50%

      (1) ↑ GFR → glucose excretion occurs in nearly all pregnant women

      (2) Thus urine dipsticks are not useful in managing pts with diabetes

      (3) However, there should be no significant ↑ in protein loss

    c. Serum creatinine and blood urea nitrogen ↓

6. Endocrine

    a. ↓ Fasting blood glucose in mother due to fetal utilization

    b. ↑ Postprandial glucose in mother due to ↑ insulin resistance

    c. Fetus produces its own insulin starting at 9–11 wks

    d. ↑ Maternal thyroid-bonding globulin (TBG) due to ↑ estrogen, ↑ total T_3 and T_4 due to ↑ TBG

    e. Free T_3 and T_4 remain the same so pregnant women are euthyroid

    f. ↑ Cortisol and cortisol-binding globulin

7. Skin

    a. Nml skin changes in pregnancy mimic liver dz due to ↑ estrogen

    b. Can see spider angiomas, palmar erythema

    c. Hyperpigmentation occurs from ↑ estrogen and melanocyte-stimulating hormone; affects umbilicus, perineum, face (chloasma), and linea (nigra)

D. Medical Conditions in Pregnancy

1. Gestational Diabetes Mellitus (GDM)

    a. GDM—glucose intolerance or DM first recognized during pregnancy

    b. **Number one medical complication of pregnancy, occurs in 2% of pregnancies**

    c. GDM risk factors: previous Hx of GDM, maternal age ≥30 yrs, obesity, FHx of DM, previous Hx of infant weighing 4,000 g at birth, Hx of repeated spontaneous abortions or unexplained stillbirths

d. GDM caused by placental-released hormone, human placental lactogen (HPL), which antagonizes insulin

e. GDM worsens as pregnancy progresses because ↑ amounts of HPL are produced as placenta enlarges

f. Maternal complications = hyperglycemia, ketoacidosis, ↑ risk of UTIs, **2-fold ↑ in PIH**, retinopathy (can occur very quickly and dramatically)

g. Fetal complications

   (1) Macrosomia (≥4,500 g), neonatal hypoglycemia due to abrupt separation from maternal supply of glucose, hyperbilirubinemia, polycythemia, polyhydramnios (amniotic fluid volume ≥2,000 mL)

   (2) **Abruption and PTL** due to ↑ uterine size and postpartum uterine atony, **3- to 4-fold ↑ in congenital anomalies** (often cardiac and limb deformities), spontaneous abortion, and respiratory distress

h. Dx = 1-hr Glucola screening test at 24–28 wks or at the onset of prenatal care in pt with known risk factors; confirm with 3-hr glucose tolerance test

i. Tx = strict glucose control, which significantly ↓ complications

   (1) Insulin is not required if the pt can adhere to a proper diet

   (2) **Oral hypoglycemics are contraindicated** because they cross the placenta and can result in fetal and neonatal hypoglycemia

   OB Pearl—White Classification of Diabetes Class A₁: gestational diabetes, diet controlled; and Class A₂: gestational diabetes, insulin controlled

j. Delivery

   (1) Route of delivery determined by estimated fetal weight

   (2) If 4,500 g, consider C-section; if 5,000 g, C-section recommended

   (3) Postpartum 95% of GDM pts return to nml glucose levels

   (4) Glucose tolerance screening recommended 2–4 mo postpartum to pick up those few women who will remain diabetic and require Tx

2. Thromboembolic Dz

   a. Incidence during pregnancy is 1%–2%, usually occurs postpartum (80%)

b. Si/Sx for superficial thrombophlebitis = swelling, tenderness, erythema, warmth (four cardinal signs of inflammation), may be a palpable cord

c. Deep venous thrombosis (DVT) occurs postpartum due to spread of uterine infxn to ovarian veins

d. Si/Sx of DVT = persistent fever, uterine tenderness, palpable mass, but often aSx

e. Dx
   (1) Doppler Utz is first line, sensitivity and specificity >90%
   (2) Gold standard is venography, but this is invasive

f. Tx
   (1) Superficial thrombophlebitis → leg elevation, rest, heat, NSAIDs
   (2) DVT → heparin to maintain partial thromboplastin time (PTT) 1.5–2.5 × baseline
   (3) **Warfarin (Coumadin) contraindicated in pregnancy** because it crosses the placenta, is teratogenic early, and causes fetal bleeding later

g. Px
   (1) 25% of untreated DVT progress to pulmonary embolism (PE)
   (2) Anticoagulation ↓ progression to 5%
   (3) PEs in pregnancy are treated identically to DVT

3. PIH
   a. Epidemiology
      (1) Develops in 5%–10% of pregnancies, 30% of multiple gestations
      (2) Causes 15% of maternal deaths
      (3) Risk factors = nulliparity, age >40 yrs, FHx of PIH, chronic HTN, chronic renal dz, diabetes, twin gestation
   b. Types (Table 3.4)
   c. Other Si/Sx seen in preeclampsia or eclampsia
      (1) Pts have rapid weight gain (2° to edema)
      (2) Peripheral lower-extremity edema is common in pregnancy; however, persistent edema unresponsive to rest and leg elevation or edema involving the upper extremities or face is not nml
      (3) Hyperreflexia and clonus are noted
   d. Tx
      (1) Only cure for PIH is delivery of the baby; decision to deliver depends on severity of preeclampsia and maturity of fetus

Table 3.4 Types of Pregnancy-Induced Hypertension

Dz	Characteristics
Preeclampsia	• HTN (>140/90 or ↑ SBP >30 mm Hg or DBP >15 mm Hg compared to previous) • New-onset proteinuria and/or edema • Generally occurring at ≥20 wk
Severe preeclampsia	• SBP >160 mm Hg or DBP >110 mm Hg • Marked proteinuria (>1 g/24-hr collection or >11 on dip), oliguria, ↑ creatinine • CNS disturbances (e.g., headaches or scotomata) • Pulmonary edema or cyanosis • Epigastric or right upper quadrant pain, hepatic dysfunction
Eclampsia	• **Convulsions** in a woman with preeclampsia • 25% occur before labor, 50% during labor, and 25% in first 72 hr postpartum

DBP, diastolic blood pressure; SBP, systolic blood pressure.

   (2) Mild pre-eclampsia + immature fetus → bed rest, prefer-
       ably in left lateral decubitus position to maximize blood
       flow to uterus; close monitoring; tell pt to return to ER
       if preeclampsia worsens
   (3) Severe preeclampsia/eclampsia → delivery when pos-
       sible, magnesium sulfate to prevent seizure, antihyper-
       tensives to maintain BP <140/100
  e. Complication of severe PIH = HELLP syndrome
   (1) **HELLP** = **H**emolysis, **E**levated **L**iver enzymes, **L**ow
       Platelets
   (2) Occurs in 5%–10% of women with severe preeclampsia
       or eclampsia, more frequently in multiparous, older pts
   (3) Tx = delivery (the only cure), transfuse blood, platelets,
       fresh-frozen plasma as needed, IV fluids and pressors as
       needed to maintain BP
4. Cardiac Dz
  a. Pts with congenital heart dz have ↑ risk (1%–5%) of having
     a fetus with a congenital heart dz
  b. Pts with pulmonary HTN and ↑ right-sided pressures (e.g.,
     Eisenmenger's complex) have poor Px with pregnancy
  c. Tx of preexisting cardiac dz = supportive, e.g., preven-
     tion and/or prompt correction of anemia, aggressive Tx of
     infxns, ↓ physical activity/strenuous work, adherence to a
     low-sodium diet, and proper weight gain

d. Peripartum cardiomyopathy
   (1) Rare but severe pregnancy-associated condition
   (2) Occurs in last mo of pregnancy or first 6 mo postpartum
   (3) Risk factors = African-American, multiparous, age >30 yrs, twin gestation, or preeclampsia
   (4) Tx = bed rest, digoxin, diuretics, possible anticoagulation, consider post-delivery heart transplant especially in those whose cardiomegaly has not resolved 6 mos after Dx

5. Group B Streptococcus (GBS = *Streptococcus agalactiae*)
   a. aSx cervical colonization occurs in up to 30% of women
   b. 50% of infants become colonized, clinical infxn in <1%
   c. Intrapartum prophylaxis with penicillin is reserved for the following situations:
      (1) PTL (<37 wks) or prolonged ROM (>18 hrs) or fever in labor regardless of colonization status
      (2) Women identified as colonized with GBS through screening at 35–37 wks of gestation
      (3) Women with GBS bacteriuria or with previous infant with GBS dz
      (4) Pts with severe PCN allergies may consider clindamycin or erythromycin if no GBS resistance noted
      (5) Broader spectrum antibiotics may be needed if chorioamnionitis occurs

6. Hyperemesis Gravidarum
   a. ↑ nausea and vomiting that, unlike "morning sickness," persists past wk 16 of pregnancy
   b. Causes = ↑ hCG levels, thyroid, or GI hormones
   c. Si/Sx = excessive vomiting, dehydration, hypochloremic metabolic alkalosis
   d. Dx = clinical, rule out other cause
   e. Tx = fluids, electrolyte repletion, antiemetics (IV, IM, or suppositories)
   f. Some pts require feeding tubes and parenteral nutrition

E. Fetal Assessment and Intrapartum Surveillance
   1. Fetal Growth
      a. Measure by fundal height; if 2-cm deviation from expected fundal height during wks 18–36 → repeat measurement and/or Utz
      b. Utz is most reliable tool for assessing fetal growth

    c. In early pregnancy, measurement of gestational sac and crown–rump length correlate very well with gestational age

    d. Later in pregnancy, four measurements are done because of wide deviation in nml range: biparietal diameter of skull, abd circumference, femur length, and cerebellar diameter

2. Fetal Well-Being

    a. ≥4 fetal movements per hour generally indicate fetal well-being

    b. Nonstress test (NST)

        (1) Measures response of fetal heart rate (FHR) to movement

        (2) Nml (i.e., reactive) NST occurs when FHR ↑ by 15 bpm for 15 sec following fetal movement

        (3) Two such accelerations within 20 min are considered nml

        (4) Nonreactive NST → further assessment of fetal well-being

        (5) Test has a high false-positive rate (test suggests fetus is in trouble, but fetus actually is healthy), so the result must be interpreted in the context of other tests and often is repeated within 24 hrs to verify results

    c. Biophysical profile

        (1) Measures of fetal well-being, each rated on a scale from 0–2

            (a) Fetal breathing → ≥1 fetal breathing movement in 30 min lasting at least 30 sec

            (b) Gross body movement → ≥3 discrete movements in 30 min

            (c) Fetal tone → ≥1 episode of extension with return to flexion of fetal limbs/trunk OR opening/closing of hand

            (d) Qualitative amniotic fluid volume → ≥1 pocket of amniotic fluid at least 1 cm in two perpendicular planes

            (e) Reactive FHR → reactive NST

        (2) Final score of 8–10 is nml, score of 6 is equivocal and requires further evaluation, score of ≤4 is abnormal and usually requires immediate intervention

3. Tests of Fetal Maturity

    a. Respiratory system is last fetal system to mature, so decisions regarding when to deliver a premature infant often depend on tests that assess the maturity of this system

b. Phospholipid production (collectively known as "surfactant") remains low until 32–33 wks of gestation, but this is highly variable

c. Lack of surfactant → neonatal respiratory distress syndrome (RDS)

d. Phospholipids enter amniotic fluid from fetal breathing and are obtained by amniocentesis and tested for maturity

e. Tests for fetal maturity
   (1) Lecithin/sphingomyelin (L:S) ratio
      (a) Lecithin is major phospholipid found in surfactant and ↑ as fetal lungs become mature
      (b) Sphingomyelin production remains constant throughout pregnancy
      (c) Ratio >2.0 is considered mature
   (2) Phosphatidylglycerol appears late in pregnancy; its presence generally indicates maturity

4. Intrapartum Fetal Assessment
   a. Causes of nonreassuring fetal status
      (1) Uteroplacental insufficiency
         (a) Placenta impaired or unable to provide oxygen and nutrients while removing products of metabolism and waste
         (b) Causes = placenta previa or abruption, placental edema from hydrops fetalis or Rh isoimmunization, postterm pregnancy, intrauterine growth retardation (IUGR), uterine hyperstimulation
         (c) Fetal response to hypoxia → shunting of blood to brain, heart, and adrenal glands
         (d) If unrecognized, can progress to metabolic acidosis with accumulation of lactic acid and damage to vital organs
      (2) Umbilical cord compression due to oligohydramnios, cord prolapse or knot, anomalous cord, or abnormal cord insertion
      (3) Fetal anomalies include IUGR, prematurity, postterm, sepsis, congenital anomalies
   b. FHR monitoring
      (1) Nml FHR is 120–160 bpm
      (2) Tachycardia = FHR >160 bpm for ≥10 min
         (a) Most common cause is maternal fever (which may signal chorioamnionitis)

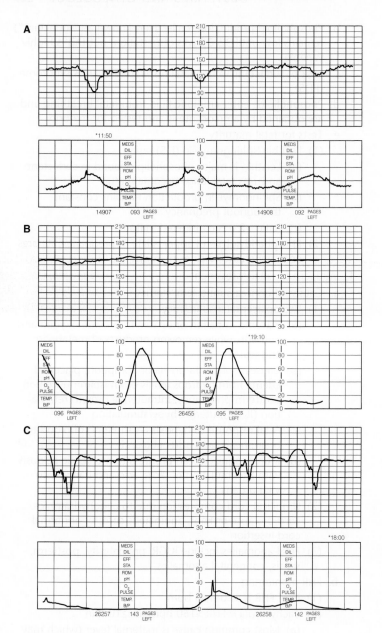

(b) Other causes = fetal hypoxia, immaturity, tachyar-rhythmias, anemia, infxn, maternal thyrotoxicosis, or Tx with sympathomimetics

(3) Bradycardia = FHR <120 bpm for ≥10 min, caused by congenital heart block, fetal anoxia (e.g., from placental separation), and maternal Tx with β-blockers

(4) FHR variability

(a) Fetal heart rate variability is the normal irregular changes and fluctuations in the fetal heart rate that show as an irregular heart rate seen on the tracing instead of a smooth line

(b) Reliable indicator of fetal well-being, suggesting sufficient CNS oxygenation

(c) ↓ Variability associated with fetal hypoxia/acidosis, depressant drugs, fetal tachycardia, CNS or cardiac anomalies, prolonged uterine contractions, prematurity, and fetal sleep

c. Accelerations

(1) Types and patterns of accelerations play a role in intra-partum evaluation of the fetus

(2) Accelerations

(a) ↑ FHR of at least 15 bpm above baseline for 15–20 sec

(b) This pattern indicates a fetus unstressed by hypoxia or acidemia → reassuring and suggests fetal well-being

(3) Early decelerations (Figure 3.1)

(a) ↓ FHR (not <100 bpm) that mirrors a uterine contraction (i.e., begins with onset of contraction, dips at peak of contraction, returns to baseline with end of contraction)

(b) Results from pressure on fetal head → vagus nerve stimulated reflex response to release acetylcholine at fetal sinoatrial node

(c) Considered physiologic and not harmful to fetus

(4) Variable decelerations (see Figure 3.1)

(a) Do not necessarily coincide with uterine contraction

←

FIGURE 3.1

A. Early deceleration pattern is depicted in this fetal heart rate (FHR) tracing. Note that each deceleration returns to baseline before the completion of the contraction. The remainder of the FHR tracing is reassuring. **B.** Repetitive late decelerations in conjunction with ↓ variability. **C.** Variable decelerations are the most common periodic change of the FHR during labor. Repetitive mild-to-moderate variable decelerations are present. Baseline is nml.

        (b) Characterized by rapid dip in FHR, often <100 bpm with rapid return to baseline

        (c) Also reflex-mediated due to umbilical cord compression

        (d) Can be corrected by shifting maternal position or amnioinfusion if membranes have ruptured and cord compression is 2° to oligohydramnios

    (5) Late decelerations (see Figure 3.1)

        (a) Begin after contraction has already started, dip after peak of contraction, return to baseline after contraction is over

        (b) Viewed as potentially dangerous, associated with uteroplacental insufficiency

        (c) Causes include placental abruption, PIH, maternal diabetes, maternal anemia, maternal sepsis, postterm pregnancy, and hyperstimulated uterus

        (d) Repetitive late decelerations require intervention

5. Isoimmunization

  a. Development of maternal immunoglobulin G (IgG) antibodies following exposure to fetal RBC antigens

  b. Exposure commonly occurs at delivery but can occur during pregnancy

  c. In subsequent pregnancies (rarely late in the same pregnancy), these antibodies can cross the placenta → attach to fetal RBCs and hemolyze them → fetal anemia

  d. Can occur with any blood group, but most often occurs when mother is Rh-negative and fetus is Rh-positive

  e. Extent to which fetus is affected depends on amount of IgG antibodies crossing placenta and ability of fetus to replenish destroyed RBCs

  f. Worst-case scenario is hydrops fetalis

    (1) Significant transfer of antibodies across placenta → fetal anemia

    (2) Liver attempts to make new RBCs (fetal hematopoiesis occurs in liver and bone marrow) at the expense of other necessary proteins → ↓ oncotic pressure → fetal ascites and edema

    (3) High-output cardiac failure associated with severe anemia

  g. Maternal IgG titer ≥1:16 is sufficiently high to pose risk to the fetus

    h. Tx = RhoGAM
- (1) Administration of antibody to the Rh antigen (Rh immune globulin = RhoGAM) within 72 hrs of delivery prevents active antibody response by the mother in most cases
- (2) Risk of subsequent sensitization ↓ from 15% to 2%
- (3) When RhoGAM is also given at 28 wks of gestation, risk of sensitization is further reduced to 0.2%

    i. RhoGAM given to Rh-negative mother if baby's father is Rh-positive or unknown
- (1) At 28 wks of gestation
- (2) Within 72 hrs of delivery of Rh-positive infant
- (3) Other times maternal–fetal blood mixing can occur
  - (a) At time of amniocentesis
  - (b) After an abortion
  - (c) After an ectopic pregnancy

6. Genetic Testing
- a. Chromosomal abnormalities account for 50%–60% of spontaneous abortion, 5% of stillbirths, 2%–3% of couples with multiple miscarriages
- b. 0.6% of all live births have a chromosomal abnormality
- c. Indications for prenatal genetic testing
  - (1) Most common is advanced maternal age (AMA)
    - (a) Trisomy 21 (Down's syndrome) incidence ↑ 10-fold from age 35–45 yrs, other polysomies ↑ similarly
    - (b) New Practice Bulletin by American College of Obstetricians and Gynecologist (ACOG) January, 2007, states that "All pregnant women, regardless of their age, should be offered screening for Down's syndrome"
  - (2) Prior child with chromosome or single gene abnormality
  - (3) Known chromosomal abnormality such as balanced translocation or single gene disorder in parent(s)
  - (4) Abnormal results from screening tests such as the triple-marker screen or quadruple-marker screen

F. Labor and Delivery
1. Initial Presentation
- a. Labor = progressive effacement and dilation of uterine cervix resulting from contractions of uterus
- b. **Braxton Hicks contractions** (false labor) = uterine contractions without effacement and dilation of cervix
- c. 85% of pts undergo spontaneous labor and delivery between 37 and 42 wks of gestation

d. Pts are told to come to hospital for regular contractions q5min for at least 1 hr, ROM, significant bleeding, ↓ fetal movement

e. Initial exam upon arrival

(1) Auscultation of fetal heart tones

(2) Leopold maneuvers help determine fetal lie (relation of long axis of fetus with maternal long axis), fetal presentation (i.e., breech vs. cephalic), and position of presenting part with respect to right or left side of maternal pelvis

(3) Vaginal examination

(a) Check for ROM, cervical effacement, and cervical dilation (in cm)

(b) Fetal station (level of fetal presenting part relative to ischial spines) measured from −3 (presenting part palpable at pelvic inlet) to +3 (presenting part palpable beyond pelvic outlet)

(c) 0 station = presenting part palpable at ischial spines, significance of 0 station is that biparietal diameter (biggest diameter of fetal head) has negotiated pelvic inlet (smallest part of pelvis)

2. Labor divided into four stages (Figure 3.2)

a. Stage 1

(1) Interval between onset of labor and full cervical dilation (10 cm)

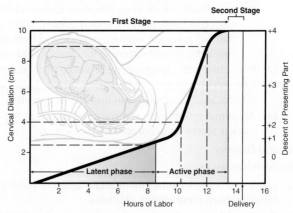

FIGURE 3.2

Schematic illustration of progress of rotation of occipitoanterior presentation in the successive stages of labor. Note the relationship between changes in cervical dilation and phases of labor.

    (2) Further subdivided into:
        (a) Latent phase = cervical effacement and early dilation
        (b) Active phase = more rapid cervical dilation occurs, usually beginning at 3–4 cm
    (3) In Stage 1, continuous monitoring of FHR, either via Doppler or internal monitoring via fetal scalp electrode
    (4) Monitoring of uterine activity by
        (a) External tocodynamometer measures frequency and duration of contractions but not intensity, OR
        (b) Intrauterine pressure catheter (IUPC) measures intensity by measuring intrauterine pressure
    (5) Analgesic (typically meperidine) and/or anesthetic (typically an epidural block that provides both continuous analgesia and anesthesia) can be given—agents usually not given until active stage of labor

b. Stage 2 = interval between complete cervical dilation and delivery of infant
    (1) Maternal effort (i.e., pushing) accelerates delivery of fetus (↑ intra-abd pressure assists fetal descent down birth canal)
    (2) Delivery should be well controlled with protection of the perineum
    (3) If used, episiotomies usually are cut midline, no longer indicated if you can slow delivery and allow to tear in a controlled fashion
    (4) After head is delivered, bulb suction of nose and mouth is performed and neck is evaluated for the presence of nuchal cord
    (5) Shoulders are delivered by applying gentle downward pressure on head to deliver anterior shoulder followed by easy upward force to deliver posterior shoulder
    (6) Delivery of body follows, cord is clamped and cut, and infant is given to mother or placed in warmer
    (7) Blood from umbilical cord sent for ABO and Rh testing as well as arterial blood gases

c. Stage 3 = interval between delivery of infant and delivery of placenta
    (1) Three signs of placenta separation
        (a) Uterus rises in abdomen signaling that placenta has separated

        (b) Gush of blood

        (c) Lengthening of umbilical cord

    (2) Excessive pulling on placenta should be avoided because of the risk of uterus inversion with associated profound hemorrhage and retained placenta

    (3) Gentle traction should be applied at all times

    (4) May take up to 30 min for placenta to be expulsed

  d. Stage 4 = immediate postpartum period lasting 2 hrs, during which pt undergoes significant physiologic changes

    (1) Systematic evaluation of cervix, vagina, vulva, perineum, and periurethral area for lacerations

    (2) Likelihood of serious postpartum complications is greatest in first 1–2 hr postpartum

3. Abnormal Labor

  a. Dystocia = difficult labor

    (1) Cause detected by evaluating the **3 Ps**

      (a) **Power**

        (i) Refers to strength, duration, and frequency of contractions

        (ii) Measured by using tocodynamometer or IUPC

        (iii) For cervical dilation to occur, ≥ 3 contractions in 10 min must be generated

        (iv) During active labor maternal effort comes into play as maternal exhaustion, effects of analgesia/anesthesia, or underlying dz may prolong labor

      (b) **Passenger**

        (i) Refers to estimates of fetal weight + evaluation of fetal lie, presentation, and position

        (ii) Occiput posterior presentation, face presentation, and hydrocephalus are associated with dystocia

      (c) **Passage**

        (i) Difficult to measure pelvic diameters

        (ii) Adequacy of pelvis often unknown until progress (or no progress) is made during labor

        (iii) Distended bladder, adnexal or colon masses, and uterine fibroids can all contribute to dystocia

    (2) Dystocia divided into prolongation disorders

      (a) Prolonged latent phase

        (i) Latent phase >20 hrs in primigravid or >14 hrs in multigravid pt is prolonged and abnormal

   (ii) Causes include ineffective uterine contractions, fetopelvic disproportion, and excess anesthesia

   (iii) Prolonged latent phase → no harm to mother or fetus

  (b) Prolonged active phase

   (i) Active phase >12 hrs or rate of cervical dilation, <1.2 cm/hr in primigravid, or <1.5 cm/hr in multigravid

   (ii) Causes include excess anesthesia, ineffective contractions, fetopelvic disproportion, fetal malposition, ROM before onset of active labor

   (iii) Prolonged active phase → ↑ risk of intrauterine infxn and ↑ risk of C-section

 b. Arrest disorders

  (1) 2° arrest occurs when cervical dilation during active phase ceases for ≥2 hrs

  (2) Suggests either cephalopelvic disproportion or ineffective uterine contractions

 c. Management of abnormal labor

  (1) Labor induction = stimulation of uterine contractions before spontaneous onset of labor

  (2) Augmentation of labor = stimulation of uterine contractions that began spontaneously but have become infrequent, weak, or both

  (3) Induction trial should occur only if cervix is prepared or "ripe"

  (4) Bishop score used to try to quantify cervical readiness for induction (Table 3.5)

 d. Indications for induction = suspected fetal compromise, fetal death, PIH, premature ROM, chorioamnionitis, postdates pregnancy, maternal medical complication

Table 3.5 Bishop Score

Factor	Points			
	0	1	2	3
Dilation (cm)	Closed	1–2	3–4	≥5
Effacement (%)	0–30	40–50	60–70	≥80
Station	−3	−2, −1	0	≥+1
Position		Posterior	Mid	Anterior

Score from 9–13 is associated with highest likelihood of successful induction.
Score from 0–4 is associated with highest likelihood of failed induction.

    e. Contraindications for induction include placenta previa, active genital herpes, abnormal fetal lie, cord presentation

    f. If cervix not "ripe," prostaglandin E_2 gel can be used to attempt to ripen cervix; biggest risk is uterine hyperstimulation → uteroplacental insufficiency

    g. Another method is insertion of laminaria or rods inserted into the internal os that absorb moisture and expand, slowly dilating cervix; risks include failure to dilate, laceration, ROM, and infxn

    h. Prolonged latent phase can be managed with rest, augmentation of labor with oxytocin, and/or amniotomy that may allow for fetal head to provide greater dilating force

    i. During active phase of labor, fetal malposition and cephalopelvic disproportion must be considered and may warrant C-section versus augmentation

    j. If fetus has descended far enough, forceps or vacuum can be used; if not, C-section is performed

    k. Risks of prolonged labor include infxn, exhaustion, lacerations, uterine atony with hemorrhage

    l. Breech presentation occurs in 2%–4% of pregnancies and risk ↑ in cases of multiple gestations, polyhydramnios, hydrocephaly, anencephaly, and uterine anomalies (see Figure 3.3)

4. Postpartum Hemorrhage

    a. Defined as blood loss >500 mL associated with delivery

    b. Causes = uterine atony (most common), lacerations, retained placenta

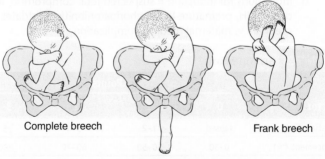

Complete breech   Frank breech

Footling breech

FIGURE 3.3

Different breech presentations.

c. **Uterine atony**

(1) Normally uterus quickly contracts following delivery of placenta, muscle contraction compresses down on spiral arteries and prevents excessive bleeding

(2) If contraction does not occur → postpartum hemorrhage

(3) Risk factors for uterine atony = multiple gestations, hydramnios, multiparity, macrosomia, previous Hx of postpartum hemorrhage, fibroids, magnesium sulfate, general anesthesia, prolonged labor, amnionitis

(4) Dx based on clinical exam of soft, "boggy" uterus

(5) Tx

    (a) Start with uterine massage to stimulate contractions

    (b) IV fluids and transfusions as needed, cervix and vagina visualized for lacerations

    (c) Medical Tx = oxytocin, methylergonovine maleate (Methergine; potent uterotonic always given IM; if given, IV can cause severe HTN), or prostaglandins → uterine contractions

    (d) If these measures are unsuccessful, surgical interventions are used and include ligation of uterine arteries, ligation of internal iliac arteries, selective arterial embolization, or hysterectomy as last resort

d. Retained placenta

(1) Occurs when separation of placenta from uterine wall or expulsion of placenta is incomplete

(2) Risk factors include previous C-section, fibroids, and prior uterine curettage

(3) Placental tissue that abnormally implants into uterus can result in retention

(4) Placenta accreta: placental villi abnormally adhere to superficial lining of uterine wall

(5) Placenta increta: placental villi penetrate into uterine muscle layer

(6) Placenta percreta: placental villi completely invade uterine muscle layer

e. Disseminated intravascular coagulation (DIC)

(1) Rare cause of postpartum hemorrhage

(2) Severe preeclampsia, amniotic fluid embolism, and placental abruption are associated with DIC

(3) Tx aimed at correcting coagulopathy

G. Postpartum Care

1. Lactation and Breast-Feeding

   a. Engorgement occurs approximately 3 days postpartum

   b. Three causes of tender, enlarged breasts postpartum are engorgement, mastitis, and plugged duct

   c. Treat engorgement with continued breast-feeding, mastitis with antibiotics (nursing can be continued), and plugged duct with warm packs

   d. Advantages of breastfeeding = ↑ bonding between mother and child, convenience, ↓ cost, protection against infxn and allergies

   e. Breast milk provides all vitamins except vitamin K

2. Contraception

   a. Contraception should be discussed with all pts prior to discharge

   b. Approximately 15% of women are fertile 6 wk postpartum

   c. OCPs are not contraindicated in breastfeeding women, postpartum tubal ligation should be discussed as well

3. Postpartum Immunizations

   a. Rubella nonimmune women should be immunized (they can continue to breastfeed)

   b. Rh-negative woman who has given birth to an Rh-positive baby should receive RhoGAM

4. Postpartum Depression

   a. Recurrence rate for pts with previous postpartum depression is 25%

   b. Postpartum depression ranges from the "blues," which affects 50% of women and typically occurs on Days 2–3 and resolves in 1–2 wks, to postpartum depression, which affects 10% of women, to suicidal ideation, which occurs more rarely

   c. Especially worrisome is a mother who has estranged herself from her newborn or has become indifferent

   d. Tx depends on severity of Sx and may range from simple telephone contact to psychotherapy and medication to inpt hospitalization

5. Postpartum Uterine Infxn

   a. Incidence of infxn ranges from 10%–50% depending on population, mode of delivery (C-section > vaginal delivery), and risk factors

b. Risk factors = maternal obesity, immunosuppression, chronic dz, vaginal infxn, amnionitis, prolonged labor, prolonged ROM, multiple pelvic examinations during labor, internal fetal monitoring or IUPC, C-section

c. **Most common infxn post C-section is metritis** (uterine infxn)

d. Si/Sx = fever on first or second postpartum day, uterine tenderness, ↓ bowel sounds, leukocytosis (difficult to interpret because of nml leukocytosis in puerperium)

e. DDx = same as postsurgical, see Chapter 2.III.C.2.a

f. Metritis usually polymicrobial with aerobic and anaerobic organisms present

g. Dx = clinical

h. Tx = first-generation cephalosporin, broaden antibiotics if no response within 48–72 hrs

i. Prophylactic antibiotic Tx (one-time dose) at time of C-section delivery significantly reduces incidence of postpartum infxn

H. Obstetrical Complications

1. Abortion

a. Termination of a pregnancy before viability, usually at ≤20 wks, occurs spontaneously in 15% of all pregnancies

b. Risk factors = ↑ parity, AMA, ↑ paternal age, conception within 3 mos of a live birth

c. Single pregnancy loss does not significantly ↑ risk of future loss

d. Chromosomal abnormalities cause 50% of early spontaneous abortions, mostly trisomies (the longer a pregnancy goes before undergoing spontaneous abortion, the less likely the fetus is chromosomally abnormal)

e. Other causes = endocrine dz (e.g., thyroid), structural abnormalities (e.g., fibroids, incompetent cervix), infxn (e.g., *Listeria; Mycoplasma; Toxoplasma;* Rubella, Cytomegalovirus, Herpes Simplex Virus, and Syphilis [ToRCHs]), chronic dz (e.g., DM, systemic lupus erythematosus, renal or cardiac dz), environmental factors (e.g., toxins, radiation, smoking, alcohol)

f. Vaginal bleeding in first half of any pregnancy is presumed to be a threatened abortion unless another Dx, such as ectopic pregnancy, cervical polyps, cervicitis, or molar pregnancy, can be made

g. Types (Table 3.6)

Table 3.6 Types of Abortions

Threatened	• Si/Sx = vaginal bleeding in first 20 wks of pregnancy without passage of tissue or ROM, with cervix closed • Occurs in 25% of pregnancies (half go on to spontaneously abort) • ↑ Risk preterm labor and delivery, low birth weight, perinatal mortality • Dx = Utz to confirm early pregnancy is intact • If no cardiac activity by 9 wks → consider D&C procedure • hCG levels are used to identify viable pregnancies at various stages of development
Inevitable	• Si/Sx = threatened abortion with dilated cervical os and/or ROM, usually accompanied by cramping with expulsion of products of conception (POC) • Pregnancy loss is unavoidable • Tx = surgical evacuation of uterine contents and RhoGAM if mother is Rh-negative
Completed	• Si/Sx = documented pregnancy that spontaneously aborts all POCs • POCs should be grossly examined and submitted to pathology to confirm fetal tissue and/or placental villi; if none is observed, must rule out ectopic pregnancy • Pts may require curettage because of ↑ likelihood that abortion was incomplete (suspected if β-hCG levels plateau or fail to decline to zero) • RhoGAM given to Rh-negative women
Incomplete	• Si/Sx = cramping, bleeding, passage of tissue, with dilated cervix and visible tissue in vagina or endocervical canal • Curettage usually needed to remove remaining POCs and control bleeding • Rh-negative pts are given RhoGAM • Hemodynamic stabilization may be required if bleeding is very heavy
Missed	• Failure to expel POC • Si/Sx = lack of uterine growth, lack of fetal heart tones, and cessation of pregnancy Sx • Evacuation of uterus required after confirmation of fetal death, suction curettage recommended for first-trimester pregnancy, dilation and evacuation (D&E) recommended for second-trimester pregnancies • DIC is serious but rare complication • Rh-negative pts receive RhoGAM
Recurrent	• Si/Sx = ≥2 consecutive or total of 3 spontaneous abortions • If early, often due to chromosomal abnormalities → karyotyping for both parents to determine if they carry a chromosomal abnormality • Examine mother for uterine abnormalities • Incompetent cervix is suspected by Hx of painless dilation of cervix with delivery of nml fetus between 18 and 32 wks of gestation • Tx = surgical cerclage procedures to suture cervix closed until labor or rupture of membranes occurs

2. Ectopic Pregnancy
   a. Implantation outside of uterine cavity
   b. ↑ Incidence recently because of ↑ in pelvic inflammatory dz (PID), second leading cause of maternal mortality
   c. Risk factors = previous ectopic pregnancy, previous Hx of salpingitis (scarring and adhesions impede transport of ovum down the tube), age ≥35 yrs, >3 prior pregnancies, sterilization failure
   d. Si/Sx = abd/pelvic pain, referred shoulder pain from hemo-peritoneal irritation of diaphragm, amenorrhea, vaginal bleeding, cervical motion or adnexal tenderness, nausea, vomiting, orthostatic changes
   e. DDx = surgical abdomen, abortion, salpingitis, endometrio-sis, ruptured ovarian cyst, ovarian torsion
   f. Ectopic pregnancy should be suspected in any reproductive-age woman who presents with abd/pelvic pain, irregular bleeding, and amenorrhea—lag in Tx is a significant cause of mortality
   g. Dx
      (1) ⊕ Pregnancy test with Utz to determine intrauterine versus extrauterine pregnancy
      (2) Very low progesterone level strongly suggests nonviable pregnancy that may be located outside the uterine cav-ity; higher levels suggest viable pregnancy
   h. Tx
      (1) Surgical removal now commonly done via laparoscopy with maximum preservation of reproductive organs
      (2) Methotrexate can be used early, especially if pregnancy is <3.5 cm in diameter, with no cardiac activity on Utz
      (3) Regardless of technique used, post-Tx serial β-hCG levels must be followed to ensure proper falloff in level
      (4) Rh-negative women should receive RhoGAM to avoid Rh sensitization
3. Third-Trimester Bleeding
   a. Occurs in approximately 5% of all pregnancies
   b. Half of these are due to placenta previa or placental abrupti-on, others due to vaginal/vulvar lacerations, cervical polyps, cervicitis, cervical CA
   c. In many cases, no cause of bleeding is found
   d. Comparison of placenta previa and placental abruption (Table 3.7)

Table 3.7 Comparison of Placenta Previa and Placental Abruption

	Placenta Previa	Placental Abruption
Abnormality	Placenta implanted over internal cervical os (completely or partially)	Premature separation (complete or partial) of normally implanted placenta from decidua
Epidemiology	↑ Risk grand multiparas and prior C-section	↑ Risk preeclampsia, previous Hx of abruption, rupture of membranes in a pt with hydramnios, cocaine use, cigarette smoking, and trauma
Time of onset	20–30 wks	Any time after 20 wks
Si/Sx	Sudden, **painless** bleeding	**Painful** bleeding, can be heavy and painful, and frequent uterine contractions
Dx	Utz → placenta abnormal location	Clinical, based on presentation of painful vaginal bleeding, frequent contractions, and fetal distress. **Utz not useful**
Tx	Hemodynamic support, expectant management, deliver by C-section when fetus is mature enough	Hemodynamic support, urgent C-section or vaginal induction if pt is stable and fetus is not in distress
Complications	Associated with 2-fold ↑ in congenital malformations, so evaluation for fetal anomalies should be undertaken at Dx	↑ Risk of fetal hypoxia/death, DIC may occur as a result of intravascular and retroplacental coagulation

4. Preterm Labor (PTL)
   a. Regular uterine contractions at ≤10-min intervals, lasting ≥30 sec, between 20 and 36 wks of gestation, accompanied by cervical effacement, dilation, and/or descent of fetus into the pelvis
   b. Major cause of preterm birth → significant perinatal morbidity and mortality
   c. Risk factors = premature rupture of membranes (PROM), infxn (UTI, vaginal, amniotic), dehydration, incompetent cervix, smoking, fibroids, placenta previa, placental abruption, many cases are idiopathic
   d. Si/Sx = cramps, dull low-back pain, abd/pelvic pressure, vaginal discharge (mucous, water, or bloody), and contractions (often painless)

e. Dx = external fetal monitoring to quantify frequency and duration of contractions, vaginal exam → extent of cervical dilation/effacement

f. Utz to confirm gestational age, amniotic fluid volume (helps determine if ROM has occurred), fetal presentation, and placental location

g. Tx focused on delaying delivery if possible until fetus is mature

(1) 50% of pts have spontaneous resolution of preterm uterine contractions

(2) IV hydration important because dehydration causes uterine irritability

(3) Empiric antibiotic Tx is given for suspected chorioamnionitis or vaginal infxn

(4) Tocolytic regimens

(a) Magnesium sulfate, β_2-agonists such as terbutaline and ritodrine, Ca^{2+} blockers such as nifedipine or indomethacin may be instituted, although they have never been shown to substantially prolong delivery for more than several days

(b) Contraindications to tocolysis = advanced labor (cervical dilation >3 cm), mature fetus, chorioamnionitis, significant vaginal bleeding, anomalous fetus, acute fetal distress, severe preeclampsia or eclampsia

(5) From 24 to 34 wks, steroids such as betamethasone are generally used to enhance pulmonary maturity

(6) Management of infants at 34–37 wks is individualized; survival rates for infants born at 34 wk is within 1% of the survival rate for infants born at ≥37 wk; assessment of fetal lung maturity may help decide who to deliver between 34 and 37 wks

h. Common complications include death, RDS and subsequent bronchopulmonary dysplasia, sepsis, intraventricular hemorrhage, necrotizing enterocolitis, developmental delays, and seizures

5. PROM

a. Rupture of chorioamnionic membrane before onset of labor, occurs in 10%–15% of all pregnancies

b. Labor usually follows PROM; 90% of pts and 50% of preterm pts go into labor within 24 hrs after rupture

c. Biggest risk is labor and delivery of preterm infant with associated morbidities/mortality, second biggest complication is infxn (chorioamnionitis)

d. PROM at ≤26 wk of gestation is associated with pulmonary hypoplasia

e. Dx = vaginal exam with testing of nonbloody fluid from the vagina

   (1) Nitrazine test: uses pH to distinguish alkaline amniotic fluid (pH >7.0) with more acidic urine and vaginal secretions. (*Note:* false-positive result seen with semen, cervical mucus, *Trichomonas* infxn, blood, unusually basic urine.)

   (2) Fern test: amniotic fluid placed on slide that is allowed to dry in room (up to 30 min); branching fern leaf pattern that results when the slide is completely dry is caused by sodium chloride precipitates from amniotic fluid

   (3) Utz confirms Dx by noting oligohydramnios, labor is less likely to occur if sufficient fluid remains

f. Tx

   (1) If intrauterine infxn is suspected, empiric broad-spectrum antibiotics are started

   (2) Otherwise treat as for PTL above

6. Multiple Gestations

a. 1 in 90 incidence in the US; incidence slightly higher in black women, slightly lower in white women.

b. **Dizygotic twins occur when two separate ova are fertilized by two separate sperm, incidence ↑ with ↑ age and parity**

c. Monozygotic twins represent division of the fertilized ovum at various times after conception

d. Multiple gestations are considered high-risk pregnancies because of the disproportionate ↑ in perinatal morbidity and mortality as compared with a singleton gestation

   (1) Spontaneous abortions and congenital anomalies occur more frequently in multiple pregnancies as compared with singleton pregnancies

   (2) Maternal complications = anemia, hydramnios, eclampsia, PTL, postpartum uterine atony and hemorrhage, ↑ risk for C-section

   (3) Fetal complications: congenital anomalies, spontaneous abortion, IUGR, prematurity, PROM, umbilical cord prolapse, placental abruption, placenta previa, and malpresentation

e. Average duration of gestation ↓ with ↑ number of fetuses (twins deliver at 37 wk, triplets deliver at 33 wk, quadruplets deliver at 29 wk)

f. Twin–twin transfusion syndrome

    (1) Occurs in 10% of twins sharing a chorionic membrane

    (2) Occurs when blood flow is interrupted by a vascular anastomoses such that one twin becomes the donor twin and can have impaired growth, anemia, hypovolemia, and the other twin (recipient twin) can develop hypervolemia, HTN, polycythemia, and congestive heart failure as a result of ↑ blood flow from one twin to the other

g. Dx of twins usually suspected when uterine size exceeds calculated gestational age and can be confirmed with Utz

h. DDx = incorrect dates, fibroids, polyhydramnios, and molar pregnancy

i. Delivery method largely depends on presentation of twins; usually if first fetus is in vertex presentation, vaginal delivery is attempted; if not, C-section is often performed

j. Important to watch for uterine atony and postpartum hemorrhage because overdistended uterus may not clamp down normally

k. ↑ Incidence of multiple gestations also seen in females taking fertility meds

II. Gynecology

A. Benign Gynecology

  1. Menstrual Cycle (Figure 3.4)

    a. Due to hypothalamic pulses of gonadotropin-releasing hormone (GnRH), pituitary release of follicle-stimulating hormone (FSH) and luteinizing hormone (LH), and ovarian sex steroids estradiol and progesterone

    b. ↑ Or ↓ of any of these hormones → irregular menses or amenorrhea

    c. At birth, the human ovary contains approximately 1 million primordial follicles, each with an oocyte arrested in the prophase stage of meiosis

    d. Process of ovulation begins in puberty = follicular maturation

      (1) After ovulation, the dominant follicle released becomes the corpus luteum, which secretes progesterone to prepare the endometrium for possible implantation

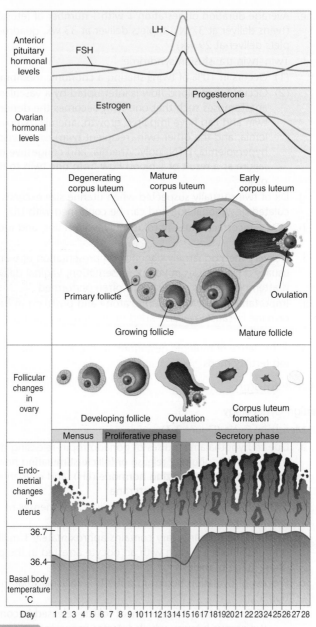

FIGURE 3.4

Nml menstrual cycle. (From Premkumar K. *The massage connection anatomy and physiology.* Baltimore, MD: Lippincott Williams & Wilkins, 2004.)

Table 3.8 Phases of the Menstrual Cycle (see Figure 3.4)

Follicular Phase (Proliferative Phase)	Ovulatory Phase	Luteal Phase (Secretory Phase)
Days 1–13 of cycle: Estradiol-induced negative feedback on FSH and ⊕ feedback on LH in anterior pituitary leads to LH surge on Days 11–13	Days 13–17 of cycle: Dominant follicle secretion of estradiol→ ⊕ feedback to anterior pituitary FSH and LH, ovulation occurs 30–36 hrs after the LH surge, small FSH surge also occurs at time of LH surge	Day 15 to first day of menses: Marked by change from estradiol to progesterone predominance, corpus luteal progesterone acts on hypothalamus, causing negative feedback on FSH and LH, resulting in ↓ to basal levels prior to next cycle; if fertilization and implantation do not occur → rapid ↓ in progesterone

    (2) If the ovum is not fertilized, the corpus luteum undergoes involution, menstruation begins, and cycle repeats

  e. Phases of the menstrual cycle (Table 3.8). First day of menstrual bleeding is Day 1 of the cycle

2. Contraception

  a. OCPs = combination estrogen and progestin

    (1) Progestin is major contraceptive by suppressing LH and thus ovulation, also thickens cervical mucus so it is less favorable to semen

    (2) Estrogen participates by suppressing FSH, thereby preventing selection and maturation of a dominant follicle

    (3) Estrogen and progesterone together inhibit implantation by thinning endometrial lining, also resulting in light or missed menses

    (4) Monophasic pills deliver a constant dose of estrogen and progestin

    (5) Phasic OCPs alter this ratio (usually by varying the dose of progestin) that slightly ↓ the total dose of hormone per mo but also has slightly ↑ rate of breakthrough bleeding between periods

    (6) Pts usually resume fertility once OCPs are discontinued; **however, 3% may have prolonged postpill amenorrhea**

    (7) Risks and benefits (Table 3.9)

    (8) Absolute contraindications to use of OCPs = pregnancy, DVT or thromboembolic dz, endometrial CA,

Table 3.9 Risks and Benefits of Oral Contraceptives

Advantages	Disadvantages

• Highly reliable, failure rate <1% (failure usually related to missing pills)
• Protect against endometrial and ovarian CA
• ↓ Incidence of pelvic infxns and ectopic pregnancies
• Menses are more predictable, lighter, less painful
	• Require daily compliance
	• Does not protect against sexually transmitted dz
	• 10%–30% have breakthrough bleeding
	• Side effects:
	  ◊ Estrogen → bloating, weight gain, breast tenderness, nausea, headaches
	  ◊ Progestin → depression, acne, HTN[a]

[a]Try lower-dose progesterone pill if HTN does not resolve. Discontinue OCPs—pts with pre-existing HTN can try OCPs if they are ≤35 yrs and under good medical control.

cerebrovascular or coronary artery dz, breast CA, cigarette smoking in women >35 yrs old, hepatic dz/neoplasm, abnormal vaginal bleeding, hyperlipidemia
(9) Alternatives to standard OCPs (Table 3.10)
3. Pap Smear
   a. Current ACOG recommendations are: women from ages 21–30 are to be screened every two years with either a standard Pap smear or liquid-based cytology.
   b. Women 30 yrs and older who have had three consecutive negative cervical cytology test results can be screened once every 3 yrs with either Pap smear or liquid-based cytology. If multiple risk factors exist, then screen more frequently, i.e. HIV, immunosuppressed, exposed to diethylstilbesterol (DES) in utero, or previously for cervical intraepithelial neoplasia (CIN) or cervical cancer.
   c. Reliability depends on presence/absence of cervical inflammation, adequacy of specimen, and prompt fixation of specimen to avoid artifact
   d. If Pap → mild- or low-grade atypia → repeat Pap—atypia may spontaneously regress
   e. Recurrent mild atypia or high-grade atypia → more intensive evaluation
      (1) Colposcopy
         (a) Allows for magnification of cervix so that subtle areas of dysplastic change can be visualized, optimizing selection of Bx sites

Table 3.10 Alternatives to Oral Contraceptives

Method	Indication	Advantage	Disadvantage
Progestin-only pills ("mini pills")	• **Lactating women**	• Can start immediately postpartum • No impact on milk production or on the baby	• ↑ Failure rate than OCP (ovulation continues in 40%) • Requires strict compliance—low dose of progesterone requires that pill be taken at the same time each day
Drospirenone and ethinyl estradiol	• Contraception for 1 mo	• Drospirenone is a synthetic progestin, has antimineralo-corticoid activity that diminishes salt retention versus standard progestins • One pill once per mo	• Risk of hyperkalemia
Depo-Provera (medroxy-progesterone)	• Contraception for ≥1 yr • Noncompliance with daily OCPs • Breastfeeding	• **IM injection** maintained for 14 wks	• Irregular vaginal bleed[a] • 50% pts infertile for 10 mos after last injection • Risk of abortion[b]
Norplant	• Long-term contraception	• Subcutaneous implants provide **contraception for 5 yr** • Prompt fertility following D&C	• 30% of breakthrough pregnancies are ectopic
Patch	• Contraception for 1 mo	• Patch worn on skin like Band-Aid; slowly releases estrogen/progestin • Wear for 3 wks, then take off for 1 wk • 99% effective	• Does not protect against STDs • Less effective (92%) for women ≥198 pounds
Intrauterine device	• For those at low risk for STDs	• Inserted into endometrial cavity, left in place for several years	• Contraindicated cervical or vaginal infxn, Hx of PID or infertility • Spontaneous expulsion, menstrual pain, ↑ rate of ectopic pregnancy, septic abortion, and pelvic infxns

(continued)

Table 3.10 *Continued*			
Method	**Indication**	**Advantage**	**Disadvantage**
Vaginal contraceptive ring	• Contraception for 1 mo	• Flexible ring inserted into vagina, releases estrogen/progestin locally • Wear for 3 wks, take out for 1 wk	• If ring is expelled and stays out for ≥3 hrs, must use another birth control method until new ring is in place for 7 days
Postcoital	• Emergency contraception	• **Progestin/estrogen taken within 72 hrs of intercourse,** repeat in 12 hrs • Allows for early termination of unwanted pregnancy	• Follow pt to ensure withdrawal bleeding occurs within 5 days • Nausea

*aOral estrogen or NSAIDs can ↓ bleeding, bleeding ↓ with each use, 50% pts are amenorrheic in 1 yr.
bInjection given within first 5 days of menses (ensuring pt not pregnant).
STD, sexually transmitted dz.

    (b) Cervix washed with acetic acid solution; white areas, abnormally vascularized areas, and punctate lesions are selected for Bx

  (2) Endocervical curettage (ECC) → sample of endocervix obtained at the same time of colposcopy so that dz further up in endocervical canal may be detected

  (3) Cone Bx

    (a) Cone-shaped specimen encompassing squamocolumnar junction and any lesions on ectocervix removed from cervix by knife, laser, or wire loop

    (b) Allows for more complete ascertainment of extent of dz, in many cases is therapeutic as well as diagnostic

    (c) Indications = ⊕ ECC, unsatisfactory colposcopy = entire squamocolumnar junction not visualized, and discrepancy between Pap and colposcopy Bx

  f. Tx = excision of premalignant or malignant lesions—if CA, see Section D. for appropriate adjunctive modalities

4. Human Papilloma Virus (HPV) Vaccine

  a. Vaccination protects against HPV 16 and 18, which cause 70% of cervical CA, and 6 and 11, which cause 90% of genital warts

    b. Vaccination appears to be 100% effective at preventing genital warts and precancerous lesions of cervix, vulva, and vagina caused by the targeted HPV serotypes

    c. Vaccination is less effective once the virus is already contracted, so must vaccinate prior to contracting HPV

    d. Official recommendation is to vaccinate all 11–12-yr-old girls (can be given to girls as young as 9) and also recommended for 13–26-yr-old girls/women who have not yet received or completed the vaccine series

5. Vaginitis

    a. 50% of cases due to *Gardnerella* ("bacterial vaginosis"), 25% due to *Trichomonas,* 25% due to *Candida* (↑ frequency in diabetics, women who are pregnant or have HIV)

    b. Most common presenting Sx in vaginitis is discharge

    c. Rule out noninfectious causes, including chemical or allergic sources

    d. Dx by pelvic examination with microscopic examination of discharge

    e. DDx of vaginitis (Table 3.11)

6. Endometriosis

    a. Affects 1%–2% of women (up to 50% in infertile women), peak age = 20s–30s

    b. Endometrial tissue in extrauterine locations, most commonly ovaries (60%) but can be anywhere in the peritoneum and rarely extraperitoneal

OBSTETRICS AND GYNECOLOGY

Table 3.11 Differential Diagnosis of Vaginitis (Figure 3.5)

	Candida	Trichomonas	Gardnerella
Vaginal pH	4–5	>6	>5
Odor	None	Rancid	"Fishy" on KOH prep
Discharge	Cheesy white	Green, frothy	Variable
Si/Sx	Itchy, burning erythema	Severe itching	Variable to none
Microscopy	Pseudohyphae, more pronounced on 10% KOH prep	Motile organisms with flagellae	Clue cells (large epithelial cells covered with dozens of small dots)
Tx	Fluconazole	Metronidazole— treat partner also	Metronidazole

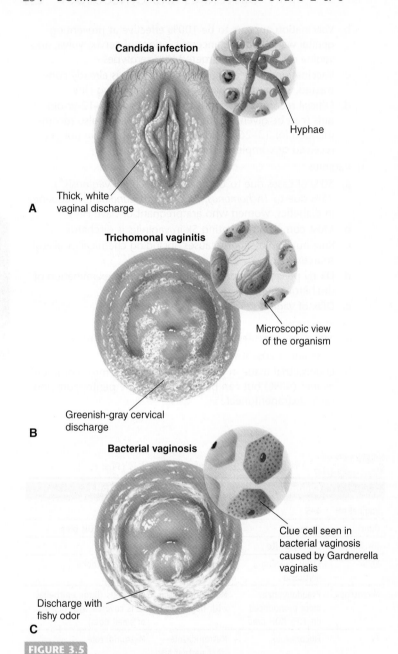

Candida infection

Hyphae

Thick, white
A vaginal discharge

Trichomonal vaginitis

Microscopic view
of the organism

Greenish-gray cervical
discharge
B

Bacterial vaginosis

Clue cell seen in
bacterial vaginosis
caused by Gardnerella
vaginalis

Discharge with
fishy odor
C

FIGURE 3.5

Vaginitis. **A.** *Candida* vaginitis. **B.** *Trichomonas* vaginitis. **C.** Bacterial vaginosis.
All assets provided by Anatomical Chart Co.

   c. Adenomyosis = endometrial implants within the uterine wall

   d. Endometrioma = endometriosis involving an ovary with implants large enough to be considered a tumor, filled with chocolate-appearing fluid (old blood) that gives them their name of "chocolate cysts"

   e. Si/Sx = **the 3 Ds = dysmenorrhea, dyspareunia, dyschezia** (painful defecation), pelvic pain, infertility, uterosacral nodularity palpable on rectovaginal exam; severity of Sx often do not correlate with the extent of dz

   f. Dx requires direct visualization via laparoscopy or laparotomy with histologic confirmation

   g. Tx

     (1) Start with NSAIDs, can add combined estrogen and progestin pills, allowing maintenance without withdrawal bleeding and dysmenorrhea

     (2) Can use progestin-only pills, drawback is breakthrough bleeding

     (3) GnRH agonists inhibit ovarian function → hypoestrogen state

     (4) Danazol inhibits LH and FSH midcycle surges; side effects include hypoestrogenic and androgenic (hirsutism, acne) states

     (5) Conservative surgery involves excision, cauterization, or ablation of endometrial implants with preservation of ovaries and uterus

     (6) Recurrence after cessation of medical Tx is common, definitive Tx requires hysterectomy, ⊕ oophorectomy (total abd hysterectomy with bilateral salpingo-oophorectomy [TAH/BSO]), lysis of adhesions, and removal of endometrial implants

     (7) Pts can take estrogen replacement Tx following definitive surgery, risk of reactivation of endometriosis is very small compared to risk of prolonged estrogen deficiency

B. Reproductive Endocrinology and Infertility

   1. Amenorrhea

     a. Definitions

       (1) Amenorrhea = absence of menstruation

       (2) 1° amenorrhea = woman who has never menstruated

       (3) 2° amenorrhea = menstrual-age woman who has not menstruated in 6 mos

    b. Causes of amenorrhea

      (1) **Pregnancy = most common cause,** thus every evaluation should begin with an exclusion of pregnancy before any further workup

      (2) Asherman's syndrome

         (a) Scarring of the uterine cavity after a dilatation and curettage (D&C) procedure

         (b) **Most common anatomic cause of 2° amenorrhea**

      (3) Hypothalamic deficiency due to weight loss, excessive exercise (e.g., marathon runner), obesity, drug-induced (e.g., marijuana, tranquilizers), malignancy (prolactinoma, craniopharyngioma), psychogenic (chronic anxiety, anorexia)

      (4) Pituitary dysfunction results from either ↓ hypothalamic pulsatile release of GnRH or ↓ pituitary release of FSH or LH

      (5) Ovarian dysfunction

         (a) Ovarian follicles are either exhausted or resistant to stimulation by FSH and LH

         (b) Si/Sx = those of estrogen deficiency = hot flashes, mood swings, vaginal dryness, dyspareunia, sleep disturbances, skin thinning

         (c) **Note that estrogen deficiency 2° to hypothalamic—pituitary failure does not cause hot flashes, whereas ovarian failure does**

         (d) Causes = inherited (e.g., Turner's syndrome), premature natural menopause, autoimmune ovarian failure (Blizzard's syndrome), alkylating chemotherapies

      (6) Genital outflow tract alteration, usually the result of congenital abnormalities (e.g., imperforate hymen or agenesis of uterus/vagina)

    c. Tx

      (1) Hypothalamic → reversal of underlying cause and induction of ovulation with gonadotropins

      (2) Tumors → excision or bromocriptine for prolactinoma

      (3) Genital tract obstruction → surgery if possible

      (4) Ovarian dysfunction → exogenous estrogen replacement

2. Dysfunctional Uterine Bleeding

    a. Irregular menstruation without anatomic lesions of the uterus

b. **Usually due to chronic estrogen stimulation** (vs. amenorrhea, an estrogen deficient state), more rarely to genital outflow tract obstruction

c. Abnormal bleeding = bleeding at intervals <21 days or >36 days, lasting >7 days, or blood loss >80 mL

d. Menorrhagia (excessive bleeding) usually due to anovulation

e. Dx

   (1) Rule out anatomic causes of bleeding, including uterine fibroids, cervical or vaginal lesions or infxn, cervical and endometrial CA

   (2) Evaluate stress, exercise, weight changes, systemic dz such as thyroid, renal, or hepatic dz and coagulopathies, and pregnancy

f. Tx

   (1) Convert proliferative endometrium into secretory endometrium by administration of a progestational agent for 10 days

   (2) Alternative is to give OCPs that suppress the endometrium and establish regular, predictable cycles

   (3) NSAIDs ⊕ iron used in pts who want to preserve fertility

   (4) **Postmenopausal bleeding is CA until proven otherwise**

3. Hirsutism and Virilization (Table 3.12)

   a. Hirsutism = excess body hair, usually associated with acne, most commonly due to polycystic ovarian dz or adrenal hyperplasia

   b. Virilization = masculinization of a woman, associated with marked ↑ testosterone, clitoromegaly, temporal balding, voice deepening, breast involution, limb–shoulder girdle remodeling

4. Menopause

   a. Defined as the cessation of menses, **average age in US is 51 yrs**

   b. Suspect when menstrual cycles are not regular and predictable and when cycles are not associated with any premenstrual Sx

   c. Si/Sx = rapid onset hot flashes and sweating with resolution in 3 min, mood changes, sleep disturbances, vaginal dryness/atrophy, dyspareunia (painful intercourse), and osteoporosis

Table 3.12 Differential Diagnosis of Hirsutism and Virilization

Dz	Characteristics	Tx
Polycystic ovarian dz	• **#1 cause of androgen excess and hirsutism** • Etiology likely related to LH overproduction • Si/Sx = oligomenorrhea or amenorrhea, anovulation, infertility, hirsutism, acne • Labs →↑ **LH/FSH**, ↑ **testosterone**	• Break feedback cycle with OCPs → ↓ LH production • Weight loss may allow ovulation, sparing fertility • Refractory pts may require clomiphene to ovulate
Sertoli-Leydig cell tumor	• Ovarian tumors secreting testosterone, usually in women age 20–40 yrs • Si/Sx = **rapid onset** of hirsutism, acne, amenorrhea, virilization • Labs →↓ **LH/FSH**, ↑↑↑ **testosterone**	• Removal of involved ovary (tumors usually unilateral) • 10-yr survival = 90%–95%
Congenital adrenal hyperplasia	• Usually due to 21-α-hydroxylase defect • Autosomal recessive, variable penetrance • When severe → virilized newborn, milder forms can present at puberty or later • Labs →↑ **LH/FSH**, ↑ **DHEA**	• Glucocorticoids to suppress adrenal androgen production

DHEA, dehydroepiandrosterone.

    d. Dx = irregular menstrual cycles, hot flashes, and ↑ FSH level (>30 mIU/mL)

    e. Depending on clinical scenario, other labs should be conducted to exclude other Dx that can cause amenorrhea, such as thyroid dz, hyperprolactinemia, pregnancy

    f. Tx

       (1) **First line is estrogen hormone replacement Tx (HRT)**

       (2) HRT can consist of continuous estrogen with cyclic progestin to allow controlled withdrawal bleeding or daily administration of both estrogen and progestin, which does not cause withdrawal bleeding

       (3) HRT now is known to ↑ the risk of cardiovascular events (stroke and myocardial infarction) and may ↑ the risk of breast CA

    (4) Raloxifene

       (a) Second-generation tamoxifen-like drug = mixed estrogen agonist/antagonist, Food and Drug Administration (FDA) approved to prevent osteoporosis

       (b) Raloxifene shown to act like estrogen in bones (good), ↓ serum low-density lipoprotein (good), but does not stimulate endometrial growth (good; unlike tamoxifen and estrogen alone), also ↓ the risk of breast CA

    (5) Calcium supplements are not a substitute for estrogen replacement

5. Infertility

  a. Defined as failure to conceive after 1 yr of unprotected sex

  b. Affects 10%–15% of reproductive-age couples in the US

  c. Causes = abnormal spermatogenesis (40%), anovulation (30%), anatomic defects of the female reproductive tract (20%), unknown (10%)

  d. Dx

    (1) Start workup with male partner not only because it is the most common cause, but because the workup is simpler, noninvasive, and more cost-effective than infertility workup of the female

    (2) Nml semen excludes male cause in >90% of couples

    (3) Workup of female partner should include measurement of basal body temperature, which is an excellent screening test for ovulation

       (a) Temperature drops at time of menses, then rises 2 days after LH surge at the time of progesterone rise

       (b) Ovulation probably occurs 1 day before first temperature elevation and temperature remains elevated for 13–14 days

       (c) Temperature elevation >16 days suggests pregnancy

    (4) Anovulation

       (a) Hx of regular menses with premenstrual Sx (breast fullness, ↓ vaginal secretions, abd bloating, mood changes) strongly suggests ovulation

       (b) Sx such as irregular menses, amenorrhea episodes, hirsutism, acne, galactorrhea, suggest anovulation

       (c) FSH measured at Days 2–3 is best predictor of fertility potential in women, FSH >25 IU/L correlates with poor Px

    (d) Dx confirm with basal body temperature, serum progesterone ($\uparrow$ postovulation, >10 ng/mL → ovulation), endometrial Bx

   (5) Anatomic disorder

    (a) **Most commonly results from an acquired disorder, especially acute salpingitis 2° to *Neisseria gonorrhoeae* and *Chlamydia trachomatis***

    (b) Endometriosis, scarring, adhesions from pelvic inflammation or previous surgeries, tumors, and trauma can disrupt nml reproductive tract anatomy

    (c) Less commonly, a congenital anomaly such as septate uterus or reduplication of the uterus, cervix, or vagina is responsible

    (d) **Dx with hysterosalpingogram**

 e. Tx

  (1) Anovulation → restore ovulation with use of ovulation-inducing drugs

   (a) First line = clomiphene, an estrogen antagonist that relieves negative feedback on FSH, allowing follicle development

   (b) Anovulatory women who bleed in response to progesterone are candidates for clomiphene, as are women with irregular menses or midluteal progesterone levels <10 ng/mL

   (c) 40% get pregnant, 8%–10% $\uparrow$ rate of multiple births, mostly twins

   (d) If no response, FSH can be given directly → pregnancy rates of 60%–80%, multiple births occur at $\uparrow$ rate of 20%

  (2) Anatomic abnormalities → surgical lysis of pelvic adhesions

  (3) If endosalpinx is not intact and transport of ovum is not possible, an assisted fertilization technique, such as in vitro fertilization, may be used with 15%–25% success

C. Urogynecology

 1. Pelvic Relaxation and Urinary Incontinence

  a. $\uparrow$ Incidence with age, birth trauma, obesity, chronic cough

  b. Si/Sx = prolapse of urethra (urethrocele), uterus, bladder (cystocele), or rectum (rectocele), pelvic pressure and pain, dyspareunia, bowel and bladder dysfunction, and urinary incontinence

  c. Types of urinary incontinence (Figure 3.6)

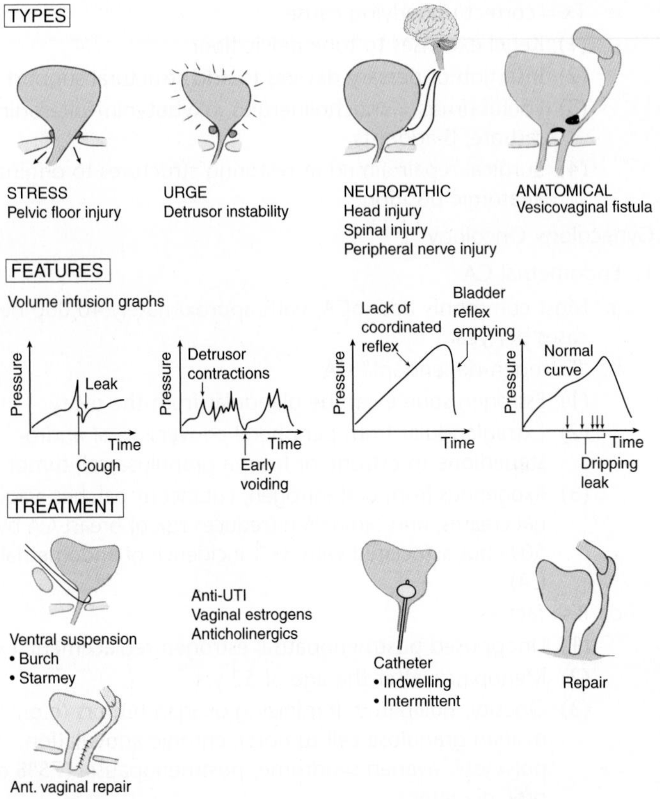

TYPES

STRESS
Pelvic floor injury

URGE
Detrusor instability

NEUROPATHIC
Head injury
Spinal injury
Peripheral nerve injury

ANATOMICAL
Vesicovaginal fistula

FEATURES

Volume infusion graphs

Cough

Detrusor
contractions

Early
voiding

Lack of
coordinated
reflex

Bladder
reflex
emptying

Normal
curve

Dripping
leak

TREATMENT

Ventral suspension
• Burch
• Starmey

Ant. vaginal repair

Anti-UTI
Vaginal estrogens
Anticholinergics

Catheter
• Indwelling
• Intermittent

Repair

FIGURE 3.6
Urinary incontinence.

OBSTETRICS AND
GYNECOLOGY

(1) Stress incontinence = bladder pressure exceeds ure-
thral pressure briefly at times of strain or stress, such as
coughing or laughing

(2) Urge incontinence and overflow incontinence result
from neuropathic bladder resulting in loss of control of
bladder function, resulting in involuntary bladder contraction (urge) or bladder atony (overflow)

d. Dx = urodynamic testing, assess for underlying medical conditions such as diabetes, neurologic dz, genitourinary surgery, pelvic irradiation, trauma, and medications that may
account for Sx

    e. Tx = correct underlying cause
      (1) Kegel exercises to tone pelvic floor
      (2) Insertion of pessary devices to add structural support
      (3) Useful drugs = anticholinergics, oxybutynin/tolterodine tartrate, β-agonists
      (4) Surgical repair aimed at restoring structures to original anatomic position

D. Gynecology Oncology
  1. Endometrial CA
    a. Most commonly adenoCA, with approximately 40,000 new cases per year
    b. "Estrogen-dependent" CA
      (1) Estrogen source can be glandular from the ovary
      (2) Extraglandular from peripheral conversion of androstenedione to estrone or from a granulosa cell tumor
      (3) Exogenous from oral estrogen, cutaneous patches, vaginal creams, and tamoxifen (reduces risk of breast CA by 50% but associated with 3× ↑ incidence of endometrial CA)
    c. Risk factors
      (1) Unopposed postmenopausal estrogen replacement Tx
      (2) Menopause after the age of 52 yrs
      (3) Obesity, nulliparity, feminizing ovarian tumors (e.g., ovarian granulosa cell tumors), chronic anovulation, polycystic ovarian syndrome, postmenopausal (75% of pts), diabetes
    d. Si/Sx = abnormal uterine bleeding, especially postmenopausal—any woman >35 yrs with abnormal uterine bleeding should have a sample of endometrium taken for histologic evaluation
    e. DDx = endometrial hyperplasia
      (1) Abnormal proliferation of both glandular and stromal elements, can be simple or complex
      (2) Atypical hyperplasia
        (a) Significant numbers of glandular elements that exhibit cytologic atypia and disordered maturation
        (b) Analogous to CA in situ (CIS) → 20%–30% risk for malignancy
    f. Dx
      (1) **Pap smear is NOT reliable in Dx of endometrial CA; however, if atypical glandular cells of undetermined**

significance (AGCUS) are found on the smear, then endometrial evaluation is mandatory

    (2) Bimanual exam for masses, nodularity, induration, and immobility

    (3) Endometrial Bx by ECC, D&C, hysteroscopy with directed Bx

  g. Tx

    (1) Simple or complex hyperplasia → progesterone to reverse hyperplastic process promoted by estrogen (e.g., Provera for 10 days)

    (2) Atypical hyperplasia → hysterectomy because of likelihood that it will become invasive endometrial CA

    (3) Endometrial CA

      (a) TAH/BSO, lymph node dissection

      (b) Adjuvant Tx may include external-beam radiation

      (c) Tx for recurrence is high-dose progestins (e.g., Depo-Provera)

  h. Px

    (1) **Most important prognostic factor is histologic grade**

    (2) G1 is highly differentiated, G2 is moderately differentiated, G3 is predominantly solid or entirely undifferentiated CA

    (3) **Depth of myometrial invasion is second most important Px factor**

    (4) Pt with G1 tumor that does not invade the myometrium has a 95% 5-yr survival, pt with G3 tumor with deep myometrial invasion has 5-yr survival rate closer to 20%

2. Uterine Leiomyomas = Fibroids

  a. Benign tumors, growth related to estrogen production, usually most rapid growth occurs perimenopausally

  b. Most common indication for hysterectomy (30% of cases)

  c. Si/Sx = bleeding (usually menorrhagia or ↑ amount and duration of flow), pelvic pressure, pelvic pain often manifested as dysmenorrhea

  d. Dx = Utz, confirm with tissue sample by either D&C or Bx (especially in postmenopausal pts)

  e. Tx

    (1) If Sx are mild → reassurance and observation

    (2) Medical Tx → estrogen inhibitors such as GnRH agonists shrink uterus, resulting in a simpler surgical

procedure or can be used as a temporizing measure until natural menopause occurs

    (3) Surgery → myomectomy indicated in young pts who want to preserve fertility (risk of intraoperative and post-operative hemorrhage ↑ compared to hysterectomy); hysterectomy is considered definitive Tx but should be reserved for symptomatic women who have completed childbearing

3. Leiomyosarcoma
   a. Rare malignancy accounting for only 3% of CA involving uterine corpus
   b. ↑ Suspicion for postmenopausal uterine enlargement
   c. Si/Sx suggestive of sarcoma = postmenopausal bleeding, pelvic pain, and ↑ vaginal discharge
   d. Tx = hysterectomy with intraoperative lymph node Bx
   e. Surgical staging same as that for endometrial adenoCA
   f. Survival rate is much lower than that for endometrial CA, only 50% of pts survive at 5 yr
   g. Adjunctive therapies are of minimal benefit

4. Cervical CA
   a. Pap smear and liquid-based cytology are the most impor-tant screening tools available to detect dz
   b. Risk factors = early sexual intercourse, multiple sexual partners, HPV infxn (especially Types 16, 18), cigarette smoking, early childbearing, and immunocompromised pts
   c. Average age at Dx = 50 yrs but can occur much earlier
   d. 85% are of squamous cell origin, 15% are adenoCA arising from endocervical glands
   e. Si/Sx = postcoital bleeding, but there is no classic presenta-tion for cervical CA
   f. Dx = Pap screening, any visible cervical lesion should be Bx
   g. Tx
       (1) Local dz → hysterectomy + lymph node dissection—ovaries may remain → survival >70% at 5 yr
       (2) Extensive or metastatic dz → pelvic irradiation → survival <40% at 5 yr
   h. Prevention—see HPV vaccine, Section II.A.4

5. Ovarian Neoplasms (Table 3.13)

Table 3.13 Ovarian Neoplasms

Neoplasm	Characteristics	Tx
Benign Cysts	• Functional growth resulting from failure of nml follicle to rupture • Si/Sx = pelvic pain or pressure, rupture of cyst → acute severe pain and hemorrhage mimicking acute abdomen • Confirm cyst with Utz	• Typically self-limiting • Rupture may require laparotomy to stop bleeding
Benign Tumors: (more common than malignant, but risk of malignancy ↑ with age)		
Epithelial cell	• Serous cystadenoma most common type, almost always benign unless bilateral →↑ risk of malignancy • Other types = mucinous, endometrioid, Brenner tumors, all rarely malignant • Dx = clinical, can see on CT/MRI	• Surgical excision
Germ cell	• Teratoma is most common (also called "dermoid cyst") • Very rarely malignant, contain differentiated tissue from all three embryologic germ layers • Si/Sx = unilateral cystic, mobile, nontender adnexal mass, often aSx • Dx confirmed with Utz	• Excision to prevent ovarian torsion or rupture
Stromal cell	• Functional tumors secreting hormones • Granulosa tumor makes estrogens → gynecomastia, loss of body hair, etc. • Sertoli–Leydig cells make androgens, virilize females	• Excision
Malignant Tumors		

• Usually occur in women >50 yr
• Risk factors = low parity, ↓ fertility, delayed childbearing—**OCP use is a protective factor**
• Ovarian is the most lethal gynecologic CA due to lack of early detection →↑ rate of metastasis (60% at Dx)
• Dz typically are aSx until extensive metastasis has occurred
• Can follow dz with CA-125 marker, not specific enough for screening
• Yearly pelvic exams remain most effective screening tool
• Si/Sx = vague abd/pelvic complaints, e.g., distention, early satiety, constipation, pelvic pain, urinary frequency; shortness of breath due to pleural effusion may be only presenting Sx
• Tx = debulking surgery with chemotherapy and radiotherapy

(continued)

OBSTETRICS AND GYNECOLOGY

Table 3.13	Continued	
Neoplasm	**Characteristics**	**Tx**
Malignant Tumors (continued)		
Epithelial cell	• Cause 90% of all ovarian malignancies • Serous cystadenocarcinoma is most common, often originate from benign precursors • Others = endometrioma and mucinous cystadenoma	• Excision
Germ cell	• Most common ovarian CA in women <20 yrs • Can produce hCG or AFP, useful as tumor markers • Subtypes = dysgerminoma, which is very radiosensitive, and immature teratoma	• Radiation first-line • Chemotherapy second-line • 5-yr survival >80% for both
Stromal cell	• Granulosa cell makes estrogen, can result in 2° endometriosis or endometrial CA • Sertoli-Leydig tumor makes androgens	• Total hysterectomy with oophorectomy

6. Vulvar and Vaginal CA
   a. Vulvar intraepithelial neoplasia (VIN)
      (1) VIN I and II = mild and moderate dysplasia, ↑ risk progressing to advanced stages and then CA
      (2) VIN III = CIS
      (3) Si/Sx = pruritus, irritation, presence of raised lesion
      (4) Dx = Bx for definitive Dx
      (5) DDx includes Paget's dz, malignant melanoma
      (6) Tx = excision, local for VIN I and II and wide for VIN III
   b. Vulvar CA
      (1) 90% are squamous
      (2) Usually presents postmenopausally
      (3) Si/Sx = pruritus, with or without presence of ulcerative lesion
      (4) Tx = excision
      (5) 5-yr survival rate is 70%–90% depending on nodal status; if deep pelvic nodes are involved, survival is a dismal 20%
   c. Vaginal CIS and CA are very rare
      (1) 70% of pts with vaginal CIS have either previous or coexistent genital tract neoplasm

       (2) Tx = radiation, surgery reserved for women with extensive dz

7. Gestational Trophoblastic Neoplasia (GTN) = Hydatidiform Mole or Molar Pregnancy

   a. Rare variation of pregnancy in which a neoplasm is derived from abnormal placental tissue (trophoblastic) proliferation

   b. Usually a benign dz called a "molar pregnancy"

      (1) A complete mole (90%) has no fetus and is 46 XX

      (2) An incomplete mole has a fetus and molar degeneration, and is 69 XXY

   c. Persistent or malignant dz develops in 20% of pts (mostly in complete moles)

   d. Si/Sx = exaggerated pregnancy Sx, with missing fetal heart tones and enlarged uterus (size > dates), painless bleeding commonly occurs in early second trimester

   e. Pts can present with PIH

   f. Dx = Utz and ↑↑↑ hCG levels

   g. Tx = removal of uterine contents by D&C and suction curettage

   h. Non-metastatic persistent GTN is treated with methotrexate

   i. Follow-up = check that hCG levels are appropriately dropping

   j. Contraception is recommended during first year of follow-up

4. PEDIATRICS

I. Development

A. **Developmental Milestones** (see Table 4.1)

B. **Puberty** (see Table 4.2)

II. Infections

A. **ToRCHS** (see Table 4.3)

B. **Infant Botulism**

1. Acute, flaccid paralysis caused by *Clostridium botulinum* neurotoxin that irreversibly blocks acetylcholine release from peripheral neurons

2. Dz acquired via **ingestion of spores in honey** or via inhalation of spores

3. 95% cases in infants aged 3 wks to 6 mos, peak 2–4 mos

4. Si/Sx = constipation, lethargy, poor feeding, weak cry, ↓ spontaneous movement, hypotonia, drooling, ↓ gag and suck reflexes, as dz progresses → **loss of head control and respiratory arrest**

5. Dx = clinical, **based on acute onset of flaccid descending paralysis with clear sensorium, without fever or paresthesias,** can confirm by demonstrating botulinum toxin in serum or toxin/organism in feces

6. Tx = intubate, supportive care, no antibiotics or antitoxin needed in infants

C. **Exanthems** (see Table 4.4)

D. **Vaccinations** (see Figure 4.1)

III. Respiratory Disorders

A. **Otitis Media (OM)**

1. Defined as inflammation of middle ear space

   a. Dx = fever, erythema of tympanic membrane (TM), bulging of the pars flaccida portion of the TM, opacity of the TM, otalgia

Text continues on page 271

Table 4.1 Developmental Milestones

Age	Gross Motor	Fine Motor	Language	Social/ Cognition
Newborn	Head side to side, **Moro (startle) and grasp reflex**			
2 mos	Holds head up	Swipes at object	Coos	Social smile
4 mos	Rolls front to back	**Grasps object**	Orients to voice	Laughs
6 mos	Rolls back to front, **sits upright**	Transfers object	Babbles	**Stranger anxiety, sleeps all night**
9 mos	Crawl, pull to stand	**Pincer grasp, eats with fingers**	**Mama-dada (non-specific)**	Waves bye-bye, responds to name
12 mos	**Stands**	**Mature pincer**	**Mama-dada (specific)**	Picture book
15 mos	**Walks**	Uses cup	4–6 words	**Temper tantrum**
18 mos	Throws ball, walks up stairs	Uses spoon for solids	Names common objects	**Toilet training may begin**
24 mos	Runs, up/down stairs	Uses spoons for semisolids	**2-word sentence** (2 words at 2 yrs)	Follows 2-step command
36 mos	Rides tricycle	Eats neatly with utensils	**3-word sentence** (3 words at 3 yrs)	Knows first and last names

Table 4.2 Tanner Stages

Boys	Girls
Testicular enlargement at 11.5 yrs[a]	Breast buds at 10.5 yrs[a]
↑ in genital size	Pubic hair
Pubic hair	Linear growth spurt at 12 yrs
Peak growth spurt at 13.5 yrs[a]	Menarche at 12.5 yrs[a]

[a]Yrs represent population averages.

Table 4.3 The ToRCHS

Dz	Characteristics
Toxoplasmosis	• Acquired in mothers via ingestion of poorly cooked meat or through contact with cat feces • Carriers common (10%–30%) in population, only causes neonatal dz if acquired during pregnancy (1%) • One-third of women who acquire during pregnancy transmit infxn to fetus, and one-third of fetuses are clinically affected • Sequelae = intracerebral calcifications, hydrocephalus, chorioretinitis, microcephaly, severe mental retardation, epilepsy, intrauterine growth retardation (IUGR), hepatosplenomegaly • Screening is useless because acquisition prior to birth is common and clinically irrelevant • Pregnant women should be told to avoid undercooked meat, wash hands after handling cat, do not change litter box • If fetal infxn established → Utz to determine major anomalies and provide counseling regarding termination if indicated
Rubella	• First-trimester maternal rubella infxn → 80% chance of fetal transmission • Second trimester → 50% chance of transmission to fetus; third trimester → 5% • Si/Sx of fetus = IUGR, cataracts, glaucoma, chorioretinitis, PDA, pulmonary stenosis, atrial or ventricular septal defect, myocarditis, microcephaly, **hearing loss, "blueberry muffin rash,"** mental retardation • Dx confirmed with IgM rubella antibody in neonate's serum or viral culture • Tx = prevention by universal immunization of all children against rubella; there is no effective therapy for active infxn
Cytomegalovirus (CMV)	• Number one congenital infxn, affecting 1% of births • Transmitted through bodily fluids/secretions, infxn often aSx • 1° seroconversion during pregnancy →↑ risk of severely affected infant, but congenital infxn can occur if mother reinfected during pregnancy • Approximately 1% risk of transplacental transmission of infxn, approximately 10% of infected infants manifest congenital defects of varying severity • Congenital defects = microcephaly, intracranial calcifications, severe mental retardation, chorioretinitis, IUGR • 10%–15% of aSx, but exposed infants develop later neurologic sequelae

Table 4.3 *Continued*	
Dz	**Characteristics**
Herpes simplex virus	• **C-section delivery for pregnant women with active herpes** • Vaginal → 50% chance that the baby will acquire the infxn and is associated with significant morbidity and mortality • Si/Sx = vesicles, seizures, respiratory distress can cause pneumonia, meningitis, encephalitis → impaired neurologic development after resolution • Tx = acyclovir (↓ mortality)
Syphilis	• Transmission from infected mother to infant during pregnancy nearly 100%, **occurs after the first trimester in the vast majority of cases** • Fetal/perinatal deaths in 40% of affected infants • Early manifestations in first 2 yrs, later manifestations in next two decades • Si/Sx of early dz = jaundice,↑ liver function tests, hepatosplenomegaly, hemolytic anemia, rash followed by desquamation of hands and feet, wartlike lesions of mucous membranes, **blood-tinged nasal secretions (snuffles), diffuse osteochondritis, saddle nose (2° to syphilitic rhinitis)** • Si/Sx of late dz = **Hutchinson teeth** (notching of permanent upper two incisors), mulberry molars (both at 6 yrs), bone thickening (frontal bossing), **anterior bowing of tibia (saber shins)** • Dx = Rapid plasma regain/Venereal Dz Research Laboratory (RPR/VDRL) and fluorescence treponemal antigen (FTA) serologies in mother with clinical findings in infant • Tx = Procaine Penicillin G 50,000 units/kg dose IM × 10 days

b. Effusions can also be seen as meniscus of fluid behind the TM indicative of poor pressure equalization by eustachian tubes

c. OM with effusion common in young children because of their eustachian tubes being smaller and more horizontal, making drainage and pressure equalization more difficult

d. Pathogens = *Streptococcus pneumoniae, Hemophilus influenzae, Moraxella catarrhalis*

e. Also commonly caused by viral pathogens

f. Tx = amoxicillin or azithromycin (first line), augmented penicillins or TMP-SMX (second line)

Text continues on page 275

Table 4.4 Viral Exanthems

Dz/Virus	Si/Sx
Measles (Rubeola)/ Paramyxovirus	• Erythematous maculopapular rash, **erupts 5 days after onset of prodromal Sx, begins on head and spreads to body, lasting 4–5 days,** resolving from head downward • **Koplik spots (white spots on buccal mucosa) are pathognomonic** but leave before rash starts, so often not found when pt presents • **Dx = fever and Hx of the 3 Cs: cough, coryza, conjunctivitis**
Rubella (German measles)/ Togavirus	• **Suboccipital lymphadenopathy** (very few dzs do this) • Maculopapular rash begins on face then generalizes • Rash lasts 5 days, fever may accompany rash on first day only • May find reddish spots of various sizes on soft palate
Hand, foot, and mouth dz/ Coxsackie A virus	• Vesicular rash on hands and feet with ulcerations in mouth • Rash clears in approximately 1 wk • Contagious by contact
Roseola infantum (Exanthem subitum)/HHV-6	• **Abrupt high fever persisting for 1–5 days even though child has no physical Sx to account for fever and does not feel ill** • When fever drops, macular or maculopapular rash appears on trunk and then spreads peripherally over entire body, lasts 24 hrs
Erythema infectiosum (fifth dz)/ Parvovirus B19	• **Classic sign = "slapped cheeks,"** erythema of the cheeks • Subsequently an erythematous maculopapular rash spreads from arms to trunk and legs, forming a reticular pattern • **Dz is dangerous in sickle cell pts (and other anemias) because of tendency of parvovirus B19 to cause aplastic crises** • **Beware of exposure to pregnant mothers because of high risk of fetal complications**
Varicella (chickenpox)/ Varicella zoster virus (VZV)	• Highly contagious, crops of pruritic "teardrop" vesicles that break and crust over, start on face or trunk (centripetal) and spread to extremities • New lesions appear for 3–5 days and typically take 3 days to crust over, so rash persists for approximately 1 wk • **Lesions are contagious until they crust over** • Zoster (shingles) = reactivation of old varicella infxn, painful skin eruptions are seen along the distribution of dermatomes that correspond to the affected dorsal root ganglia

Dx = clinical for all; Tx = supportive for all.
HHV-6, human herpes virus 6.

Recommended Immunization Schedule for Persons Aged 0 Through 6 Years—United States • 2011

For those who fall behind or start late, see the catch-up schedule

Vaccine ▼ Age ▶	Birth	1 month	2 months	4 months	6 months	12 months	15 months	18 months	19–23 months	2–3 years	4–6 years
Hepatitis B[1]	HepB	HepB			HepB						
Rotavirus[2]			RV	RV	RV[2]						
Diphtheria, Tetanus, Pertussis[3]			DTaP	DTaP	DTaP	see footnote[3]	DTaP				DTaP
Haemophilus influenzae type b[4]			Hib	Hib	Hib[4]	Hib					
Pneumococcal[5]			PCV	PCV	PCV	PCV				PPSV	
Inactivated Poliovirus[6]			IPV	IPV		IPV					IPV
Influenza[7]						Influenza (Yearly)					
Measles, Mumps, Rubella[8]						MMR		see footnote[8]			MMR
Varicella[9]						Varicella		see footnote[9]			Varicella
Hepatitis A[10]						HepA (2 doses)				HepA Series	
Meningococcal[11]										MCV4	

Range of recommended ages for all children

Range of recommended ages for certain high-risk groups

This schedule includes recommendations in effect as of December 21, 2010. Any dose not administered at the recommended age should be administered at a subsequent visit, when indicated and feasible. The use of a combination vaccine generally is preferred over separate injections of its equivalent component vaccines. Considerations should include provider assessment, patient preference, and the potential for adverse events. Providers should consult the relevant Advisory Committee on Immunization Practices statement for detailed recommendations: http://www.cdc.gov/vaccines/pubs/acip-list.htm. Clinically significant adverse events that follow immunization should be reported to the Vaccine Adverse Event Reporting System (VAERS) at http://www.vaers.hhs.gov or by telephone, 800-822-7967. Use of trade names and commercial sources is for identification only and does not imply endorsement by the U.S. Department of Health and Human Services.

FIGURE 4.1

Immunization schedules. (Courtesy of www.cdc.gov/vaccines/recs/schedules.) (continued)

Recommended Immunization Schedule for Persons Aged 7 Through 18 Years—United States • 2011

For those who fall behind or start late, see the schedule below and the catch-up schedule

Vaccine ▼ Age ▶	7–10 years	11–12 years	13–18 years
Tetanus, Diphtheria, Pertussis[1]		Tdap	Tdap
Human Papillomavirus[2]	see footnote 2	HPV (3 doses)(females)	HPV Series
Meningococcal[3]	MCV4	MCV4	MCV4
Influenza[4]		Influenza (Yearly)	
Pneumococcal[5]		Pneumococcal	
Hepatitis A[6]		HepA Series	
Hepatitis B[7]		Hep B Series	
Inactivated Poliovirus[8]		IPV Series	
Measles, Mumps, Rubella[9]		MMR Series	
Varicella[10]		Varicella Series	

Range of recommended ages for all children

Range of recommended ages for catch-up immunization

Range of recommended ages for certain high-risk groups

This schedule includes recommendations in effect as of December 21, 2010. Any dose not administered at the recommended age should be administered at a subsequent visit, when indicated and feasible. The use of a combination vaccine generally is preferred over separate injections of its equivalent component vaccines. Considerations should include provider assessment, patient preference, and the potential for adverse events. Providers should consult the relevant Advisory Committee on Immunization Practices statement for detailed recommendations: **http://www.cdc.gov/vaccines/pubs/acip-list.htm**. Clinically significant adverse events that follow immunization should be reported to the Vaccine Adverse Event Reporting System (VAERS) at **http://www.vaers.hhs.gov** or by telephone, **800-822-7967.**

FIGURE 4.1 *(continued)*

g. If chronic effusions or repeated infxns are present, surgical placement of pressure equalization tubes may be indicated

h. Note: Adults with unilateral serous effusion need to have a nasopharyngeal mass ruled out

i. Complication of OM and mastoiditis

(1) Intracranial-subdural abscess, epidural abscess, temporal lobe abscess, lateral sinus thrombosis, meningitis

(2) Extracranial-facial paralysis, labrynthitis, and subperiosteal abscess

(3) Subperiosteal abscess

(a) Bezold's abscess = infxn penetrates tip of mastoid and pus travels along sternocleidomastoid muscle and forms an abscess in posterior triangle of neck

(b) Postauricular abscess = most common subperiosteal abscess, occurs posterior to auricle, displacing ear forward

(4) Ear, nose, and throat (ENT) consult for surgical drainage and IV antibiotics

2. Bullous Myringitis

a. Associated with *Mycoplasma* infxn

b. Presents with large blebs on tympanic membrane

c. Tx = Azithromycin

3. Unilateral Serous OM

a. Presents in adults, caused by nasopharyngeal masses obstructing the Eustachian tube

b. Dx = MRI of head, endoscopic visualization, and bx

B. **Bronchiolitis**

1. Commonly seen in children age <2 yrs, peak incidence at 6 mos

2. **50% because of respiratory syncytial virus (RSV);** others include parainfluenzae and adenovirus

3. Si/Sx = mild rhinorrhea and fever progress to cough, wheezing with crackles, tachypnea, nasal flaring, ↓ appetite

4. Dx by culture or antigen detection of nasopharyngeal secretions

5. Tx = bronchodilators, oxygen (O_2) as needed

C. **Upper Respiratory Dz** (see Table 4.5; Figures 4.2 and 4.3A)

D. **Pneumonia**

1. Common etiologies vary with age

a. Newborns get *Streptococcus agalactiae* (group B *Streptococcus*), Gram-negative rod, *Chlamydia trachomatis*

Text continues on page 278

Table 4.5 Pediatric Upper Respiratory Disorders

Dz	Cause	Si/Sx	Labs	Tx
Croup (Laryngotracheo-bronchitis)	Para-influenza, influenza, RSV, *Mycoplasma*	**Presents in fall and winter, 3 mos to 3 yrs old, barking cough, inspiratory stridor, Sx worse at night,** hoarse voice, preceded by URI	**Neck X-ray → "steeple sign"** (Figure 4.2)	O₂, cool mist, racemic epinephrine (Epi) and steroids if severe, ribavirin may be used for immuno-compromised
Pertussis	*Bordetella pertussis*	**Pertussis presents with 3 stages:** (1) Catarrhal stage = 1–2 wks of cough, rhinorrhea, wheezing; (2) Paroxysmal stage = 2–4 wks of paroxysmal cough with **"whoops";** (3) convales-cent stage = 1–2 wks of persistent chronic cough; can also cause chronic cough in adults	DFA or serology, culture on Bordet–Gengou medium	Macrolide to shorten infectious period, does not affect duration of Sx, otherwise supportive

Table 4.5 *Continued*

Dz	Cause	Si/Sx	Labs	Tx
Epiglottitis	*H. influenzae* type B	**Medical emergency! Fulminant inspiratory stridor, drooling, sits leaning forward** (Figure 4.3A), dysphagia, "hot potato" voice—very rare now in the era of vaccination	**"Thumb print" sign on lateral neck film** (Figure 4.3B), cherry-red epiglottitis on endoscopy	**Examine pt in OR,** intubate as needed, ceftriaxone
Bacterial tracheitis	*Staphylococcus* and *Streptococcus.* spp.	Inspiratory stridor, high fever, toxic appearing	Leukocytosis	Vancomycin or ceftriaxone
Foreign-body aspiration		**Usually presents after age 6 mos** (need to grasp object to inhale it) with **inspiratory stridor** (chronic) wheeze, ↓ breath sounds, dysphagia, unresolved pneumonia	CXR → hyperinflation on affected side	Endoscopic or surgical removal

URI, upper respiratory infxn.

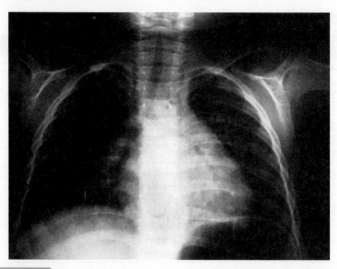

FIGURE 4.2

The "steeple sign" in the soft tissue of the neck on X-ray in a child with croup. (From Harwood-Nuss A, Wolfson AB, Linden CH, et al. *The clinical practice of emergency medicine*, 3rd Ed. Philadelphia, PA: Lippincott Williams & Wilkins, 2001.)

  b. Infants get *S. pneumoniae, H. influenzae, Chlamydia, Staphylococcus aureus, Listeria monocytogenes,* and viral

  c. Preschoolers get RSV, other viruses, and *Mycoplasma*

  d. Adolescents get *S. pneumoniae, Mycoplasma,* and *Chlamydia*

 2. Si/Sx = cough (productive in older children), fevers, nausea/ vomiting, diarrhea, tachypnea, grunting, retractions, crackles

 3. *Chlamydia* causes classic "staccato cough" and conjunctivitis, pts afebrile

 4. RSV causes wet cough, often with audible wheezes

 5. *Staphylococcus* infxns may be associated with skin lesions

 6. Dx = rapid antigen detection or culture of secretions, CXR → infiltrates

 7. Tx = infants get hospitalized, bronchodilators and O_2 for RSV, erythromycin for atypical dz (e.g., *Chlamydia, Mycoplasma*), cefuroxime for bacteria

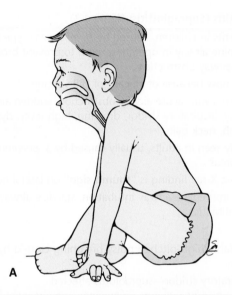

A

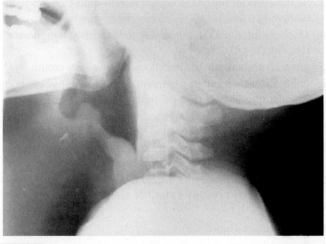

FIGURE 4.3

A. Classic posture of a child with epiglottitis, sitting forward on hands, mouth open, tongue out, head forward and tilted up in a sniffing position in an effort to relieve the acute airway obstruction. (From Nettina SM. *The Lippincott manual of nursing practice,* 7th Ed. Lippincott Williams & Wilkins, 2001.)
B. Epiglottitis on lateral neck X-ray. Note the classic "thumb print" sign below the jaw. (From Harwood-Nuss A, Wolfson AB, Linden CH, et al. *The clinical practice of emergency medicine,* 3rd Ed. Philadelphia, PA: Lippincott Williams & Wilkins, 2001.)

E. **Epiglottitis (Supraglottitis;** Figure 4.3)

1. Presents in children, caused by *H. influenzae* type B (HiB). Examine airway in operating room to prevent bronchospasm and airway obstruction

2. Rare now because of efficacy of HiB vaccine

3. Presents with acute airway obstruction, sudden airway emergency, inspiratory stridor, drooling, high fever, dysphagia, no cough, neck pain

4. Rarely seen in adults, usually caused by *S. pneumoniae* or *S. aureus*

5. Classic X-ray finding is **"thumb sign"** on lateral neck film

6. Tx = immediate airway intubation, stabilize airway and observe, IV antibiotics

F. **Stridor**

1. Laudable high-pitched noisy breathing caused by air turbulence

2. Inspiratory stridor—supraglottis affected

3. Biphasic stridor (inspiratory/expiratory)—glottic or subglottic narrowing

4. Most common pediatric noninfectious cause—laryngomalacia (see Figure 4.4)

5. Most common pediatric infectious cause is viral croup

6. Other causes—subglottic hemangioma, polyps, foreign body, vascular rings. Vocal cord paralysis

7. Tx = stabilize airway. Humidified O_2, steroids, and nebulized racemic epinephrine as needed

8. ENT consult, X-ray, lateral neck and chest X-ray, and airway fluoroscopy, to evaluate airway if stable

9. Immediate stabilization of airway if unstable, direct laryngoscopy and bronchoscopy to further evaluate airway once pt stabilized

G. **Adenoiditis** (see Figure 4.5)

1. Commonly seen in young children

2. Si/Sx = frequent OM episodes, snoring at night, constant mouth breathers, constant nasal congestion, and hypernasal voice

3. Pts develop adenoid facies from always having mouth open

4. Tx = surgical removal of adenoids

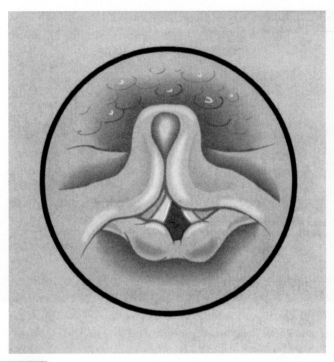

FIGURE 4.4

Laryngomalacia.

IV. Musculoskeletal

A. **Genu valgum** (Figure 4.6)

1. Commonly called **"knock-knees"**

2. A condition where the knee angle in and touch one another when the legs are straightened.

3. Mild genu valgum can be seen in children from ages 2–5, and is often corrected naturally as children grow.

4. Most mild cases will self-correct in young children but braces can be used.

5. If condition persists to adulthood, corrective orthopedic surgery may be indicated.

B. **Genu varum**

1. Commonly called **"bow-leggedness"**

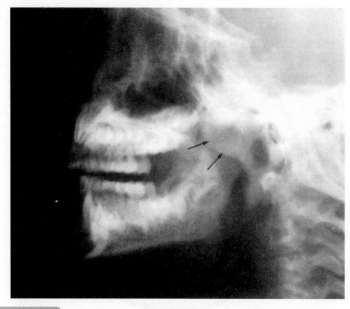

FIGURE 4.5
A lateral soft-tissue X-ray showing adenoid enlargement.

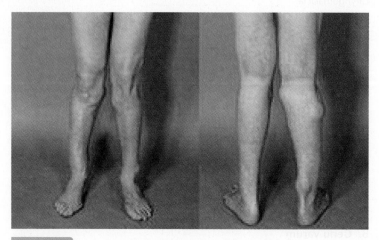

FIGURE 4.6
Genu valgum.

2. A condition where the physical deformity marked by (outward bowing) of the leg in relation to the thigh, giving the appearance of an archer's bow

3. Can be caused by Rickets

4. Treatment: Treat underlying disease if any. Can be a normal variant in children <4 yrs old. If persists past 4 yrs old may require splints or braces. Consider orthopedic surgery referral if persists despite conservative management.

C. **Limp**

1. Painful limp usually is acute onset, may be associated with fever and irritability, toddlers may refuse to walk

2. DDx painful limp (see Table 4.6; Figure 4.7)

3. Painless limp usually has insidious onset, may be because of weakness or deformity of limb 2° to developmental hip dysplasia, cerebral palsy, or leg-length discrepancy

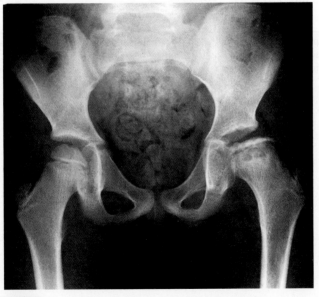

FIGURE 4.7

X-ray film of the hips of a 5-yr-old child with Legg–Calvé–Perthes dz. Note the ↑ density, flattening, and fragmentation of the left capital femoral epiphysis.

Table 4.6 Pediatric Painful Limp

Dz	Characteristics	Tx
Septic arthritis	• Number one **cause of painful limp in 1–3 yrs old** • Usually monoarticular hip, knee, or ankle • Causes = S. aureus **(most common)**, H. influenzae, Neisseria gonorrhoeae • Si/Sx = **acute-onset pain**, arthritis, fever, ↓ range of motion, child may lie still and refuse to walk or crawl, ↑ **WBC**, ↑ **ESR** • X-ray → joint space widening • Dx = joint aspiration → **WBC ≥10,000 with neutrophil predominance,** low glucose	Tx = drainage, antibiotics appropriate to Gram stain or cultures
Toxic synovitis	• Most common in boys who are 5–10 yrs old, may precede viral URI • Si/Sx = **insidious onset pain**, low-grade fever, **WBC and ESR nml** • **Typically no tenderness, warmth, or joint swelling** • X-ray → usually nml • Dx → technetium scan → ↑ **uptake of epiphysis**	Rest and analgesics synovitis for 3–5 days
Aseptic avascular necrosis	• Legg–Calvé–Perthes dz = head of femur, Osgood–Schlatter = tibial tubercle, Köhler's bone dz = navicular bone • Legg–Calvé–Perthes → usually 4–9 yrs old (boys/girls = 5:1), bilateral in 10%–20% of cases, ↑ incidence with delayed growth and ↓ birth weight • Si/Sx = **afebrile, insidious-onset hip pain, inner thigh, or knee,** ↑ pain with movement, ↓ with rest, antalgic gait, **nml WBC and ESR** • X-ray → **femoral head sclerosis** ↑ width of femoral neck (see Figure 4.7) • Dx → technetium scan → ↓ **uptake in epiphysis**	↓ Weight bearing on affected side over long time

Table 4.6 *Continued*		
Dz	**Characteristics**	**Tx**
Slipped capital femoral epiphysis	• Often in **obese male adolescents** (8–17 yrs old), 20%–30% bilateral • 80% → slow, progressive, 20% → acute, associated with trauma • Si/Sx → **dull, aching pain** in hip or knee, ↑ pain with activity • X-ray → lateral movement of femur shaft in relation to femoral head, looks like **"ice-cream scoop falling off cone"** • Dx = clinical	Surgical pinning
Osteomyelitis	• Neonates → *S. aureus* (50%), *S. agalactiae*, *Escherichia coli* • Children → *Staphylococcus*, *Streptococcus*, *Salmonella* (sickle cell) • Si/Sx young infants → fever may be only symptom • Si/Sx older children → fever, malaise, ↓ extremity movement, edema • X-ray lags changes by 3–4 wks • Dx → neutrophilic leukocytosis, ↑ ESR (50%), blood cultures, bone scan (90% sensitive), **MRI is the gold standard**	Antibiotics for 4–6 wks

D. **Collagen Vascular Dz**

1. Juvenile Rheumatoid Arthritis
   a. Chronic inflammation of ≥1 joints in pt ≤16 yrs old
   b. Most common in children aged 1–4 yrs; females > males
   c. Three categories = systemic, pauciarticular, polyarticular (see Table 4.7)
   d. Dx = Sx persists for three consecutive months with exclusion of other causes of acute/chronic arthritis or collagen vascular dz
   e. Tx = nonsteroidal anti-inflammatory drugs (NSAIDs), low-dose methotrexate, prednisone only in acute febrile onset

2. Kawasaki's Dz (Mucocutaneous Lymph Node Syndrome)
   a. Large- and medium-vessel vasculitis in children, usually under <5 yrs, predilection for Japanese children

Table 4.7 Types of Juvenile Rheumatoid Arthritis

Systemic Still's dz (10%–20%)	• High, spiking fevers with return to nml daily, generalized lymphadenopathy • Rash of small, pale pink macules with central pallor on trunk and proximal extremities with possible involvement of palms and soles • Rash classically appears with fever and wanes as fever goes away • Joint involvement may not occur for weeks to months after fever • One-third have disabling chronic arthritis
Pauciarticular (40%–60%)	• Involves ≤4 joints, large joints primarily affected (knees, ankles, elbows, asymmetric) • Other Si/Sx = fever, malaise, anemia, lymphadenopathy, **chronic joint dz is unusual** • Divided into two types ◊ Type 1 (most common) → girls <4 yrs old, ↑ risk for chronic iridocyclitis, 90% antinuclear antibody (ANA)+ ◊ Type 2 → boys >8 yrs old, ANA2, 75% HLA-B271, ↑ risk of ankylosing spondylitis or Reiter's later in life
Polyarticular	• ≥5 joints involved, small and large, insidious onset, fever, lethargy, anemia • Two types depending on whether rheumatoid factor is present • Rheumatoid factor ⊕ → 80% girls late onset, more severe, rheumatoid nodules present, 75% ANA+ • Rheumatoid factor 2 → occurs any time during childhood, mild, rarely associated with rheumatoid nodules, 25% ANA+

  b. Dx = fever >104°F (40°C) for >5 days, unresponsive to antibiotics, ⊕ 4 of 5 of the following criteria (**mnemonic: CRASH**):
    (1) **C**onjunctivitis
    (2) **R**ash, primarily truncal
    (3) **A**neurysms of coronary arteries
    (4) **S**trawberry tongue, crusting of lips, fissuring of mouth, and oropharyngeal erythema
    (5) **H**ands and feet show induration, erythema of palms and soles, desquamation of fingers and toes
  c. Complications = cardiac involvement; 10%–40% of untreated cases show evidence of coronary vasculitis (dilation/aneurysm) within first weeks of illness

    d. Tx = IVIG to prevent coronary vasculitis, **high-dose aspi-rin—prednisone is contraindicated and will exacerbate the dz!**

    e. Px

      (1) Response to IVIG and aspirin is rapid, two-thirds of the pts afebrile within 24 hrs

      (2) Evaluate pts 1 wk after discharge, repeat echocardiography 3–6 wks after onset of fever; if baseline and repeat echo do not detect any coronary abnormalities, further imaging is unnecessary

  3. Henoch–Schönlein Purpura

    a. Immunoglobulin IgA small-vessel vasculitis, related to IgA nephropathy (Berger's dz)

    b. Si/Sx = **pathognomonic palpable purpura** on legs and but-tocks (in children), abd pain, may cause intussusception

    c. Tx = self-limited, rarely progresses to glomerulonephritis

E. **Histiocytosis X**

  1. Proliferation of histiocytic cells resembling Langerhans' skin cells

  2. Three common variants

    a. Letterer–Siwe dz

      (1) Acute, aggressive, disseminated variant, usually fatal in infants

      (2) Si/Sx = hepatosplenomegaly, lymphadenopathy, pancy-topenia, lung involvement, recurrent infxns

    b. Hand–Schüller–Christian dz

      (1) Chronic progressive variant, presents prior to age 5 yrs

      (2) **Classic triad = skull lesions, diabetes insipidus, exophthalmus**

    c. Eosinophilic granuloma

      (1) Extraskeletal involvement generally limited to lung

      (2) Has the best Px, rarely fatal, sometimes spontaneously regresses

V. Metabolic

A. **Congenital Hypothyroidism**

  1. Because of 2° agenesis of thyroid or defect in enzymes

  2. **T_4 during first 2 yrs of life is crucial for nml brain development**

  3. Birth Hx → nml Apgar score, prolonged jaundice (fi indirect bilirubin)

4. Si/Sx = presents at age 6–12 wks with poor feeding, lethargy, **hypotonia, coarse facial features, large protruding tongue,** hoarse cry, constipation, developmental delay

5. Dx = $\downarrow T_4$, $\uparrow$ thyroid-stimulating hormone

6. Tx = levothyroxine replacement

7. **If Dx delayed beyond 6 wks, child will be mentally retarded**

8. Newborn screening is mandatory by law

B. **Newborn Jaundice**

1. Physiologic jaundice is clinically benign, occurs 24–48 hrs after birth

   a. Characterized by unconjugated hyperbilirubinemia

   b. 50% of neonates have jaundice during first week of life

   c. Results from $\uparrow$ bilirubin production and relative deficiency in glucuronyl transferase in the immature liver

   d. Requires no Tx

2. **Jaundice present AT birth is ALWAYS pathologic**

3. Unconjugated Hyperbilirubinemia

   a. Caused by hemolytic anemia or congenital deficiency of glucuronyl transferase (e.g., Crigler–Najjar and Gilbert's syndromes)

   b. Hemolytic anemia can be congenital or acquired

      (1) Congenital because of spherocytosis, glucose-6-phosphate dehydrogenase (G6PD), pyruvate kinase deficiency

      (2) Acquired because of ABO/Rh isoimmunization, infxn, drugs, twin–twin transfusion, chronic fetal hypoxia, delayed cord clamping, maternal diabetes

4. Conjugated Hyperbilirubinemia (see Table 4.8)

   a. Infectious causes = sepsis, the ToRCH group, syphilis, *L. monocytogenes,* hepatitis

   b. Metabolic causes = galactosemia, a_1-antitrypsin deficiency

   c. Congenital causes = extrahepatic biliary atresia, Dubin–Johnson and Rotor syndromes

5. Tx = phototherapy with blue light (not ultraviolet (UV) light, which can harm skin and retina) to break down bilirubin pigments and Tx underlying cause

6. Tx urgently to prevent mental retardation 2° to kernicterus (bilirubin precipitation in basal ganglia)

Table 4.8	Differential Diagnosis of Neonatal Jaundice by Time of Onset
Within 24 hrs of birth	• Hemolysis (ABO/Rh isoimmunization, hereditary spherocytosis) • Sepsis
Within 48 hrs of birth	• Hemolysis • Infxn • Physiologic
After 48 hrs	• Infxn • Hemolysis • Breast milk (liver not mature to handle lipids of breast milk) • Congenital malformation (biliary atresia) • Hepatitis

C. **Reye Syndrome**

1. Acute encephalopathy and fatty degeneration of the liver associated with the **use of salicylates in children with varicella or influenza-like illness**

2. Most cases in children aged 4–12 yrs old

3. Si/Sx = biphasic course with prodromal fever → aSx interval → abrupt onset vomiting, delirium, stupor, hepatomegaly with abnormal liver function tests, may rapidly progress to seizures, coma, and death

4. Dx = clinical ⊕↑↑ liver enzymes, nml cerebrospinal fluid (CSF)

5. Tx = control of ↑ intracranial pressure because of cerebral edema (major cause of death) with mannitol, fluid restriction, give glucose because glycogen stores are commonly depleted

6. Px =↑ chance to progress into coma if ≥threefold ↑ in serum ammonia level, ↓ prothrombin not responsive to vitamin K

7. Recovery rapid in mild dz, severe dz may → neuropsychological defects

D. **Febrile Seizures**

1. Usually occurs between the age of 3 mos and 5 yrs, associated with fever without evidence of CNS infxn or other defined cause

2. Most common convulsive order in young children, rarely develops into epilepsy

PEDIATRICS

3. Risk = very high fever (≥102°F [39°C]) and FHx; seizure occurs during rise in temperature, not at the peak of temperature

4. Si/Sx = commonly tonic–clonic seizure with most lasting <10 minutes with a drowsy postictal period

5. Note: If seizure lasts >15 min, most likely because of infxn or toxic process, careful workup should follow

6. Dx = clinical, routine lab tests should be performed only to evaluate fever source, EEG not indicated unless febrile seizure is atypical (complex febrile seizure)

7. Consider lumbar puncture to rule out meningitis

8. Tx = careful evaluation for source of fever, control of fever with antipyretics, parental counseling, and reassurance to ↓ anxiety

9. Px = 33%–50% of children experience recurrence of seizure

VI. Genetic and Congenital Disorders

A. Failure to Thrive (FTT)

1. Failure of children to grow and develop at an appropriate rate

2. Because of inadequate calorie intake or inadequate calorie absorption

3. Can be idiopathic or because of gastroesophageal reflux, urinary tract infxns, cardiac dz, cystic fibrosis, hypothyroidism, congenital syndromes, lead poisoning, malignancy

4. Additional factors include poverty, family discord, neonatal problems, maternal depression

5. Dx requires three criteria

   a. Child <2 yrs old with weight <third to fifth percentile for age on more than one occasion

   b. Child <2 yrs old whose weight is <80% of ideal weight for age

   c. Child <2 yrs old whose weight crosses two major percentiles downward on a standardized growth chart

   d. Exceptions = children of genetically short stature, small-for-gestational-age infants, preterm infants, normally lean infants, "overweight" infants whose rate of height gain ↑ while rate of weight gain ↓

6. Tx

   a. Organic causes → treat underlying condition and provide sufficient caloric supplementation

    b. Idiopathic → observe the parent feeding the infant and educate parents on appropriate formulas, foods, and liquids for the infant

    c. In older infants and children, it is important to offer solid foods before liquids, ↓ distractions during meal times, and child should eat with others and not be force-fed

    d. Monitor closely for progressive weight gain in response to adequate calorie feeding

  7. Px poor in first year of life because of maximal postnatal brain growth during the first 6 mos of life—one-third of the children with nonorganic FTT are developmentally delayed

B. **Craniofacial Abnormalities**

  1. Mildest form is bifid uvula, no clinical significance

  2. Cleft Lip (Figure 4.8)

    a. Can occur unilaterally or bilaterally, because of failure of fusion of maxillary prominences

    b. **Unilateral cleft lip is the most common malformation of the head and neck**

    c. Does not interfere with feeding

    d. Tx = surgical repair

  3. Cleft Palate (Figure 4.8)

    a. Can be anterior or posterior (determined by the position relative to incisive foramen)

    b. Anterior cleft palate because of failure of palatine shelves to fuse with primary palate

    c. Posterior cleft palate because of failure of palatine shelves to fuse with nasal septum

    d. **Interferes with feeding, requiring a special nipple for the baby to feed**

    e. Tx = surgical repair, or orthodontic appliance

  4. Macroglossia

    a. Congenitally enlarged tongue seen in Down's syndrome, gigantism, hypothyroidism

    b. Can be acquired in amyloidosis and acromegaly

    c. Different from glossitis (redness and swelling, with burning sensation) seen in vitamin B deficiencies

    d. Tx is directed at underlying cause

C. **Patau's Syndrome**

  1. **Caused by trisomy 13**

  2. Si/Sx → arrhinencephaly, holoprosencephaly, "**Rocker Bottom Feet**"

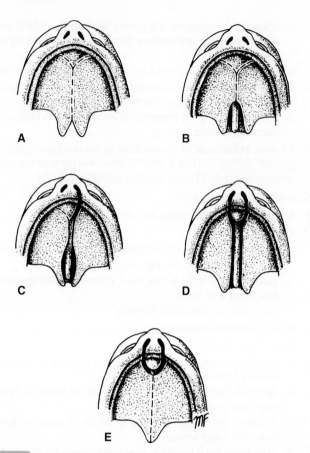

Different forms of cleft palate: **A.** Cleft uvula. **B.** Cleft soft and hard palate. **C.** Total unilateral cleft palate and cleft lip. **D.** Total bilateral cleft palate and cleft lip. **E.** Bilateral cleft lip and jaw. (From Snell RS. *Clinical anatomy,* 7th Ed. Lippincott Williams & Wilkins, 2003.)

D. **Edward's Syndrome**

   1. **Caused by trisomy 18**

   2. Si/Sx → arrhinencephaly, corpus callosum agenesis, **microcephaly and micrognathia**

E. **Down's Syndrome**

   1. **Invariably caused by trisomy 21, ↑ risk if maternal age >35 yrs**

   2. Si/Sx → cardiac septal defects, psychomotor retardation, classic Down's facies, ↑ risk of leukemia, premature Alzheimer's dz

3. Down's facies (Figure 4.9) = flattened occiput (brachycephaly), **epicanthal folds, up-slanted palpebral fissures, speckled irises (Brushfield spots),** protruding tongue, small ears, redundant skin at posterior neck, **hypotonia, simian crease in palms (50%)**

4. Px = typically death in 30s–40s

F. **Turner's Syndrome**

1. **Number one cause of 1° amenorrhea,** because of XO genotype

2. Si/Sx = newborns have ↑ skin at dorsum of neck **(neck webbing)** (Figure 4.10), lymphedema in hands and feet, as they develop → short stature, ptosis, **coarctation of aorta, amenorrhea but uterus is present,** juvenile external genitalia, bleeding because of GI telangiectasias, no mental retardation

3. Tx = hormone replacement to allow 2° sex characteristics to develop

G. **Fragile X Syndrome**

1. X-linked dominant trinucleotide repeat expansion disorder

2. **Number one cause of mental retardation in boys**

3. Si/Sx = long face, prominent jaw, large ears, enlarged testes (postpubertal), developmental delay, mental retardation

4. Tx = none

H. **Arnold–Chiari Malformation**

1. Congenital disorder

2. Si/Sx = caudally displaced cerebellum, elongated medulla passing into foramen magnum, flat skull base, hydrocephalus, meningomyelocele, and aqueductal stenosis

3. Px = death as neonate or toddler

I. **Neural Tube Defects**

1. Associated with ↑ α-fetoprotein levels in maternal serum

2. **Preventable by folic acid supplements during pregnancy**

3. Si/Sx = spina bifida (posterior vertebral arches do not close) and meningocele (no vertebrae cover lumbar cord)

4. Tx = prevention; neurologic deficits often remain after surgical correction

J. **Fetal Alcohol Syndrome**

1. Seen in children born to alcoholic mothers

2. Si/Sx = characterized by facial abnormalities and developmental defects (mental and growth retardation), **smooth philtrum of lip,** microcephaly, atrial septal defect (ASD)

3. Tx = prevention

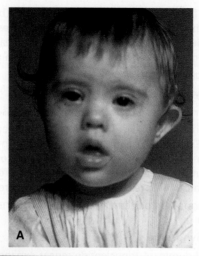

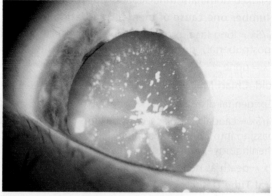

FIGURE 4.9

A. Typical facial features of the child with Down's syndrome. (From Bickley LS, Szilagyi P. *Bates' guide to physical examination and history taking,* 8th Ed. Philadelphia: Lippincott Williams & Wilkins, 2003.) **B.** Discrete flakes in the anterior and posterior cortex in a 26-yr-old man with Down's syndrome. An incomplete, cortical, star-shaped opacity is also evident. (From Tasman W, Jaeger E. *The Wills eye hospital atlas of clinical ophthalmology,* 2nd Ed. Philadelphia, PA: Lippincott Williams & Wilkins, 2001.)

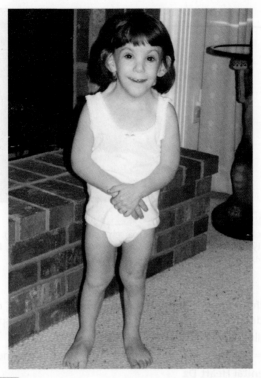

FIGURE 4.10

Neck webbing in a 3-yr-old girl with Turner's syndrome. (From Nettina SM. *The Lippincott manual of nursing practice,* 7th Ed. Lippincott Williams & Wilkins, 2001.)

K. **Tuberous Sclerosis**

1. Autosomal-dominant multinodular proliferation of multinucleated astrocytes

2. Forms small tubers = white nodules in cortex and periventricular areas

3. Characterized by seizures and mental retardation in infancy

4. Classic physical finding is "adenoma sebaceum" = small adenomas on the face in a distribution similar to acne (Figure 4.11)

5. Associated with rhabdomyosarcoma in children

L. **Congenital Pyloric Stenosis**

1. Causes projectile vomiting in first **2 wks to 2 mos of life**

2. More common in boys and in first-born children

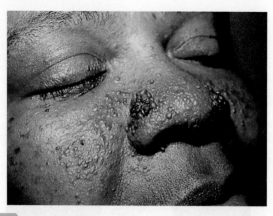

Tuberous sclerosis. This pt has adenoma sebaceum (angiofibromas). Note the similarity to acne lesions. (Hall J. *Sauer's manual of skin diseases,* 8th Ed. Philadelphia, PA: Lippincott Williams & Wilkins, 2000.)

3. **Pathognomonic physical finding is palpable "olive" nodule in midepigastrium,** representing hypertrophied pyloric sphincter
4. If olive is not present, diagnosis made by Utz
5. Tx = longitudinal surgical incision in hypertrophied muscle

M. **Congenital Heart Dz**

1. ASD (Atrial Septal Defect)
   a. Usually aSx, often found on routine preschool physicals
   b. Predispose to congestive heart failure (CHF) in second and third decades, also predispose to stroke because of embolus bypass tract (Eisenmenger's complex)
   c. Si/Sx = loud S_1, **wide fixed-split S_2,** midsystolic ejection murmur
   d. Dx = Echocardiography
   e. Tx = surgical patching of bypass, more important for females because of eventual ↑ cardiovascular stress of pregnancy

2. Ventricular Septal Defect (VSD)
   a. **Most common congenital heart defect,** 30% of small-to-medium defects close spontaneously by age 2 yrs
   b. Si/Sx = small defects may be completely aSx throughout entire life, large defects → CHF, ↓ development/growth, frequent pulmonary infxns, holosystolic murmur over entire precordium, maximally at fourth left intercostal space

    c. Eisenmenger's complex = R → L shunt 2° to pulmonary HTN
       (1) Right ventricular (RV) hypertrophy → flow reversal through the shunt, so that an R → L shunt develops
       (2) Causes cyanosis 2° because of lack of blood flow to lung
       (3) Allows venous thrombi (e.g., deep venous thrombosis [DVT]) to bypass lung, causing systemic paradoxical embolization
    d. Dx = echocardiography
    e. Tx = complete closure for simple defects

3. Tetralogy of Fallot
    a. Four physical defects comprising the tetralogy (Figure 4.12A)
       (1) VSD
       (2) Pulmonary outflow obstruction
       (3) RV hypertrophy
       (4) Overriding aorta (aorta inlet spans both ventricles)
    b. Si/Sx = acyanotic at birth, ↑ cyanosis over first 6 mo, **"Tet spell"** = acute cyanosis and panic in child, child adopts a squatting posture to improve blood flow to lungs, **CXR shows classic boot-shaped contour** because of RV enlargement (Figure 4.12B)
    c. Dx = echocardiography
    d. Tx = surgical repair of VSD, repair of pulmonary outflow tracts

4. Transposition of the Great Arteries
    a. Aorta comes off right ventricle, pulmonary artery off left ventricle
    b. Must have persistent arteriovenous communication or dz is incompatible with life (can be via patent ductus arteriosus [PDA] or persistent foramen ovale)
    c. Si/Sx = marked cyanosis at birth, early digital clubbing, often no murmur, **CXR → enlarged egg-shaped heart** and ↑ pulmonary vasculature
    d. Dx = echocardiography
    e. Tx = surgical switching of arterial roots to nml positions with repair of communication defect
    f. Px = invariably fatal within several mos of birth without Tx

5. Coarctation of the Aorta
    a. Congenital aortic narrowing, often aSx in young child
    b. Si/Sx = ↓ BP in legs with nml BP in arms, **continuous murmur over collateral vessels in back, classic CXR sign = rib notching**

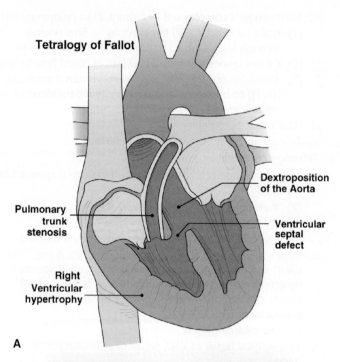

Tetralogy of Fallot

Dextroposition of the Aorta

Pulmonary trunk stenosis

Ventricular septal defect

Right Ventricular hypertrophy

A

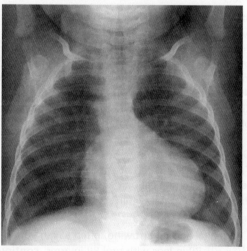

   c. Dx confirmed with aortogram or CT
   d. Tx = surgical resection of coarctation and reanastomosis
6. PDA
   a. ↑ Incidence with premature births, predisposes pt to endo-
      carditis and pulmonary vascular dz
   b. Si/Sx = **continuous machinery murmur heard best at
      second left interspace, wide pulse pressure,** hypoxia
   c. Dx = echocardiography or cardiac catheterization
   d. Tx = indomethacin (block prostaglandins, induces closure)
      for infants, surgical repair for older children

VII. Trauma and Intoxication

A. **Child Abuse** (see Figure 4.13)
   1. Can be physical trauma, emotional, sexual, or neglect
   2. Nutritional neglect is the most common etiology for under-
      weight infants
   3. Most common perpetrator of sexual abuse is family member or
      family friends; 97% of reported offenders are males
   4. **Physicians are required by law to report suspected child
      abuse or neglect (law provides protection to mandated
      reporters who report in good faith); clinical and lab
      evaluations are allowed without parental/guardian
      permission**
   5. Epidemiology
      a. 85% of the children reported to Child Protective Services
         (CPS) are <5 yrs old, 45% are <1 yr old
      b. 10% of the injuries to the children <5 yrs old seen in the
         emergency room (ER) are because of abuse, and 10% of
         abuse cases involve burns
      c. **High-risk children** = premature infants, children with
         chronic medical problems, colicky babies, those with behav-
         ioral problems, children living in poverty, children of teen-
         age parents, single parents, or substance abusers
   6. Si/Sx = injury is unexplainable or not consistent with Hx,
      bruises are the most common manifestation
      a. Accidental injuries seen on shins, forearms, hips
      b. Less likely to be accidental, are bilateral and symmetric, seen
         on buttocks, genitalia, back, back of hands, different color
         bruises (repeat injuries over time)
      c. Fractures highly suspicious for abuse: those because of pull-
         ing or wrenching, causing damage to the metaphysis

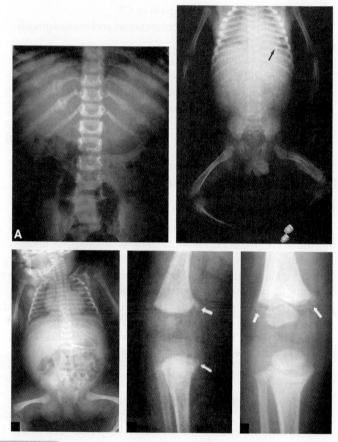

FIGURE 4.13

Skeletal survey in child abuse. **A.** Infant with multiple old rib injuries and gastric distension. (From Reece RM, Ludwig S, eds. *Child abuse: medical diagnosis and management,* 2nd Ed. Philadelphia, PA: Lippincott Williams & Wilkins, 2001, with permission.) **B.** Radiograph of the trunk and extremities of a victim of child abuse showing healed misaligned fracture of the left femur and healing rib fractures (*arrow*) on the left. (From Jones NL. *Atlas of forensic pathology.* Philadelphia, PA: Lippincott Williams & Wilkins, 1996, with permission.) **C.** "Babygram": a single frontal radiograph of the long bones and axial skeleton may mask subtle injuries because of geometric distortion and exposure variation. **D.** Frontal radiograph of the knee showing a characteristic metaphyseal "corner" fracture of the distal femur (*arrows*). **E.** Another infant's knee demonstrating the typical and highly specific "bucket-handle" fracture of the distal femur (*arrows*). (A–E: courtesy of Evan Geller. From Greenberg MI, Hendrickson RG, Silverberg M, et al. *Greenberg's text-atlas of emergency medicine.* Philadelphia, PA: Lippincott Williams & Wilkins, 2004, with permission.)

7. **Classic Findings**
   a. Chip fracture, where the corner of metaphysis of long bone is torn off with damage to epiphysis
   b. Periosteum spiral fracture before infant can walk
   c. Rib fractures
8. Dating fracture can be done by callus formation (callus appears in 10–12 days)
9. Burns
   a. Shape/pattern of burn may be diagnostic
   b. **Cigarette** → circular, punched out lesions of similar size, hands and feet common
   c. **Immersion** → most common in infants, affecting buttocks and perineum (hold thighs against abdomen), or with scalded line clearly demarcated on thighs or waist without splash marks
   d. Stocking-glove burn on hands or feet
10. Injury to head is the most common cause of death from physical abuse; infants can present with convulsions, apnea, ↑ intracranial pressure, subdural hemorrhages, retinal hemorrhages (marker for acceleration/deceleration injuries), or in a coma
11. Sexual abuse
    a. Child may talk to mother or teacher, friend, relative about situation
    b. Si/Sx = vaginal, penile, or rectal pain; erythema; discharge; bleeding; chronic dysuria; enuresis; constipation; encopresis
    c. Behaviors = sexualized activity with peers or objects, seductive behavior
12. Dx
    a. Labs → prothrombin time/partial thromboplastin time (PT/PTT) and platelets to screen for bleeding diathesis
    b. Consider bone survey in children <2 yrs old, plain films or MRI for severe injuries or refusal/inability to communicate
    c. For sexual abuse, collect specimens of offender's sperm, blood, and hair; collect victim's nail clippings and clothing, obtain *Chlamydia* and *Gonorrhea* cultures from mouth, anus, and genitalia
    d. Dx is tentatively based on H&P, record all information, photograph when appropriate
13. Tx
    a. Medical, surgical, psychiatric Tx for injuries
    b. Report immediately, do not discharge before talking to CPS

    c. Admit pt if injuries are severe enough, if Dx is unclear, or if no other safe placement is available

B. **Poisonings**

  1. Accidental, seen in younger children momentarily left unsupervised, usually a single agent ingested or inhaled (plants, household products, medications)

  2. Intentional, seen in adolescents/adults, toxic substances for recreational purposes or overdose taken with intent to produce self-harm

  3. Epidemiology

    a. Nearly 50% of the cases occur in children <6 yrs old, as a result of an accidental event or as abuse

    b. 92% occur at home; 60% with nonpharmacologic agent; 40% with pharmacologic agent

    c. Ingestion occurs in 75% of the cases, 8% dermal, 6% ophthalmic, 6% inhalation

  4. Hx is crucial during initial contact with pt or guardian

    a. Evaluation of severity (aSx, Sx)

    b. Age and weight

    c. Time, type, amount, and route of exposure

    d. Past medical Hx

  5. Si/Sx (see Table 4.9)

  6. Tx

    a. Syrup of ipecac no longer indicated by American Academy of Pediatrics.

    b. Gastric lavage usually unnecessary in children, but may be useful with drugs that ↓ gastric motility

Table 4.9 Pediatric Toxicology

Si/Sx	Possible Toxin
Lethargy/coma	Ethanol, sedative-hypnotics, narcotics, antihistamines, antidepressants, neuroleptic
Seizures	Theophylline, cocaine, amphetamines, antidepressants, antipsychotics, pesticides
Hypotension (with bradycardia)	Organophosphate pesticides, β-blockers
Arrhythmia	Tricyclic antidepressants, cocaine, digitalis, quinidine
Hyperthermia	Salicylates, anticholinergics

c. Charcoal may be the most effective and safest procedure to prevent absorption, repeat doses every 2–6 hrs with cathartic for first dose; ineffective in heavy metal or volatile hydrocarbon poisoning

VIII. Adolescence

A. Epidemiology

1. Injuries
   a. 50% of all deaths in adolescents attributed to injuries
   b. Many occur under the influence of alcohol and other drugs
   c. Older adolescents more likely to be killed in motor vehicle accidents, whereas younger adolescents are at the risk for drowning and fatal injuries with weapons
   d. Homicide rate is 5× higher for African-American males than Caucasian males

2. Suicide
   a. Second leading cause of adolescent death
   b. Females more likely to attempt than males, but males are 5× more likely to succeed than females
   c. Pts with pre-existing psychiatric problems or those who abuse alcohol and drugs more likely to attempt suicide

3. Substance Abuse
   a. Major cause of morbidity in adolescents
   b. Average age at first use is 12–14 yrs
   c. One of every two adolescents has tried an illicit drug by high school graduation
   d. Survey of high school seniors (1994–1995) noted that 90% had experience with alcohol and ≥40% had tried marijuana

4. Sex
   a. 61% of all male and 47% of all female high school students have had sex
   b. Health risks of early sexual activity are unwanted pregnancies and sexually transmitted dz (STDs) such as *Gonorrhea, Chlamydia,* and HIV
   c. 86% of all STDs occur among adolescents and young adults aged 15–29 yrs old
   d. More than one million adolescent girls become pregnant yearly; 33% are <15 yrs old—this is the second major cause of morbidity in adolescents

    5. Eating Disorders

      a. Anorexia nervosa occurs in 0.5% of adolescent girls and bulimia in 1%–3%

      b. Si/Sx = cardiovascular symptoms, fluid and electrolyte abnormalities, amenorrhea, ↓ bone density, anemia, parotid gland enlargement, tooth decay, constipation (hallmark of anorexia)

      c. Adolescents with anorexia lose 15% of ideal body weight and appear sick, but those with bulimia may look well nourished

      d. Anorexia nervosa is seen at two peak ages (14.5 yrs and 18 yrs), but 25% of girls with anorexia may be <13 yrs old

B. Confidentiality

    1. Most issues revealed by adolescents to physicians in an interview are confidential

    2. **Exceptions** include suicidal or homicidal behavior or sexual or physical abuse

    3. Physicians are strongly encouraged to inform adolescents about confidentiality at the beginning of the interview to help develop a trusting relationship between adolescent and physician

C. Screening

    1. Annual risk behavior screening in every adolescent is strongly recommended

    2. **HEADSSS** assessment allows physicians to evaluate critical areas in each adolescent's life that may be detrimental to growth and development

      a. **H**ome environment → who does adolescent live with? any recent changes? quality of parental interaction (if applicable)? has she/he ever run away from home?

      b. **E**mployment and **E**ducation → is child in school? favorite subjects? academic performance? are friends in school? any recent changes? does child have a job? future plans?

      c. **A**ctivities → what does child like to do in spare time? who does the child spend time with? involved in any sports/exercise? hobbies? attends parties or clubs?

      d. **D**rugs → has child ever used tobacco? alcohol? marijuana? other illicit drugs? If so, when was the child's last use? how often? do friends or family members use drugs? who does the child use these substances with?

      e. **S**exual activity → sexual orientation? is child sexually active? number of sexual partners? does the child use condoms or other forms of contraception? any Hx of STDs or pregnancy?

f. **S**uicide → does the child ever feel sad, tired, or unmotivated? has the child ever felt that life was not worth living? any feelings of wanting to harm self? If so, does the child have a plan? has the child ever tried to harm self in the past? does the child know anyone who has attempted suicide?

g. **S**afety → does the child use a seat belt or bike helmet? does the child enter into high-risk situations? does the child have access to a firearm?

FAMILY MEDICINE

I. Headache

A. **Si/Sx and DDx** (Table 5.1)

B. **Dx**

1. **Temporal arteritis Dx requires temporal artery Bx**

2. **Trigeminal neuralgia Dx requires head CT or MRI** to rule out sinusitis, cerebellopontine angle neoplasm, multiple sclerosis, or herpes zoster

3. **Subarachnoid hemorrhage requires** confirmation by CT scan or lumbar puncture to detect CSF blood or xanthochromia (can be detected 6 hrs after onset of headache)

4. Suspect intracranial lesion causing headache in **pts >50 or pts with headaches immediately upon waking up**

5. **Suspect ↑ intracranial pressure (ICP) in pts awakened in middle of night by headache, who have projectile vomiting, or who have focal neural deficits; obtain head CT**

C. **Tx** (Table 5.2)

II. Ears, Nose, and Throat

A. **Otitis Externa**

1. **Ear pain, itchy, draining ear, pulling on pinna, or pushing on tragus causes pain** (Figure 5.1)

   a. **Bacterial**

      (1) *Pseudomonas* is usual cause in swimmers, diabetics, or pts with eczema of external auditory canal

      (2) Tx = antibiotic ear drops, keep water out of ears, may need wick placed in canal to facilitate distribution of ear drops within external auditory canal and prevent closure of canal

      (3) For malignant otitis externa caused by *Pseudomonas* (typically in a diabetic), aggressive IV antibiotics, with surgical debridement if necessary, to prevent progression to mastoiditis

   b. **Fungal**

      (1) Otomycosis is commonly caused by *Candida* or *Aspergillus*

Table 5.1 Summary of Headaches

Type	Epidemiology	Characteristics
Tension	Usually after age 20 yrs (rarely after age 50 yrs)	• Most common headache type • **Bilateral, band-like, dull in quality** • Worse with stress; not aggravated by activity • Chronic headache associated with depression
Cluster	**Male/ female = 6:1** Mean age 30 yrs	• **Unilateral,** stabbing peri/retro-orbital pain, lasting 15 min to 3 hrs • Seasonal attacks occur in series (6×/day) lasting weeks, followed by months of remission • **Associated with ipsilateral lacrimation (85%), ptosis, nasal congestion, and rhinorrhea** • Often occurs within 90 min of onset of sleep
Migraine	80% have positive FHx **Female/ male = 3:1**	• Classically, headache is **unilateral (60%)** with **aura (only 15%);** pt looks for quiet place to rest • Visual aura: **Scotoma** (blind spots), **teichopsia** (jagged zigzag lines), **photopsias** (shimmering lights), or **rhodopsias** (colors) • Accompanied by **nausea and photophobia** • Triggered by stress, odors, certain foods, alcohol, menstruation, or sleep deprivation
Temporal arteritis (giant cell)	**Female/ male = 2:1** Age >50 yrs	• **Unilateral temporal** headache • **Associated with jaw claudication, temporal artery tenderness with palpation, ESR ≥50** • 50% also have polymyalgia rheumatica • If not treated leads to optic neuritis and **blindness** • Screen by ESR; Dx with temporal artery Bx
Trigeminal neuralgia	Peak age at 60 yrs	• Episodic, severe pain shooting from side of mouth to ipsilateral ear, eye, or nose
Withdrawal headache		• Common cause of frequent headaches • Can be withdrawal from various drugs
Subarachnoid hemorrhage		• Head trauma is most common cause • Spontaneous: Usually berry aneurysm rupture • Classically the "worst headache of my life"
Temporal mandibular joint (TMJ) disorders	Can be related to osteoarthritis or previous trauma to TMJ	• Medical and dental conditions affecting the TMJ and/or the muscles of mastication • Si/Sx = chronic ear pain, headache, jaw stiffness, facial pain, pain with chewing, jaw joint pain, jaw joint noises, and grinding (Bruxism) or clenching one's teeth

Table 5.2 Treatment of Headache

Headache	Treatment
Tension	• NSAIDs or acetaminophen • Prophylaxis with antidepressants or β-blockers
Cluster	• Acutely 100% O$_2$ or a triptan,^{a} or second-line dihydroergotamine • Prophylaxis with verapamil, lithium, methysergide, or ergotamine
Migraine	• Acutely with a triptan,^{a} NSAIDs, or second-line dihydroergotamine and/or anti-emetics • Prophylaxis with **β-blockers** (first line) or calcium blockers
Temporal arteritis	• Start treatment with corticosteroids as soon as suspected to avoid blindness • Never delay Tx while awaiting confirmatory biopsy results
Trigeminal neuralgia	• Carbamazepine (first line) or phenytoin, clonazepam, valproic acid
Withdrawal	• NSAIDs
Subarachnoid hemorrhage	• Immediate neurosurgical evaluation and nimodipine to reduce incidence of post-rupture vasospasm and ischemia
Temporal mandibular joint (TMJ) disorders	• NSAIDs/relaxation techniques/stress reduction • Muscle relaxants • Dental appliance (mouth guard) • Provide muscle relaxation and support for the jaw joints (TMJ) • Refer to dental/oral surgery

^{a}Triptans include sumatriptan, zolmitriptan, eletriptan, naratriptan, rizatriptan, frovatriptan, almotriptan; these are all contraindicated with known coronary dz or ergot drugs taken within 24 hrs.

    (2) Tx = acetic acid ear drops, nystatin and triamcinilone ointment to canal, water precautions

  c. **Viral**

    (1) Ramsay Hunt syndrome (herpes zoster oticus) caused by reactivation of Varicella Zoster Virus (VZV) in the geniculate ganglia (CN VII)

    (2) Si/Sx = painful vesicles in external auditory meatus

    (3) Tx = acyclovir to prevent progression to meningitis and facial nerve palsy

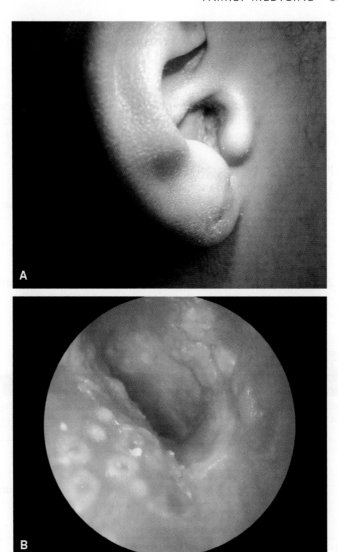

FIGURE 5.1

Otitis externa. **A.** View of infected ear. (Courtesy of Christy Salvaggio. From Greenberg MI, Hendrickson RG, Silverberg M, et al. *Greenberg's text-atlas of emergency medicine.* Philadelphia, PA: Lippincott Williams & Wilkins, 2004, with permission.) **B.** External auditory canal. (From Benjamin B, Hawke M, Stammberger H. *A color atlas of otorhinolaryngology.* Philadelphia, PA: JB Lippincott, 1995, with permission.)

2. In diabetics, get CT/MRI of temporal bone to rule out osteo-myelitis and malignant otitis externa, which requires surgical debridement

3. Gradenigo Syndrome
   a. Can be a complication of otitis media and/or mastoiditis
   b. Consists of osteomyelitis of petrous apex bone causing ipsi-lateral otorrhea, eye pain, abducens paralysis (CN VI), and diplopia, requiring emergency referral to Neurosurgery or Neuro-otology

B. **Inner Ear Dz**

1. Tinnitus (Ringing in the Ears)
   a. Causes = foreign body in external canal, pulsating vascular tumors, medications (aspirin), or hearing loss
   b. Dx = obtain audiogram to assess hearing thresholds
   c. Tx underlying cause, hearing aids may help with hearing loss related tinnitus

2. Vertigo is the feeling that the surroundings are spinning when eyes are open, whereas in dizziness, the pt feels as if she/he, not the surroundings, is spinning (Table 5.3)

Table 5.3 Causes of Vertigo

Disease	Characteristics
Benign positional vertigo	• Sudden, episodic vertigo with head movement lasting for seconds • Tx = Epley maneuver
Ménière's disease	• Dilation of membranous labyrinth resulting from excess endolymph • **Classic triad = aural fullness (hearing loss), tinnitus, and episodic vertigo lasting several hours** • Tx = low sodium, low caffeine diet, medications (thiazides, anticholinergics, antihistamines), and surgery as a last resort
Viral labyrinthitis	• Preceded by viral respiratory illness • Vertigo lasting days to weeks • Tx = meclizine
Acoustic neuroma	• CN VIII schwannoma, commonly affects vestibular portion but can also affect cochlea • Si/Sx = vertigo, sudden deafness, tinnitus • Dx = MRI of cerebellopontine angle • Tx = local radiation or surgical excision

C. **Hearing Loss**
1. Sensorineural Hearing Loss
   a. 2° to sensory damage of the organ of corti in the cochlea or retrocochlear damage such as from an acoustic neuroma or other CN VIII nerve damage
   b. May be of sudden onset, but most often slowly progressive
      (1) Presbycusis—gradual loss of high frequency hearing as a person ages
      (2) Sudden hearing loss is an emergency and immediate ENT referral should be made for appropriate Dx and Tx
      (3) Bilateral hearing loss commonly associated with drugs, i.e., loop diuretics, aminoglycosides, salicylates, and cisplatin
   c. Potential causes include idiopathic, acoustic neuroma, congenital genetic, autoimmune, infxn, inheritance, trauma, or toxins affecting nerve or cochlea
   d. Alport's syndrome
      (1) Sensorineural hearing loss, lens dislocation, hematuria
      (2) Most likely X-linked dominant inheritance
      (3) Thinning glomerular basement membrane and glomerulonephritis resulting in hematuria
   e. Congenital—refers to sensorineural hearing loss at birth, does not specify etiology
      (1) Etiologies include genetic, infectious, i.e., exposure of fetus to CMV, rubella, or syphilis in utero
      (2) Tx = hearing aids, cochlear implants, and steroids commonly used. ENT consult recommended
2. Conductive Hearing Loss
   a. Due to damage or obstruction affecting middle ear or external ear
   b. Examples include otitis media, excess cerumen, otosclerosis, cholesteatoma, or perforated tympanic membrane
   c. Mixed hearing loss (sensorineural and conductive) can be seen in chronic middle ear infxn
   d. Usually correctable with surgery or appropriate Tx
   e. Pts often benefit from hearing aids
3. Diagnostic Hearing Tests
   a. Weber's test
      (1) Vibrating tuning fork (512 Hz) is placed midline on top of head

    (2) Lateralization of hearing to one ear more than the other indicates ipsilateral conductive loss or contralateral sensorineural loss

  b. Rinne's test (comparison of air conduction to bone conduction)

    (1) Vibrating tuning fork (512 Hz) placed next to ear, then when no longer heard placed against mastoid process until no longer heard

    (2) Normally air conduction should persist twice as long as bone conduction

    (3) Positive Rinne = air conduction is heard longer and louder than bone conduction (this is the nml finding)

    (4) Negative Rinne = bone conduction is heard longer than air conduction, indicating a conductive hearing loss in that ear

  c. Audiogram

    (1) A graphic representation of a pt's pure-tone responses to various auditory frequency stimuli (250–8000 Hz)

    (2) Should be obtained in all pts with changes in hearing or new onset tinnitus or vertigo

    (3) Hearing is considered normal when hearing thresholds are <20 decibels

    (4) Air–bone gaps (a difference between the air conduction and the bone conduction lines) exist when there is a conductive hearing loss

    (5) Asymmetric hearing loss may be indicative of an acoustic neuroma and further testing is needed with auditory brain response measurements and/or MRI with gadolinium

D. **Epistaxis**

 1. Most commonly involve nasal septum

 2. Ninety percent of bleeds occur at Kiesselbach's plexus in the anterior nasal septum

 3. Posterior bleeding more common in elderly

 4. **No. 1 cause of epistaxis in children is trauma (induced by exploring digits)**

 5. Also precipitated by rhinitis, nasal mucosa dryness, septal deviation and bone spurs, alcohol, antiplatelet medication, bleeding diathesis, cocaine abuse, chronic HTN, and hereditary hemorrhagic telangiectasia

6. Tx
  a. Direct pressure, topical nasal vasoconstrictors, i.e., oxy-metazoline, phenylephrine, silver nitrate cautery (do not cauterize same location on both sides of septum to prevent septal perforation)
  b. Consider anterior nasal packing if unable to stop
  c. Five percent originate in posterior nasal cavity requiring packing—pts with posterior packing or balloon should be admitted to hospital for airway observation as they are at ↑ risk for hypoventilation and ↓ oxygen saturations
  d. Interventional radiology embolization of affected vessels
  e. Surgical ligation of internal maxillary artery, ethmoidal arteries, or affected vessels to stop bleeding
  f. Pts need to be placed on antistaphylococcal prophylaxis meds while nose is packed.
  g. Topical vasoconstrictors may be contraindicated in pts with HTN
  h. Repeat bleeding should prompt hematologic workup for bleeding diathesis, i.e., hemophilia, von Willebrand's dz, platelet function defects

E. **Sinusitis**
  1. Maxillary sinuses most commonly involved
  2. DDx (Table 5.4)
  3. Dx = clinical, can confirm CT scan showing inflammatory changes or bone destruction (Figure 5.2)
  4. Potential complications of sinusitis include meningitis, abscess formation, orbital infxn, osteomyelitis

F. **Pharyngitis** (Table 5.5)

G. **Peritonsillar Abscess (Quinsy)**
  1. Loculation of pus in the peritonsillar space (between tonsil and superior constrictor)
  2. May be related to previous tonsillar infxn, dental caries, or allergies
  3. May be caused by anaerobic bacteria, but mostly caused by same agents seen in pharyngitis and tonsillitis
  4. Si/Sx = fever, drooling, odynophagia, trismus, and a muffled voice, soft palate and uvula are displaced and peritonsillar fluctuant swelling that is extremely painful to touch
  5. Tx = airway stabilization, incision and drainage, antibiotic Tx, and fluids, tonsillectomy immediately versus wait 6 wks before performing tonsillectomy

Table 5.4 Sinusitis

	Organisms	Si/Sx	Tx
Acute bacterial (<4 wks)	*Streptococcus pneumoniae, Haemophilus influenzae, Moraxella catarrhalis*	**Purulent rhinorrhea,** headache, **pain on sinus palpation,** fever, **halitosis,** anosmia, **tooth pain**	Saline nasal lavage, decongestants, antibiotics (TMP-SMX or amoxicillin) can be considered
Chronic bacterial (>3 mos)	*Bacteroides, S. aureus, Pseudomonas, Streptococcus* spp.	Same as for acute but lasts longer, risk of progression to brain abscess or sphenoid sinus thrombophlebitis, loss of vision, and/or cavernous sinus thrombosis	Saline nasal lavage, nasal steroids if related to allergies; surgical correction of obstruction (e.g., septal deviation or nasal polyps); antibiotics controversial
Fungal	*Aspergillus*— **in diabetics watch out for mucormycosis!**	Usually seen in immunocompromised pts, black nasal turbinates	Emergent antifungal therapy, emergent surgery

H. **Lemierre's Syndrome**
   1. Thrombophlebitis of internal jugular (IJ) vein
   2. Usually 2° to oropharyngeal infxn with anaerobic gram-negative rods, most commonly *Fusobacterium necrophorum*
   3. Si/Sx = severe odynophagia, dysphagia, fevers, chills, rigors, neck swelling or pain, occasionally a palpable cord may be felt along IJ clot, septic emboli commonly metastasize to lungs forming cavitations and abscesses
   4. Tx = antibiotics targeting *F. necrophorum* and other oral faculta-tive anaerobes, and possible surgical drainage of abscesses or surgical ligation of clot if unresponsive to antibiotics and continued emboli

I. **Retropharyngeal Abscess**
   1. An abscess formed from breakdown and necrosis of enlarged lymph nodes in retropharyngeal space
   2. More common in children and usually following a severe pha-ryngeal infxn or longstanding upper respiratory infxn

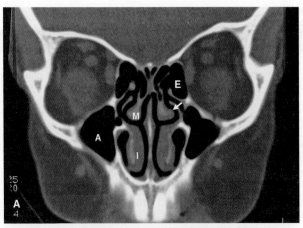

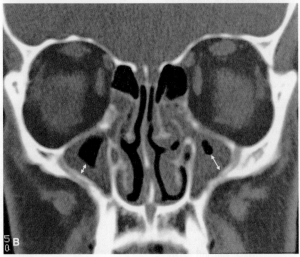

FIGURE 5.2

Coronal CT scan. **A.** Nml sinuses. Note the excellent demonstration of the bony margins. The *arrow* points to the middle meatus into which the maxillary antrum and frontal, anterior, and middle ethmoid sinuses drain. A, maxillary antrum; E, ethmoid sinus; I, inferior turbinate; M, middle turbinate.
B. Sinusitis. Mucosal thickening prevents drainage of the sinuses. Both antra are almost opaque. The *arrows* indicate mucosal thickening in the antra. (From Armstrong P, Wastie ML. *Diagnostic imaging,* 4th Ed. Oxford: Blackwell Scientific, 1998, with permission.)

Table 5.5 Pharyngitis

Disease	Si/Sx	Dx	Tx
Group A Strep throat	High fever, severe throat pain without cough, edematous tonsils with white or yellow exudate, cervical adenopathy	• H&P 50% accurate • Rapid antigen test for point-of-care screening • Throat swab culture is gold standard	Penicillin to prevent acute rheumatic fever
Membranous (diphtheria)	High fever, dysphagia, drooling, **can cause respiratory failure** (airway occlusion)	• **Pathognomonic gray membrane on tonsils extending into throat**	**STAT antitoxin**
Fungal (*Candida*)	Dysphagia, sore throat with white, cheesy patches in oropharynx (oral thrush), **seen in AIDS, diabetics, steroids, and small children**	• Clinical or endoscopy	Fluconazole
Adenovirus	**Pharyngoconjunctival fever (fever, red eye, sore throat)**	• Clinical	Supportive
Mononucleosis (Epstein–Barr virus [EBV])	Generalized lymphadenopathy, exudative tonsillitis, palatal petechiae, splenomegaly	• ⊕ **Heterophile antibody and other more specific EBV serologies** • **Skin rash** in pts given ampicillin	Supportive. Pt should avoid contact sports to avoid splenic rupture due to splenomegaly
Herpangina (coxsackie A)	Fever, pharyngitis, body ache, tender vesicles along tonsils, uvula, and soft palate	• Clinical	Supportive

3. Si/Sx = toxic appearing, drooling stridor, high fever, head tilted to one side, dysphagia, odynophagia. Unilateral bulging noted within oropharynx

4. Dx = CT scan with contrast, lateral neck, airway fluoroscopy

5. Tx = Stabilize airway, IV antibiotics, ENT consult and surgery if Sx do not improve or pt unstable

J. Dental Infections

1. Ludwig's Angina—Severe cellulitis that usually originates in an infected tooth root and spreads along the floor of the mouth and eventually into neck causing airway compromise

2. Severe swelling in neck and floor of mouth, trismus, fever, and pain in oral cavity and neck

3. Dx—CT scan of face and neck demonstrating drainable collection or diffuse edema and focal point of infection

4. Dental evaluation for drainage and/or removal of infected tooth, IV antibiotics to cover mouth flora (e.g., streptococcal species and anaerobes)

5. May need surgical drainage of neck if infection has spread to neck, and may require intubation or tracheotomy to protect airway until infection resolves

K. **Hoarseness (Dysphonia)**

1. Perceived rough quality of the voice (caused by structural or functional abnormalities)

2. Many causes:

   a. **Congenital**—laryngeal webs, clefts, cysts

   b. **Infectious**—papillomatosis, viral, bacterial and fungal laryngitis, tuberculosis

   c. **Inflammatory**—reflux laryngitis, rheumatoid arthritis

   d. **Latrogenic**—recurrent laryngeal nerve (RLN) damage occurring during neck or cardiothoracic surgery

   e. **Traumatic**—vocal fold nodules, polyps, arytenoid dislocation, laryngeal framework disruption (fracture), and postintubation

   f. **Endocrine**—hypothyroidism, hyperthyroidism

   g. **Connective tissue dz**—scleroderma, sarcoidosis

   h. **Neoplastic**

      (1) Benign—human papillomavirus (HPV), granuloma, laryngeal chondroma

      (2) Malignant (1°)—squamous cell CA (larynx/lung) or thyroid CA invading RLN

      (3) Malignant (metastasis)

   i. **Neurologic**—vocal fold paralysis, multiple sclerosis, viral neuronitis, spasmodic dysphonia

   j. **Senile larynx (old age)** (Hoarseness differential by Dr. Ramon Franco)

III. Outpatient Gastrointestinal Complaints

A. Dyspepsia

1. Si/Sx = upper abd pain, early satiety, postprandial abd bloating or distention, nausea, vomiting, often exacerbated by eating

2. DDx = peptic ulcer, gastroesophageal reflux dz (GERD), CA, gastroparesis, malabsorption, intestinal parasite, drugs (e.g., NSAIDs), etc.

3. Dx = clinical

4. Tx

   a. Avoid caffeine, alcohol, cigarettes, NSAIDs; eat frequent small meals; reduce stress; maintain ideal body weight; elevate head of bed

   b. H_2 blockers and antacids, or proton pump inhibitor

   c. Empiric **antibiotics for *Helicobacter pylori* are NOT indicated for nonulcer dyspepsia**

B. GERD

1. Causes = obesity, relaxed lower esophageal sphincter, esophageal dysmotility, hiatal hernia

2. Si/Sx = heartburn occurring 30–60 min postprandial and upon reclining, usually relieved by antacid self-administration, dyspepsia, postprandial burning sensation in esophagus, regurgitation of gastric contents into the mouth, cough, hoarseness, globus sensation

3. Atypical Si/Sx sometimes seen = asthma, chronic cough/laryngitis, atypical chest pain

4. Acidic beverages (soda, citrus juices), fatty foods, chocolate, spicy foods, alcohol all cause lower esophageal sphincter relaxation and exacerbate GERD symptoms

5. Eating shortly before going to sleep or lying down exacerbates symptoms

6. Dx = clinical, can confirm with ambulatory pH monitoring—EGD to screen patients with chronic GERD (e.g., >10 yrs), particularly in patients >50 yrs, for Barrett's esophagus, and if Barrett's found, consider surgical intervention to prevent transformation to esophageal adenocarcinoma

7. Tx

   a. First line = lifestyle modifications: Avoid lying down postprandial, avoid spicy foods and foods that delay gastric emptying, reduce meal size, lose weight

b. If medications, proton pump inhibitors are the most effective option long term with H$_2$ receptor antagonists useful for rapid onset and breakthrough Sx

c. Often will require maintenance Tx since Sx return upon discontinuation

d. For severe, refractory dz, can consider surgical fundoplication, relieves Sx in 90% of pts, may be more cost-effective in younger pts or those with severe dz

8. Sequelae

a. **Barrett's esophagus** (Figure 5.3)

(1) Chronic GERD → metaplasia from squamous to columnar epithelia in lower esophagus

(2) Requires close surveillance with endoscopy and aggressive Tx as 30% progress to **adenoCA**

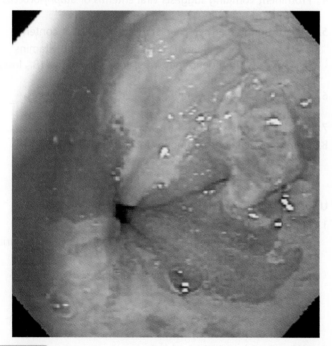

FIGURE 5.3

Barrett's esophagus with an early adenoCA identified on surveillance endoscopy. (From Yamada T, Alpers DH, Kaplowitz N, et al, eds. *Atlas of gastroenterology*, 3rd Ed. Philadelphia, PA: Lippincott Williams & Wilkins, 2003, with permission.)

      (3) Multiple FDA-approved Tx, including radiofrequency ablation, photodynamic Tx, cryotherapy, endoscopic mucosal resection

   b. Peptic stricture

      (1) Results in gradual solid food dysphagia often with concurrent improvement of heartburn Sx

      (2) Endoscopy establishes Dx

      (3) Requires aggressive proton pump inhibitor Tx and surgical opening if unresponsive

C. Diarrhea

1. Diarrhea = stool weight >300 g/day (nml = 100–300 g/day)
2. Small-bowel dz → stools typically voluminous, watery, and fatty
3. Large-bowel dz → stools smaller in volume but more frequent
4. Prominent vomiting suggests viral enteritis or *Staphylococcus aureus* food poisoning
5. Malabsorption diarrhea characterized by high-fat content
   a. Lose fat-soluble vitamins, iron, calcium, and B vitamins
   b. Can cause iron deficiency, megaloblastic anemia (B_{12} loss), and hypocalcemia
6. General Tx = oral rehydration, IV fluids, and electrolytes (supportive)
7. Specific diarrheas (Table 5.6)
8. Common infectious pathogens for diarrhea (Table 5.7)

IV. Urogenital Complaints

A. Urinary Tract Infxn (UTI)

1. Epidemiology
   a. Forty percent of females have ≥1 UTI, 8% have bacteriuria at a given time
   b. Most common in sexually active young women, elderly, posturethral catheter or instrumentation—rare in males (↑ risk with prostate dz)
   c. Usually caused by *Escherichia coli* (80%) and other gram-negative rods
2. Si/Sx = **burning during urination,** urgency, sense of incomplete bladder emptying, hematuria, lower abd pain, nocturia
3. Systemic Sx such as fever, chills, and/or flank or **back pain suggest pyelonephritis**

Text continues on page 323

Table 5.6 Diarrheas

Type	Characteristics	Dx	Tx
Infectious	• **#1 cause of acute diarrhea** • Causes include Enterovirus spp. and **Norwalk virus (cause of cruise-ship diarrhea),** which cause noninflammatory diarrhea, bacteria that cause inflammatory diarrhea (*Campylobacter* #1, *E. coli* for traveler's diarrhea, *Salmonella, Shigella, Clostridium difficile* with antibiotic exposure), and parasites (*Giardia, Entamoeba, Cryptosporidium*) • Si/Sx = vomiting, pain; blood/mucus, and fevers/chills suggest invasive dz	• Stool culture, ova and parasites (O&P) • *C. difficile* toxin test	• Fluoroquinolone • Metronidazole or oral vancomycin for *C. difficile*[a]
Osmotic	• Causes = lactose intolerance, oral Mg, sorbitol/mannitol	• ↑ Osmotic gap • Check fecal fat	• Withdraw inciting agent
Secretory	• Causes = toxins (cholera), enteric viruses, ↑ dietary fat	• Normal osmotic gap • Fasting → no change	• Supportive
Exudative	• Mucosal inflammation → plasma and serum leakage • Causes = enteritis, TB, colon CA, inflammatory bowel dz	• ↑ ESR & CRP • Radiologic imaging or colonoscopy to visualize intestine	• Varies by cause
Rapid transit	• Causes = laxatives, surgical excision of intestinal tissue	• Hx of surgery or laxative use	• Supportive

(continued)

Table 5.6 *Continued*

Type	Characteristics	Dx	Tx
Encopresis	• Oozing around fecal impaction in children or sick elderly	• Hx of constipation	• Fiber-rich diet and laxatives
Celiac sprue	• Gluten allergy (wheat, barley, rye, oats) • Si/Sx = weakness, failure to thrive, growth retardation • Classic rash = **dermatitis herpetiformis** = pruritic, red papulovesicular lesions on shoulders, elbows, and knees • 10%–15% of pts develop intestinal lymphoma	• **Antiendomysial, anti-tissue transglutaminase, and antigliadin antibodies typically positive** • **Dx confirmed by small-bowel biopsy showing pathognomonic blunting of villi**	• Avoid dietary gluten
Tropical sprue	• Diarrhea probably caused by a tropical infection • Si/Sx = glossitis, diarrhea, weight loss, steatorrhea	• Dx = clinical	• Tetracycline ⊕ folate
Whipple's disease	• GI infection by *Tropheryma whippelii* • Si/Sx = diarrhea, arthritis, rash, anemia, can also caused endocarditis and encephalitis	• Dx = intestinatl biopsy → p-aminosalicylic acid (PAS) ⊕ macrophages in intestines	• Penicillin or tetracycline
Lactase deficiency	• Most of world is lactase deficient as adults (lactase enzyme expression is lost during transition from adolescence to adulthood) • Si/Sx = abd pain, diarrhea, flatulence after ingestion of any lactose-containing product	• Dx = clinical	• Avoid lactose or take exogenous lactase

Table 5.6 *Continued*			
Type	**Characteristics**	**Dx**	**Tx**
Intestinal lymphan-giectasia	• Seen in children, congenital or acquired dilation of intestinal lymphatics leads to marked GI protein loss • Si/Sx = diarrhea, hypoproteinemia, edema	• Dx = jejunal biopsy	• Supportive
Pancreas dz	• Typically seen in pancreatitis and cystic fibrosis due to deficiency of pancreatic digestive enzymes • Si/Sx = foul-smelling steatorrhea, megaloblastic anemia (folate deficiency), weight loss	• Hx of prior pancreatic disease	• Pancrease supplementation

*Vancomycin is more effective for severe disease.
CRP, C-reactive protein.

4. Dx = **Urinalysis (UA)** → **pyuria;** ⊕ bacteria on Gram stain; ⊕ culture results

5. Tx = cephalosporin, aminoglycoside, or fluoroquinolone, narrow treatment based on cultures

6. Men with cystitis that are cured within 7 days of Tx do not warrant further workup, but **adolescents and men with pyelo-nephritis or recurrent infxn require renal US and IV pyelo-gram (IVP) to rule out anatomic etiology**

Table 5.7 Infectious Causes of Diarrhea			
	Bacterial	**Viral**	**Parasitic**
Etiology	*E. coli, Shigella, Salmonella, Campylobacter jejuni, Vibrio parahaemolyticus, Vibrio cholera, Yersinia enterocolitica*	Rotavirus Norwalk virus	*Giardia lamblia, Cryptosporidium, Entamoeba histolytica*
Tx	Fluoroquinolone	Supportive	Metronidazole

7. Bacterial prostatitis requires longer antibiotics (2 wks for acute infection, 6–12 wks for chronic)

8. aSx bacteriuria

   a. Defined as urine culture >100,000 colony-forming units (CFUs)/mL but no Sx

   b. Only Tx in (i) pregnant pts (use penicillins or nitrofuran-toin), (ii) pts with renal transplant, (iii) about to undergo genitourinary procedure, (iv) severe vesicular-ureteral reflux, or (v) struvite calculi

B. **Sexually Transmitted Dz (STDs) (Table 5.8). See Section C for AIDS.**

C. **Acquired Immunodeficiency Syndrome (AIDS)**

   1. Epidemiology

      a. AIDS is a global pandemic

      b. **Heterosexual transmission is the most common mode worldwide**

      c. Homosexual transmission is still the most common mode in the United States, but IV drug users and their sex partners are the fastest growing population of human immunodeficiency virus (HIV) ⊕ pts

   2. Dz Course

      a. In most untreated pts, AIDS is relentlessly progressive and death occurs within 10–15 yrs of HIV infxn

      b. Long-term survivors

         (1) Up to 5% of untreated pts are "long-term survivors," meaning the dz does not progress even after 15–20 yrs without Tx

         (2) This may be the result of infxn with defective virus, a potent host immune response, or genetic resistance of the host

         (3) People with homozygous deletions of CCR5 or other viral coreceptors are highly resistant to infxn with HIV, whereas heterozygotes are less resistant

      c. Death usually is caused by opportunistic infxns or malignancies

         (1) Opportunistic infxns typically onset after CD4 counts fall <200

         (2) When CD4 counts are <200, all pts should be on permanent TMP-SMX prophylaxis against *Pneumocystis* pneumonia (PCP) and *Toxoplasma* encephalitis

Text continues on page 327

Table 5.8 Sexually Transmitted Diseases

Disease	Characteristics	Tx
Herpes simplex virus (HSV)	• Most common cause of genital ulcers (causes 60%–70% of cases) • Si/Sx = **painful vesicular and ulcerated** lesions 1- to 3-mm diameter, onset 3–7 days after exposure • Lesions generally resolve over 7 days • Primary infection also characterized by malaise, low-grade fever, and inguinal adenopathy in 40% of pts • Recurrent lesions are similar appearing, but milder in severity and shorter in duration, lasting approximately 2–5 days • Dx confirmed with direct fluorescent antigen (DFA) staining, Tzanck prep, serology, HSV PCR, or culture	• Tx = acyclovir, famciclovir, or valacyclovir to ↓ duration of viral shedding and shorten initial infection
Pelvic inflammatory disease (PID)	• *Chlamydia trachomatis* and *Neisseria gonorrhoeae* are primary pathogens, but PID is polymicrobial involving both aerobic and anaerobic bacteria • PID includes endometritis, salpingitis, tubo-ovarian abscess (TOA), and pelvic peritonitis • Infertility occurs in 15% of pts after 1 episode of salpingitis, ↑ to 75% after ≥3 episodes • Risk of ectopic pregnancy ↑ 7–10 times in women with Hx of salpingitis • Dx = abd, adnexal, and cervical motion tenderness + at least one of the following: ⊕ Gram stain, temp >38°C, WBC >10,000, pus on culdocentesis or laparoscopy, TOA on bimanual or US	• Toxic pts, ↓ immunity and noncompliant should be Tx as in patients with IV antibiotics • Can use azithromycin, or fluoroquinolone + metronidazole or cephalosporin + doxycycline • Start antibiotic as soon as PID is suspected, even before culture results are available

(continued)

Table 5.8 *Continued*

Disease	Characteristics	Tx
Human papillomavirus (HPV)	• Serotypes **6 and 11** most commonly associated with **genital warts** • Serotypes **16 and 18** most commonly associated with **cervical cancer** • Incubation period varies from 6 wks to 3 mos, spread by direct skin-to-skin contact • Infection after single contact with an infected individual results in 65% transmission rate • Si/Sx = condyloma acuminata (genital warts) = soft, fleshy growths on vulva, vagina, cervix, perineum, anus • Dx = clinical, confirmed with biopsy	• Topical podophyllin or trichloroacetic acid, if refractory → cryosurgery or excision • If pregnant, C-section recommended to avoid vaginal lesions • Vaccines are approved by FDA for females and males 9–26 yrs old for the *prevention* of cervical cancer, precancerous or dysplastic lesions, and genital warts caused by HPV Types 6, 11, 16, and 18
Syphilis (*Treponema pallidum*)	• Si/Sx = **painless ulcer** with bilateral inguinal adenopathy, chancre heals in 3–9 wks • Because of lack of Sx, Dx of primary syphilis is often missed • 4–8 wks after appearance of chancre, 2° dz → fever, lymphadenopathy, maculopapular rash affecting palms and soles, condyloma lata in intertriginous areas • Dx = serologies, VDRL/RPR for screening, FTA-ABS to confirm	• Benzathine penicillin G
Male urethritis	• Typically caused by *N. gonorrhea* or *Chlamydia trachomatis,* can also be caused by *Ureaplasma urealyticum, Trichomonas vaginalis,* and HSV • Si/Sx = burning on urination and penile discharge • Dx by sampling purulent penile discharge for Gram stain to detect *N. gonorrhea,* and by nucleic acid amplification test of urine for *N. gonorrhea* and *Chlamydia*	• Third-generation cephalosporin for *N. gonorrhea,* azithromycin or doxycycline for *Chlamydia,* metronidazole for *Trichomonas,* acyclovir for HSV

Table 5.8 *Continued*

Disease	Characteristics	Tx
Lympho-granuloma venereum	• Caused by *Chlamydia trachomatis* serovars L1–L3 • Presents with a painless papule that erodes into a painless ulcer, accompanied by tender, swollen lymph nodes causing a groove along the inguinal ligament ("groove sign"), lymph nodes can cause draining sinus tracts to skin • Dx = clinical + serology	• Doxycycline or macrolide
Chancroid	• Caused by *Haemophilus ducreyi*, a gram-negative bacillus • Very rare in developed countries, typically seen in underdeveloped countries, patients have contact with commercial sex workers • Presents with painful ulcer, accompanied by painful, swollen lymph nodes which suppurate and cause destructive changes in the groin • Dx = clinical + Gram stain/culture	• Tx = macrolide, doxycycline, cephalosporin
Granuloma inguinale (Donovaniasis)	• Caused by *Klebsiella granulomatis* • A disease of underdeveloped countries • Presents with painless nodules which over time slough off, exposing large ulcers which spread and cause extensive, destructive changes in the groin • Dx = clinical + biopsy showing purple oval forms inside macrophages which stain purple by Wright stain	• Tx = macrolide or doxycycline

(3) When CD4 counts are <50, all pts should receive azithromycin prophylaxis against *Mycobacterium avium-intracellulare* complex (MAC)

(4) Kaposi's sarcoma = common skin CA found in homosexual HIV pts, caused by cotransmission of human herpes virus-8 (HHV-8)

        (5) Non-Hodgkin's lymphomas, typically high grade and aggressive, are far more common in HIV pts than non-HIV pts and are also harder to treat

        (6) Other dz found in AIDS pts include generalized wasting and dementia

3. Tx

  a. Highly Active Antiretroviral Tx (HAART)

     (1) Generally involves combination of a minimum of three active antiviral agents—now can administer one pill once per day that has three active drugs in it

     (2) Can use resistance testing to determine to which agents a pt's virus is susceptible

     (3) Initiate HAART if a pt has an AIDS-defining opportunistic infxn or CA, has symptoms related to HIV infection, or if the pt's CD4 count is <500 per µl

     (4) Give TMP-SMX prophylaxis if CD4 count is <200

     (5) Give azithromycin prophylaxis if CD4 count is <75

  b. With effective therapy in an adherent patient, HIV has become a manageable chronic disease

  c. Increasingly, patients with HIV die of chronic illnesses, such as cardiovascular dz and cancer

D. **Hematuria**

1. Can be painful or painless

  a. Painless due to 1° renal dz (tumor, glomerulonephritis), bladder tumor, prostatic dz

  b. Painful due to nephrolithiasis, renal infarction, UTI

2. DDx = myoglobinuria or hemoglobinuria, where hemoglobin dipstick is ⊕ but no RBCs are seen on microanalysis

3. Dx = finding of RBCs in urinary sediment

  a. UA → WBCs (infxn) or RBC casts (glomerulonephritis)

  b. CBC → anemia (renal failure), polycythemia (renal cell CA)

  c. Urogram will show nephrolithiasis and tumors (US → cystic versus solid)

  d. Cystoscopy only after UA and IVP; best for lower urinary tract

4. Tx varies by cause

E. **Prostate**

1. **Benign Prostatic Hyperplasia (BPH)**

  a. Hyperplasia of the periurethral prostate causing bladder outlet obstruction

b. Common after age 45 (autopsy shows that 90% of men older than 70 have BPH)

c. Does not predispose to prostate CA

d. Si/Sx urinary frequency, urgency, nocturia, ↓ size and force of urinary stream leading to hesitancy and intermittency, sensation of incomplete emptying worsening to continuous overflow incontinence or urinary retention, rectal exam → enlarged prostate (classically a rubbery versus firm, hard gland that may suggest prostate CA) with loss of median furrow

e. Labs → prostate-specific antigen (PSA) elevated in up to 50% of pts, not specific, so not a useful marker for BPH

f. Dx based on symptomatic scoring system, i.e., prostate size >30 mL (determined by US or exam), maximum urinary flow rate (<10 mL/s), and post-void residual urine volume (>50 mL)

g. Tx = α-blocker (e.g., terazosin), 5α-reductase inhibitor (e.g., finasteride); avoid anticholinergics, antihistaminergics, or narcotics

h. Refractory dz requires surgery = transurethral resection of prostate (TURP); open prostatectomy recommended for larger glands (>75 g)

2. **Prostatitis**

a. Si/Sx = fever, chills, low back pain, urinary frequency and urgency, tender, possible fluctuant and swollen prostate

b. Labs → leukocytosis, pyuria, bacteriuria

c. Dx = clinical

d. Tx = fluoroquinolone or TMP-SMX

3. **Prostate CA**

a. Most common CA in males, second most common cause of CA death (first = lung)

b. It is adenoCA histologically

c. More common in African-Americans, rare in Asians

d. PSA ↑ in 90% of adenoCA pts, but not specific, **controversy over use as a screening tool**, used to follow Tx by watching for dropping PSA levels

e. Metastasis occurs via lymph or blood, commonly causes **osteoblastic** lesions in bone

f. Tx = surgery, hormones, and/or radiation Tx

F. **Impotence**

1. Affects 30 million men in USA, strongly associated with age (approximately 40% among 40-yr-olds and 70% among 70-yr-olds)

2. Causes

   a. $1°$ erectile dysfunction = never been able to sustain erections

      (1) Psychological (sexual guilt, fear of intimacy, depression, anxiety)

      (2) ↓ testosterone $2°$ to hypothalamic–pituitary–gonadal disorder

      (3) Hypothyroidism or hyperthyroidism, Cushing's syndrome, ↑ prolactin

   b. $2°$ erectile dysfunction = acquired, **>90% from an organic cause**

      (1) Vascular dz = atherosclerosis of penile arteries and/or venous leaks cause inadequate impedance of venous outflow

      (2) Drugs = diuretics, clonidine, CNS depressants, tricyclic antidepressants, high-dose anticholinergics, antipsychotics

      (3) Neurologic dz = stroke, temporal lobe seizures, multiple sclerosis, spinal cord injury, autonomic dysfunction $2°$ to diabetes, post-TURP or open prostatic surgery

3. Dx

   a. Clinical, rule out above organic causes

   b. **Nocturnal penile tumescence** testing differentiates psychogenic from organic—nocturnal tumescence is involuntary, ⊕ in psychogenic but not in organic dz

4. Tx

   a. Cyclic GMP-specific phosphodiesterase 5 (PDE5) inhibitors

      (1) Examples include sildenafil, tadalafil, vardenafil

      (2) Inhibition of PDE5 → improves relaxation of smooth muscles in corpora cavernosa

      (3) Side effects = transient headache, flushing, dyspepsia, rhinitis, transient visual disturbances (blue hue) is very rare, drug may lower blood pressure → **use of nitrates is an absolute contraindication,** deaths have resulted from combo

   b. Vacuum-constriction devices use negative pressure to draw blood into penis with band placed at the base of penis to retain erection

    c. Intracavernosal prostaglandin injection has mean duration of approximately 60 min; risks = penile bruising/bleeding and priapism

    d. Surgery = penile prosthesis implantation; venous or arterial surgery

    e. Testosterone Tx for hypogonadism

    f. Behavioral Tx and counseling for depression and anxiety

V. Common Sports Medicine Complaints

A. Plantar Fasciitis

1. Inflamed plantar fascia band originating from the medial calcaneal tuberosity, which fans and inserts on the flexor mechanism of the toes at the metatarsal heads

2. Inflammatory condition common in runners and dancers who use repetitive, maximal plantar flexion of the ankle and dorsiflexion of the metatarsophalangeal joints

3. Si/Sx = pain in heel with first morning step (dorsiflexion), irritated and inflamed fascia is stretched causing severe pain

4. Tx = morning stretches/exercises and NSAIDs, rarely steroid injection or surgery

B. Low Back Pain

1. Eighty percent of people experience low back pain—second most common complaint in 1° care (next to common cold)

2. Fifty percent **of cases recur within the subsequent 3 yrs**

3. **Majority of cases attributed to muscle strains,** but always consider disk herniation

4. Si/Sx of disk herniation = shooting pain down leg (sciatica), pain on **straight leg raise** (>90% sensitive), and pain on **crossed straight leg raise** (>90% specific, not sensitive)

5. Dx

    a. **Always rule out RED FLAGS** (see later) with H&P exam

    b. If no red flags detected, presume Dx is muscle strain and not serious—**no radiologic testing is warranted**

    c. Dz not remitting after 4 wks of conservative Tx should be evaluated further with repeat H&P; consider radiologic studies

    d. Red Flags (Table 5.9)

6. Tx

    a. No red flags → conservative with acetaminophen (safer) or NSAIDs, **muscle relaxants have not been shown to help;** avoid narcotics

Table 5.9 Low Back Pain Red Flags

Diagnosis	Si/Sx
Fracture	• Hx of trauma (fall, car accident) • Minor trauma in elderly (e.g., strenuous lifting) • Dx with X-rays
Tumor	• **Pt age >50 yrs** (accounts for >80% of cancer cases) or <20 yrs • Prior Hx of CA • **Constitutional Sx** (fever/chills, weight loss) • Pain worse when supine or at night • Dx with MRI
Infection	• Immunosuppressed pts • Constitutional Sx • Recent bacterial infection or IV drug abuse • Dx with MRI
Cauda equina syndrome	• Acute urinary retention, saddle anesthesia, lower-extremity weakness or paresthesias and ↓ reflexes, ↓ anal sphincter tone—this is a medical emergency as it can rapidly progress to paralysis • Dx with MRI
Spinal stenosis	• Si/Sx = **pseudoclaudication** (neurogenic) with pain ↑ with walking **and standing;** relieved by sitting or leaning forward • Dx with MRI
Radiculopathy (herniation compressing spinal nerves)[a]	• Sensory loss: (**L5** → **L**arge toe/medial foot, **S1**→ **S**mall toe/lateral foot) • Weakness: (L1–L4 → quadriceps, L5 → foot dorsiflexion, S1 → plantar flexion) • ↓ Reflexes (L4 → patellar, S1 → Achilles) • Dx is **clinical**—MRI may confirm a clinical Dx but false-positive results are common (clinically insignificant disk herniation common on MRI) (See Figure 5.4)

[a]Radiculopathy ≠ herniation; radiculopathy indicates evolving spinal nerve impingement and is a more serious Dx than simple herniation indicated by straight leg testing and sciatica.

b. **Strict bed rest is NOT warranted** (extended rest shown to be debilitating, especially in older pts)—encourage return to nml activity, low-stress aerobic, and back exercises
c. Ninety percent **of cases resolve within 4 wks with conservative Tx**
d. Red flags:
   (1) Fracture → surgical consult
   (2) Tumor → urgent radiation/steroid (↓ compression), then excise

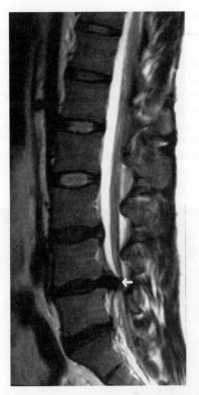

FIGURE 5.4

MRI scan showing a prolapsed disk at L4–5 with posterior deviation of the theca (*arrow*).

    (3) Infxn → abscess drainage and antibiotics per pathogen

    (4) Cauda equina syndrome → emergent surgical decompression

    (5) Spinal stenosis → complete laminectomy

    (6) Radiculopathy → anti-inflammatories, nerve root decompression with laminectomy or microdiscectomy only if (i) sciatica is severe and disabling, (ii) Sx persist for 4 wks or worsening progression, and (iii) strong evidence of specific nerve root damage with MRI correlation of level of disk herniation

C. **Shoulder Injuries**

1. Dislocation
    a. Subluxation = symptomatic translation of humeral head relative to glenoid articular surface
    b. Dislocation = complete displacement out of the glenoid
    c. Anterior instability (approximately 95% of cases) usually as a result of subcoracoid dislocation is the most common form of shoulder dislocation
    d. Si/Sx = pain, joint immobility, arm "goes dead" with over-head motion
    e. Dx = clinical, assess axillary nerve function in neurologic exam, look for signs of rotator cuff injury, confirm with X-rays if necessary (Figure 5.5)

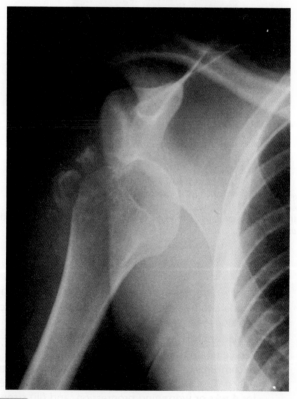

FIGURE 5.5

Anterior dislocation with a fracture of the greater tuberosity. (From Bucholz RW, Heckman JD. *Rockwood & Green's fractures in adults,* 5th Ed. Philadelphia, PA: Lippincott Williams & Wilkins, 2001.)

    f. Tx = initial reduction of dislocation by various traction—countertraction techniques, 2- to 6-wk period of immobilization (longer for younger pts), intense rehabilitation

  2. Shoulder Rotator Cuff Injury

    a. Often causes pain, but can cause just weakness in the shoulder without pain—classic symptoms are pain with overhead reach and pain at night

    b. Dx is clinical, confirm with MRI

    c. Tx for partial tears is conservative, with rest, NSAIDs, and physical therapy—complete tears require surgical repair

D. Clavicle Fracture

  1. Occurs primarily as a result of contact sports in adults

  2. Si/Sx = pain and deformity at clavicle

  3. Dx = clinical, confirm fracture with standard AP view X-ray

  4. Must rule out subclavian artery injury by checking pulses, brachial plexus injury with neurologic examination, and pneumothorax by checking breath sounds

  5. Tx = sling until range of motion is painless (usually 2–4 wks)

E. Elbow Injuries

  1. Epicondylitis (Tendonitis)

    a. Lateral epicondylitis **(tennis elbow)**

      (1) Usually in tennis player (>50%) or participants in racquetball, squash, fencing

      (2) Si/Sx = pain 2–5 cm distal and anterior to lateral epicondyle reproduced with wrist extension while elbow is extended

    b. Medial epicondylitis **(golfer's elbow)**

      (1) Commonly in golf, racquet sports, bowling, baseball, swimming

      (2) Si/Sx = acute onset of medial elbow pain and swelling 1 or 2 cm distal to medial epicondyle, pain usually reproduced with wrist flexion and pronation against resistance

    c. Tx for both = ice, rest, NSAIDs, counterforce bracing, rehabilitation

    d. Px for both varies, can become chronic condition; surgery sometimes indicated

  2. Olecranon Fracture

    a. Usually direct blow to elbow with triceps contraction after fall on flexed upper extremity

    b. Tx = long arm cast or splint in 45- to 90-degree flexion for ≥3 wks

    c. Displaced fracture requires open reduction and internal fixation

  3. Dislocation

    a. Elbow joint: Most commonly dislocated joint in children, second most in adults (next to shoulder)

    b. Fall onto outstretched hand with fully extended elbow (posterolateral dislocation) or direct blow to posterior elbow (anterior dislocation)

    c. May be seen in child after child's arm is jerked or child swung around by his arms (**nursemaid's elbow**). **Not true dislocation but a subluxation and treated with pronation of arm.**

    d. Key is associated nerve injury (ulnar, median, radial, or anterior interosseous nerve), vascular injury (brachial artery), or other structural injury (associated coronoid process fracture common)

    e. Tx = reduce elbow by gently flexing supinated arm, long arm splint, or bivalved cast applied at 90-degree flexion

  4. Olecranon Bursitis

    a. Inflammation of bursa under olecranon process

    b. Seen with direct blow to elbow by collision or fall on artificial turf

    c. Si/Sx = swollen and painful posterior elbow with restricted motion

    d. Dx = clinical, confirm with bursa aspiration to rule out septic bursitis

    e. Tx = bursa aspiration, compression dressing, and pad

F. **Wrist Injuries**

  1. Fractures

    a. Distal radius fracture (**Colles**) occurs after fall on outstretched hand (Figure 5.6)

    b. Ulnar fracture occurs after direct blow; commonly seen in hockey, lacrosse, or martial arts

    c. Dx = X-rays, H&P

    d. Tx for both = cast immobilization for 2–4 wks followed by bracing

    e. Scaphoid fracture

      (1) Usually 2° to falls; commonly misdiagnosed as a "wrist sprain"

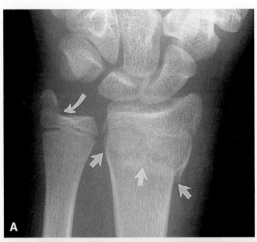

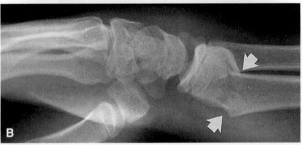

FIGURE 5.6
A. Extra-articular (Colles) distal radial fracture (*arrow*) in frontal projection associated with a fracture of the base of the ulnar styloid (*curved arrow,* A). (From Harris JH Jr, Harris WH. *The radiology of emergency medicine,* 3rd Ed. Philadelphia, PA: Lippincott-Raven, 2000, with permission.) **B.** Extra-articular (Colles) distal radial fracture (*arrow*) in lateral projection associated with a fracture of the base of the ulnar styloid (*curved arrow,* A). (From Harris JH Jr, Harris WH. *The radiology of emergency medicine,* 3rd Ed. Philadelphia, PA: Lippincott-Raven, 2000, with permission.)

FAMILY MEDICINE

      (2) Dx = clinical (pain in anatomic **snuffbox**), X-rays to confirm, bone scan or MRI for athletes who require early definitive Dx (Figure 5.7)

      (3) Tx = thumb splint for 10 wks (↑ risk of avascular necrosis)

  2. Carpal Tunnel Syndrome

    a. Si/Sx = pain and paresthesias in fingers worse at night

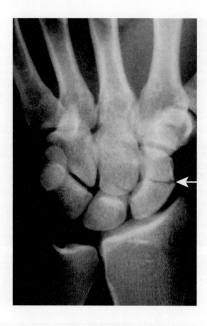

FIGURE 5.7

Scaphoid fracture. (From Bucholz RW, Heckman JD. *Rockwood & Green's fractures in adults,* 5th Ed. Philadelphia, PA: Lippincott Williams & Wilkins, 2001.)

b. Dx = **Tinel's sign** (pathognomonic) = tapping median nerve on palmar aspect of wrist producing "shooting" sensation to fingers and **Phalen's test** = wrist flexion to 60° for 30–60 sec reproduces a pt's Sx

c. Tx = avoid causative activities, splint wrist in slight extension, consider steroid injection into carpal canal; surgery for refractory dz

d. Px = may require up to 1 yr before Sx resolve even after surgery

G. **Hip Problems**

1. Trochanteric bursitis

   a. Si/Sx = pain right over the lateral aspect of the trochanter and is reproducible by pressing right over the trochanter—in contrast, pain from true hip disease refers to the groin

   b. Dx = clinical

   c. Tx = NSAIDs

2. Hip osteoarthritis
   a. Si/Sx = pain in the groin area, often worse in the morning, worse with activity/walking
   b. Dx = clinical, confirm osteoarthritis of the joint with X-rays
   c. Tx = rest, NSAIDs, ultimately joint replacement if symptoms are severe enough
3. Dislocations
   a. Requires significant trauma, usually posterior, occur in children
   b. Sciatic nerve injury may be present—do a careful neurologic exam
   c. Dx = X-rays, consider CT scan to assess any associated fractures
   d. Tx
      (1) **Orthopedic emergency requiring reduction under sedation (open reduction may be required)**
      (2) Light traction for ≥5 days is strongly recommended
      (3) No weight-bearing for 3-wk minimum, followed by 3–4 wks of light weight-bearing activities
      (4) Follow-up imaging studies required every 3–6 mos for 2 yrs
   e. Major complication is avascular necrosis of femoral head
4. Femoral Neck Fracture (Figure 5.8)
   a. Like hip dislocation, requires significant force
   b. Si/Sx = severe hip and groin pain worse with movement; leg may be externally rotated
   c. Dx = radiograph is definitive diagnosis
   d. Tx = operative reduction with internal fixation

H. **Knee Problems**
   1. Baker's cyst
      a. Posterior herniation of tense knee effusion, causing acute swelling behind the knee or down to mid-calf
      b. Often seen in patients with osteoarthritis or meniscal injuries
      c. DDx = DVT, ruled out with US
      d. Tx = conservative, NSAIDs and rest, can aspirate if pain is substantial
   2. Bursitis
      a. Prepatellar bursitis caused by kneeling on hard surfaces, causes pain over patella

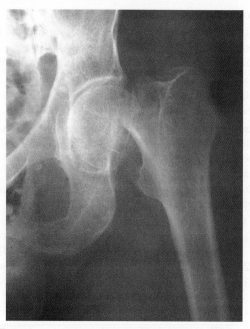

FIGURE 5.8

Femoral neck fracture. (From Bucholz RW, Heckman JD. *Rockwood & Green's fractures in adults,* 5th Ed. Philadelphia, PA: Lippincott Williams & Wilkins, 2001.)

   b. Pes anserine bursitis occurs on the medial side of the tibia, several inches below the knee joint, pain often worse going upstairs
   c. For both, rest and NSAIDs, tap the bursa if any question of infection, consider steroid injection if pain refractory
3. Ligament injuries (Table 5.10)
   a. Medial collateral and lateral collateral ligaments (MCL and LCL)
      (1) Injury results when foot is planted and a sideways force is directed at the knee
      (2) Si/Sx = pain with walking, but often little swelling
      (3) Dx = clinical, but can confirm injury by MRI
      (4) Tx = rest, ice, NSAIDs, consider knee immobilizer
   b. Anterior cruciate injury
      (1) Injury caused by planted foot with force applied to front or back of the knee

Table 5.10 Knee Injuries

Injury	Characteristics	Tx
Anterior cruciate ligament tear (ACL)	• Si/Sx = **presents with a "pop" in the knee,** pt may also complain of **knee instability or giving way** • **Lachman test** and/or anterior drawer finds pathologic anterior tibial translation and can Dx without imaging • MRI is most helpful to determine full extent of injury	Conservative or arthroscopic repair of tear
Posterior cruciate ligament tear (PCL)	• Tear seen during falls on flexed knee and dashboard injuries in motor vehicle accidents (MVAs) • X-rays to rule out associated injury or fracture • MRI useful to determine full extent of injury	Conservative or arthroscopic repair of tear
Collateral ligament tear	• **Medial collateral is the most commonly injured knee ligament** (lateral collateral is least commonly injured) • Seen after direct blow to lateral knee • **Commonly pt also injures ACL or PCL** • X-rays to rule out associated injury or fracture • MRI useful to determine full extent of injury	Hinge brace
Meniscus tear	• Acute trauma or more commonly due to degeneration seen with aging • Medial menisci injured three times more often, male > female • Dx = **McMurray test** = pt supine with hips flexed 90° and knee fully flexed, maneuver foot into abduction–adduction and external–internal rotation while palpating joint line for a click • MRI is standard diagnostic test (Figure 5.9)	Rest (fails >50% of time), consider arthroscopy

    (2) Si/Sx = pain/swelling of the knee, difficulty walking
    (3) Dx = clinical, can confirm ligament injury by MRI
    (4) Tx = rest, ice, NSAIDs, but surgical repair often required
  c. Meniscal tears
    (1) Can be from acute or chronic, repetitive injury
    (2) Si/Sx = intermittent pain and swelling, knee may "lock up" while walking, walking uphill, and climbing stairs may make the pain worse
    (3) Dx = clinical, MRI can confirm the diagnosis
    (4) Tx = rest, ice, NSAIDs, consider surgery if the symptoms are debilitating

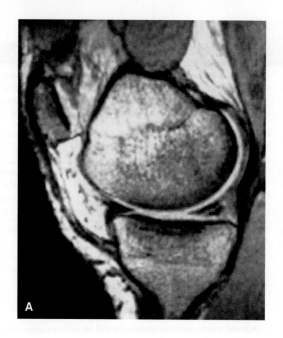

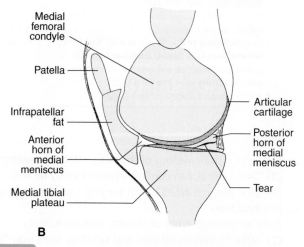

FIGURE 5.9

Tear of medial meniscus. **A.** Sagittal MRI through the medial part of the knee joint showing a tear in the posterior horn of the medial meniscus. **B.** The anterior horn appears nml. (Adapted from Armstrong P, Wastie M. *Diagnosticimaging*, 4th Ed. Oxford: Blackwell Science, 1998, with permission.)

I. **Ankle Injuries**

1. Achilles Tendonitis
   a. 2° to overuse, commonly seen in runners, gymnasts, cyclists, and volleyball players
   b. Si/Sx = swelling or erythema along Achilles tendon with tenderness proximal to calcaneus
   c. Evaluate for rupture = Thompson's test (squeezing leg with passive plantar flexion) positive only with complete tear
   d. Tx = rest, ice, NSAIDs, taping or splinting to ↓ stress and ↑ support
   e. Rupture requires short leg cast for 4 wks, short leg walking cast for 4 wks, then heel lift for 4 wks
   f. Open repair has lower re-rupture rate and is recommended with complete tears in younger pts

2. Ankle Sprains
   a. Lateral sprain occurs when ankle is plantar-flexed (90% of sprains)
   b. Anterior drawer sign is done with foot in 10- to 15-degree plantar flexion
   c. Medial sprain is rare (10%) because ligament is stronger
   d. Dx = Consider multiple view X-rays both free and weight-bearing r/o fracture
   e. **Ottawa rules used to determine need for X-rays, if a pt has pain in malleolar zone, with tenderness at posterior edge of distal 6 cm or tip of lateral malleolus, or unable to bear weight and walk four steps in ED, then obtain X-rays to r/o fracture**
   f. Tx = **RICE** = **R**est (limit activity ± crutches), **I**ce, **C**ompression (ACE bandage), **E**levation above level of heart to ↓ swelling
   g. Severe sprains may benefit from casting, open repair rarely indicated

VI. Nutrition

A. Nutritional Assessment

1. Diet history: Many methods can be used to assess a pt's nutritional status, whatever method used must start with a careful history of nutritional intake
2. Labs occasionally used:
   a. Serum albumin levels: Half-life 18–20 days, nml levels 3.5–5.5 g/dL, severe malnutrition <2.1 g/dL
   b. Serum pre-albumin levels: Half-life 2–4 days, nml levels 15.7–29.6 mg/dL, severe malnutrition <8 mg/dL

  c. Serum transferrin levels: Half-life 8–9 days, nml levels 200–400 mg/dL, severe malnutrition <100 mg/dL

  d. Serum retinal-binding protein: Half-life 12 hr, reflects very recent changes in protein and caloric intake, influenced by vitamin A intake

  e. Twenty-four hour collection for urine urea nitrogen to assess nitrogen balance before and after starting nutritional Tx—nitrogen losses are proportional to catabolic state

3. Anthropometric Measurements

 a. Ideal body weight (IBW)

  (1) Males: Height of 5 ft, ideal weight 106 lb and add 6 lb +/– 10% (frame size) for each additional inch over 5 ft

  (2) Females: Height of 5 ft, ideal weight 100 lb and add 5 lb +/– 10% (frame size) for each additional inch over 5 ft

  (3) Percent IBW = (actual weight/IBW) × 100, severely malnourished <69%, overweight >120%, morbidly obese = 200%

 b. Body mass index (BMI)

  (1) Useful in Dx of obesity, correlated with total body fat

  (2) Nml range is 19.0–26.0, pts with a BMI between 26.1 and 29.0 are considered overweight

  (3) BMI >30 is considered obese, >40 is considered morbidly obese

  (4) Formula: BMI = Weight (kg)/Height (m^2)

 c. Triceps skin fold

  (1) Measurements obtained using skin fold calipers on triceps of nondominant arm

  (2) Results compared with standardized tables and provide an estimate of overall subcutaneous fat stores.

4. Calculating Nutritional Requirements

 a. Caloric requirements: Harris–Benedict equation (kcal/kg/day) calculates resting metabolic rate

  (1) Men: 66 + 13.7 (weight [kg]) + 5 (height [cm]) – 6.9 (age [yr])

  (2) Women: 665 + 9.6 (weight) + 1.8 (height) – 4.7 (age)

 b. Estimated caloric requirements

  (1) Unstressed person: 25–35 kcal/kg/day

  (2) Hospitalized pt: 35–45 kcal/kg/day

  (3) Severely ill (ICU) pt: 50–70 kcal/kg/day

 c. Protein requirements

  (1) Maintenance: 1.0–1.5 g/kg/day

  (2) Repletion: 1.5–2.0 g/kg/day

  (3) Excessive loss: 2.0–2.5 g/kg/day

    d. Lipid requirements
- (1) Usually 25%–30% of total calories
- (2) Essential fatty acids are 2%–4% of those calories

5. Nutritional Supplements
    a. Enteral feeding is the preferred method of nutritional supplementation. Whenever possible feed the gut
- (1) Enteral feeding maintains gut integrity, reduces the risk of sepsis from gut bacteria
- (2) May be administered orally, per nasogastric, gastrostomy, or jejunostomy tube. All carry the risk of aspiration, but jejunostomy has the lowest
- (3) May be continuous or intermittent bolus feedings
- (4) Least expensive, most convenient

    b. Parenteral feeding
- (1) Useful when a pt is on bowel rest, and gut should not or cannot be fed
- (2) Total parenteral nutrition (TPN) requires central venous access. Solutions are a hyperosmolar mixture of dextrose, amino acids, vitamins, minerals, trace elements, electrolytes, and, in some institutions, fat emulsions are also directly added to mixture
- (3) Provides pts with all the necessary daily requirements
- (4) Monitor pts carefully when starting TPN. Electrolytes, liver enzymes, white count, and fluid status. These pts are at high risk for hyperglycemia, infxn, hypophosphatemia, hyponatremia, hepatic steatosis, and biliary dz
- (5) When discontinuing TPN, you should slowly taper the person off of TPN. This will prevent hypoglycemia by allowing pts' insulin levels to slowly return to nml

B. Vitamins and Nutrition

Nutrient	Deficiency	Excess
B_1 (thiamine)	**Dry beriberi** → neuropathy Wet beriberi → high-output cardiac failure Either → Wernicke–Korsakoff's syndrome	
B_2 (riboflavin)	**Cheilosis (mouth fissures)**	
B_3 (niacin)	Pellagra → dementia, diarrhea, dermatitis **Also seen in Hartnup's dz (dz of tryptophan metabolism)**	
B_5 (pantothenate)	**Enteritis, dermatitis**	

(continued)

Nutrient	Deficiency	Excess
B$_6$ (pyridoxine)	Neuropathy (frequently caused by isoniazid Tx for TB)	
B$_{12}$ (cyanocobalamin)	Pernicious anemia (lack of intrinsic factor) → neuropathy, megaloblastic anemia, glossitis	
Biotin	Dermatitis, enteritis (caused by consumption of raw eggs, due to the avidin in raw eggs blocking biotin absorption)	
Chromium	Glucose intolerance (cofactor for insulin)	
Copper	Leukopenia, bone demineralization	
Folic acid	Neural tube defects, megaloblastic anemia	
Iodine	Hypothyroidism, cretinism, goiter	
Iron	Plummer–Vinson syndrome = esophageal webs, spoon nails	Hemochromatosis → multiorgan failure (bronze diabetes)
Selenium	Myopathy (Keshan's dz, see Appendix A)	
Vitamin A	Metaplasia of respiratory epithelia (seen in cystic fibrosis due to failure of fat-soluble vitamin absorption), xerophthalmia, night blindness (lack of retinal in rod cells), acne, Bitot's spots, frequent respiratory infxns (respiratory epithelial defects)	Pseudotumor cerebri (can be caused by consuming polar bear livers), headache, nausea, vomiting, skin peeling
Vitamin C	Scurvy: Poor healing, hypertrophic bleeding gums, easy bruising, deficient osteoid mimicking rickets	
Vitamin D	Rickets in kids, osteomalacia in adults	Kidney stones, dementia, constipation, abd pain, depression
Vitamin E	Fragile RBCs, sensory and motor peripheral neuropathy	
Vitamin K	Clotting deficiency	
Zinc	Poor wound healing, ↓ taste and smell, alopecia, diarrhea, dermatitis, depression (similar to pellagra)	

Nutrient	Deficiency	Excess
Calories	Marasmus = total calorie malnutrition → pts look deceptively well but are immunosuppressed, poor wound healing, impaired growth	
Protein	Kwashiorkor = protein malnutrition → edema/ascites, immunosuppression, poor wound healing, impaired growth and development	

VII. Cancer Screening

Cancer	Screening Method
Breast	• U.S. Preventive Services Task Force (USPSTF) recommends screening mammography every 2 yrs starting at age 50 • American Cancer Society recommends annual mammography starting at age 40
Cervix	• Pap smear annually starting 3 yrs after initial sexual contact, but no later than age 21 • Switch to every 2–3 yrs for women over 30 with 3 consecutive negative smears • Stop screening at ≥65 yrs if 3 negative consecutive paps, or for patients who have had total hysterectomies
Colon	• From age ≥50 yrs, fecal occult blood testing annually or flexible sigmoidoscopy every 5 yrs or double contrast barium enemas every 5 yrs or colonoscopy every 10 yrs

6. PSYCHIATRY

I. Introduction

A. **DSM-IV (***Diagnostic & Statistical Manual of Mental Disorders, Fourth Ed.***)** (Table 6.1)

1. The DSM-IV lists current US diagnostic criteria for psychiatric conditions

2. **The United States Medical Licensing Examination (USMLE) will rely on DSM-IV diagnostic criteria, with DSM-V projected to come out in 2013; USMLE will take some time to catch up to any changes**

B. **Principles of Psychiatry for the USMLE (more complex in real life)**

1. Major psychiatric Dx requires **significant impairment in the pt's life**

2. **Always rule out drug abuse** (frequent comorbidity in psychiatric dz)

3. **Combination Tx** (pharmacology and psychotherapy) **is superior** to either alone, but **pharmacologic Tx is first line for severe dz in acute setting**

4. **Criteria for hospitalization (any single criterion is acceptable)**
   a. Danger to self (suicide)
   b. Danger to others
   c. Unable to care for self, provide food, clothing, shelter (grave disability)

5. Psychiatric dz is chronic—if asked about dz course, **"cures" are rare**

6. Px depends on Sx onset, insight, and premorbid function (Table 6.2)

Table 6.1 DSM-IV Classifications

Axis	Type of Disorder
I	Clinical psychiatric disorders
II	Personality disorders/mental retardation
III	Medical conditions
IV	Social and environmental factors
V	Level of functioning

PSYCHIATRY 349

PSYCHIATRY

Table 6.2 Prognosis of Psychiatric Disorders

Prognosis	Symptom Onset	Insight[a]	Premorbid Function
Favorable	Acute	Good	High
Unfavorable	Subacute/chronic	Poor	Low

[a]Insight refers to pt who recognizes Sx are abnormalities and is distressed by them.

II. Mood Disorders

A. Major Depressive Disorder (MDD)

1. Syndrome of **repeated major depressive episodes**
2. One of the most common psychiatric disorders, with lifetime prevalence of 15%–25%, with a greater incidence in women and elderly (often overlooked)
3. Si/Sx for depression in general
   a. Major Si/Sx = ↓ **mood** and/or **anhedonia** (inability to experience pleasure)
   b. Others = insomnia (less commonly hypersomnia), ↓ appetite/weight loss (less commonly ↑ appetite/weight gain), fatigue, ↓ concentration, irritability, guilt or feeling worthless, recurrent thoughts of death and suicide
   c. **Commonly presents with various somatic complaints and ↓ energy level rather than complaints of depression—** beware of clinical scenarios in which pts have multiple unrelated physical complaints
4. DDx = dysthymic disorder, bipolar disorder, medical dz **(classically hypothyroidism—particularly in the elderly!),** bereavement
5. Dx requires two depressive episodes to continue for ≥2 wks each, separated by ≥2 mos
6. Tx
   a. Drug therapy (Table 6.3)
   b. Psychotherapy = **psychodynamic** (understanding self/inner conflicts), **cognitive/behavioral therapy (CBT)** (recognizing negative thought or behavior and altering thinking/behavior accordingly), **interpersonal** (examines relation of Sx to negative/absent relationships with others)
   c. **Electroconvulsive Tx (ECT)** is effective for refractory cases, main side effect is short-term memory loss

Table 6.3 Pharmacologic Therapy for Depression[a]

Drug	Examples	Side Effects
SSRIs[b]	Fluoxetine, paroxetine, sertraline, citalopram, escitalopram	• Favorable profile: rare impotence
TCAs[b]	Amitriptyline, desipramine, imipramine, nortriptyline (these also may be used for neuropathic pain)	• More severe: confusion, sedation (making it useful at night for depression with insomnia), **orthostatic hypotension, prolonged QRS duration**
MAOIs[b]	Phenelzine, tranylcypromine (very rarely used now)	Very severe: classic syndromes • **Serotonin syndrome** = caused by **MAOI interaction with SSRIs, meperidine (Demerol), pseudoephedrine,** and others; presents with hyperthermia, muscle rigidity, altered mental status • **Hypertensive crisis** = malignant hypertension when ingested with foods rich in **tyramine** (wine and cheese)
SNRIs	Duloxetine, mirtazapine	• Mirtazapine associated with agranulocytosis

[a]Takes 2–6 wks for effect.
[b]Selective serotonin reuptake inhibitors (SSRIs) are first line; tricyclic antidepressants (TCAs) are second line; monoamine oxidase inhibitors (MAOIs) are third line; serotonin-norepinephrine reuptake inhibitors (SNRIs) are newest options.

B. **Dysthymic Disorder**

1. Si/Sx = as per major depressive episodes but is continuous

2. Dx = **steady Sx duration for minimum of 2 yrs**—dysthymic disorder is longer but less acute than MDD

3. If major depressive episode takes place during the 2 yrs of dysthymia, then by definition the Dx is MDD rather than dysthymic disorder

4. Tx = as per MDD

C. **Bereavement**

1. **Bereavement** is a commonly asked test question!

2. Si/Sx = in an older adult whose partner has died: feeling sad, losing weight, and sleeping poorly (depression Sx)

3. Dx: key is **how much time** has elapsed since the partner died—**if Sx persist for >2 mos, Dx is MDD** rather than nml bereavement

4. Although bereavement is nml behavior, grief management may be helpful

D. **Bipolar Disorder (Manic Depression)**

1. Seen in 1% of population, genders equally affected but **often presents in young people,** whereas **major depression is a dz of middle age (40s)**

2. Si/Sx = abrupt onset of ↑ **energy,** ↓ **need to sleep, pressured speech** (speaks quickly to the point of making no sense), ↓ attention span, impulsivity, **hypersexuality, spending large amounts of money,** engaging in outrageous activities (e.g., directing traffic at an intersection while naked)

3. DDx = cocaine and amphetamine use, personality disorders (see Section V.B, Cluster B), schizophrenia (see Section III), hypomania

4. Dx

   a. **Manic episode causes significant disability,** whereas hypomania presents with identical Sx but no significant disability

   b. Episodes **must last ≥1 wk and should be abrupt, not continuous,** which would suggest personality disorder or schizophrenia

   c. **Bipolar I** = manic episode with or without depressive episodes (pts often have depressive episodes before experiencing mania)

   d. **Bipolar II** = depressive episodes **with hypomanic episodes** but, by definition, **the absence of manic episodes**

   e. **Rapid cycling** = four episodes (depressive, manic, or mixed) in 12 mos; can be precipitated by antidepressants

5. Tx

   a. Hospitalization, often involuntary because manic pts rarely see the need

   b. **Valproate** first line, **lithium** second line

   c. Valproate and carbamazepine cause **blood dyscrasias**

   d. Lithium blood levels must be checked because of frequent toxicity, including **tremor** and polyuria resulting from **nephrogenic diabetes insipidus**

6. Px worse than major depression, episodes more frequent with age

E. **Drug-Induced Mania**

1. Cocaine and amphetamines are major culprits

2. Si/Sx = as per mania, also tachycardia, HTN, dilated pupils, **ECG arrhythmia, or ischemia in young people is highly suggestive**

3. Dx = urine or serum toxicology screen
4. Tx = calcium channel blockers for acute autonomic Sx, drug Tx programs longer term

III. Psychosis

A. Si/Sx

1. **Hallucinations and delusions** are hallmark
   a. Hallucination = false sensory perception not based on real stimulus (e.g., seeing people that aren't there and thinking they're out to get you)
   b. Delusion = false interpretation of external reality (e.g., seeing the post office person who really is standing in front of you and thinking he's an agent of the CIA who's out to get you)
   c. Can be paranoid, grandiose (thinking one possesses special powers), religious (God is talking to the pt), or ideas of reference (every event in the world somehow involves the pt)

B. DDx (Table 6.4)

C. Tx

1. Hospitalization if voices tell pts to hurt themselves or others, or if condition is disabling to the point that pts cannot care for themselves
2. Pharmacologic Tx (Table 6.5)
   a. All antipsychotics act as predominantly dopamine blockers
   b. Differences among agents relate to side effect profile (Table 6.6)
   c. Long-term compliance to drugs can be improved with **depot** form of haloperidol, which administers a 1-mo supply of drug in 1 IM injection
3. Psychotherapy can improve social functioning
   a. Behavioral Tx teaches social skills that allow pts to deal more comfortably with other people
   b. Family-oriented Tx teaches family members to act in more appropriate, positive fashion

D. Px

1. Schizophrenia is a chronic, episodic dz, recovery from each relapse typically leaves pt below former baseline function
2. Presence of negative Sx (e.g., flat affect, avolition, alogia) marks poor Px
3. High-functioning prior to psychotic break marks better Px

Table 6.4 Diagnosis of Psychotic Disorders

Disease	Characteristics
Schizophrenia	• **Presents in late teens to 20s (slightly later in women), very strong genetic predisposition** • Often accompanied by **premorbid** sign, including poor school performance, poor emotional expression, lack of friends • Positive Sx = hallucinations (**more often auditory than visual**) and delusions • Negative Sx = lack of affect, alogia (lack of speech) • Other Sx = disorganized behavior and/or speech • **Schizophrenia lasts ≥6 continuous months** • **Schizophreniform disorder lasts 1–6 mos** • **Brief psychotic disorder lasts 1 day–1 mo,** with full recovery of baseline functioning—look for acute stressor, e.g., death of a loved one
Other psychoses	• Schizoaffective disorder = meets criteria for mood disorders and schizophrenia • Delusional disorder = **non-bizarre delusions** (they could happen, e.g., pt's spouse is unfaithful, a person is trying to kill the pt, etc.), without hallucinations, disorganized speech, or disorganized behavior
Mood disorders	• Major depression and bipolar disorder can cause delusions, and, in extreme cases, hallucinations—can be difficult to differentiate from schizophrenia
Delirium	• Seen in pts with underlying illnesses, often in ICU (ICU psychosis) • **Patients are not orientated to person, place, time** • **Severity waxes and wanes even during the course of 1 day** • Resolves with treatment of underlying dz
Drugs	• LSD and PCP → predominantly visual, taste, touch, or olfactory hallucination • Cocaine and amphetamines → paranoid delusions **and classic sensation of bugs crawling on the skin (formication)** • Anabolic steroids → bodybuilder with bad temper, acne, shrunken testicles • Corticosteroids → psychosis/mood disturbances early in course of therapy
Medical	• Metabolic, endocrine, neoplastic, and seizure dz can all cause psychosis • **Look for associated Si/Sx not explained by psychosis,** including focal neurologic findings, seizure, sensory/motor deficits, abnormal lab values

LSD, lysergic acid diethylamide; PCP, phencyclidine.

Table 6.5 Antipsychotic Drugs

Drug		Adverse Effects[a]
Typical Antipsychotics[b]		
Chlorpromazine	Low potency	↑ Anticholinergic effects, ↓ movement disorders
Haloperidol	High potency	↓ Anticholinergic effects, ↑ movement disorders
Atypical Antipsychotics[b]		
Clozapine	For refractory dz	No movement disorders; 1% incidence of agranulocytosis mandates weekly CBC
Risperidone	First line	Rare movement disorders, but can occur at high doses; linked to new onset diabetes
Olanzapine, quetiapine, ziprasidone, aripiprazole	First line	No movement disorders; linked to new onset diabetes; ziprasidone and aripiprazole may cause less weight gain

[a]Anticholinergic effects = dry mouth, blurry vision (miosis), urinary retention, constipation.
[b]Atypical agents have much lower incidence of movement disorders (discussed ahead).

IV. Anxiety Disorders

A. Panic Disorder

1. Si/Sx = mimic myocardial infarction (MI): chest pain, palpitations, diaphoresis, nausea, marked anxiety, escalate for 10 min, remain for approximately 30 min (rarely >1 hr)

2. Occurs in younger pts (average age 25)—good way to distinguish from MI

3. DDx = MI, drug abuse (e.g., cocaine, amphetamines), phobias (discussed further)

4. Dx is by exclusion of true medical condition and drug abuse

5. Panic attacks are unexpected, so if pt consistently describes panic Sx in a specific setting, phobia is a more likely diagnosis

6. Tx
   a. Selective serotonin reuptake inhibitors (SSRIs) or serotonin-norepinephrine reuptake inhibitor (SNRI)
   b. Benzodiazepines work immediately, have ↑ risk of abuse

Table 6.6 Antipsychotic-Associated Movement Disorders

Disorder	Time Course	Characteristics
Acute dystonia	4 hrs → 4 days	• Sustained muscle spasm anywhere in the body but often in neck (torticollis), jaw, or back (opisthotonos) • Tx = immediate IV diphenhydramine
Parkinsonism	4 days → 4 mos	• Cog-wheel rigidity, shuffling gait, resting tremor • Tx = benztropine (anticholinergic)
Tardive dyskinesia	4 mo → 4 yrs	• Involuntary, irregular movements of the head, tongue, lips, limbs, and trunk • Tx = immediately change medication or ↓ doses because effects often are permanent
Akathisia	Any time	• Subjective sense of discomfort → restlessness: pacing, sitting down and getting up • Tx = lower medication doses
Neuroleptic malignant syndrome	Any time	• Life-threatening muscle rigidity → fever, ↑ BP/HR, rhabdo-myolysis over 1–3 days • Can be easily misdiagnosed as ↑ psychotic Sx • Labs → ↑ WBC, ↑ creatine kinase, ↑ transaminases, ↑ plasma myoglobin, as well as myoglobinuria • Tx = supportive: immediately stop drug, give dantrolene (inhibits Ca release into cells), cool pt to prevent hyperpyrexia

   c. Therefore, start benzodiazepine for immediate effects, add a TCA or SSRI, taper off the benzodiazepine as the other drugs kick in

   d. Cognitive/behavioral Tx and **respiratory relaxation training** (to help pts recognize and overcome desire to hyperventilate) are helpful

B. **Agoraphobia**

   1. Sx = fear of being in situations where escaping would be very difficult should a panic attack arise

2. Theorized that pts develop agoraphobia because they have experienced enough unexpected panic attacks to know that the attacks can come at any time

3. Dx = clinical, look for evidence of social/occupational dysfunction

4. Tx (for phobias in general)

   a. β-blockers useful for prophylaxis in phobias related to performance

   b. **Exposure desensitization** = exposure to noxious stimulus in increments while undergoing concurrent relaxation Tx

C. **Obsessive–Compulsive Disorder (OCD)**

1. **Obsessions = recurrent thought; compulsions = recurrent act**

2. Sx = obsessive thought causes anxiety, and the compulsion is a way of temporarily relieving that anxiety (e.g., pt worries whether she/he locked the door; going back to see if the door is locked relieves the anxiety), but because relief is only temporary, the pt performs compulsion repeatedly

3. Obsessions commonly involve **cleanliness/contamination** (washing hands), doubt, symmetry (elaborate rituals for entering doorways, arranging books, etc.), and counting

4. Dx = pt should be disturbed by their obsessions and **should recognize their absurdity** in contrast to obsessive–compulsive personality disorder, where pt sees nothing wrong with compulsion

5. Tx = SSRIs (first line) or clomipramine, CBT in which the pt is literally forced to overcome the behavior

D. **Posttraumatic Stress Disorder (PTSD)**

1. Dx requires a traumatic, violent incident that effectively scars the person involved; the experiences of combat veterans are emblematic of this disorder

2. Sx

   a. **Pt relives the initial incident via conscious thoughts or dreams**

   b. Due to resultant subjective and physiologic distress, the pt avoids any precipitating stimuli and **hence often avoids public places and activities**

   c. Pt may suffer restricted emotional involvement/responses and may experience a detachment from others

   d. **Depression is common; look for moodiness, diminished interest in activities, and difficulties with sleeping and concentrating**

3. DDx = **Acute Stress Disorder,** which also requires a traumatic incident, but Sx are more immediate (within 4 wks of the event) and limited in time (<4 wks) than PTSD—commonly seen in victims of sexual assault

4. Tx
   a. SSRIs are first line
   b. **Beware of giving benzodiazepines because of high association between substance abuse and PTSD!**
   c. Psychotherapy takes two approaches:
      (1) Prolonged Exposure Tx: "reliving" the experience
      (2) Cognitive Processing Therapy: Attacking the source versus controlling the Sx

5. Px = variable, abrupt Sx and strong premorbid functioning lead to better outcomes

E. **Generalized Anxiety Disorder**

1. Sx = worry for most days for at least 6 mos, irritability, inability to concentrate, insomnia, fatigue, restlessness

2. DDx = specific anxieties, including separation anxiety disorder, anorexia nervosa, hypochondriasis

3. **Dx requires evidence of social dysfunction** (e.g., poor school grades, job stagnation, or marital strains) to rule out "normal" anxiety

4. Tx = psychotherapy because of chronicity of the problem
   a. CBT = teaching pt to recognize his/her worrying and finding ways to respond to it through behavior and thought patterns
   b. **Biofeedback and relaxation** techniques, in particular, can help the pt deal with physical manifestations of anxiety, e.g., heart rate
   c. Pharmacotherapy includes buspirone or β-blockers (works for peripheral Sx, e.g., tachycardia, but not for worry itself)

V. Personality Disorders

A. **General Characteristics**

1. Sx = pervasive pattern of maladaptive behavior causing functional impairment; consistent behavior often can be traced back to childhood

2. Typically present to psychiatrists because behavior is causing significant problems for others, e.g., colleagues at work, spouse at home, **or for the medical staff in the inpt or clinic setting (typical USMLE question)**

3. **Pts usually see nothing wrong with their behavior (ego-syntonic),** contrast with pts who recognize their hallucinations as abnormal (ego-dystonic)
4. Ego Defenses
   a. Unconscious mental process that individuals resort to in order to quell inner conflicts and anxiety that are unacceptable to the ego
   b. Examples include "denial" and "projection"
5. Tx = psychotherapy, medication used for peripheral Sx (e.g., anxiety)

B. **Clusters**
   1. **Cluster A** = paranoid, schizoid, and schizotypal personalities, often thought of as **"weird"** or **"eccentric"**
   2. **Cluster B** = borderline, antisocial, histrionic, and narcissistic personalities, **"dramatic"** **"wild"** and **"aggressive"** personalities
   3. **Cluster C** = avoidant, dependent, and obsessive–compulsive personalities, **"shy"** and **"nervous"** personalities

C. **Specific Personality Disorders (Table 6.7)**

D. **Other Ego Defenses**
   1. Acting out: transforming unacceptable feeling into actions, often loud ones (tantrums)
   2. Altruism: constructive service to others that brings pleasure and personal satisfaction (Volunteering for Medical Missions)
   3. Denial: refusal to accept external reality because it is too threatening
   4. Displacement: redirection of some emotion from a real source to a substitute person or object
   5. Humor: overt expression of ideas and feelings (especially those that are unpleasant to focus on or too terrible to talk about) that gives pleasure to others (e.g., Jokes about someone close to you just dying)
   6. Identification: patterning behavior after someone else's
   7. Intellectualization: explaining away the unreasonable in the form of logic
   8. Introjection: identifying with some idea or object so deeply that it becomes a part of that person
   9. Projection: attributing unacceptable thoughts, feelings, behaviors, and motives to others

Table 6.7	Specific Personality Disorders
Disorder	**Characteristics**
Paranoid (Cluster A)	• Negatively misinterpret the actions, words, intentions of others • Often use **projection** as ego defense (attributing to other people impulses and thoughts that are unacceptable to their own selves) • **Do not hold fixed delusions** (delusional disorder) **or experience hallucinations** (schizophrenia)
Schizoid (Cluster A)	• Socially withdrawn, introverted, little external affect • Do not form close emotional ties with others (often feel no need) • Can recognize reality
Schizotypal (Cluster A)	• **Believe in concepts not considered real by the rest of society (magic, clairvoyance)**, display the prototypical ego defense: **fantasy** • Not necessarily psychotic (can have brief psychotic episodes) • Like schizoids, they are often quite isolated socially • **Often related to schizophrenics (unlike other Cluster A disorders)**
Antisocial (Cluster B)	• Violate the rights of others, break the law (e.g., theft, substance abuse) • Can be quite seductive (particularly with the opposite sex) • **For Dx, pt must have exhibited the behavior by a certain age (15—think truancy) but must be of a certain age (at least 18—adult)** • **Popular USMLE topic; you may have to differentiate it from conduct disorder (bad behavior, but Dx of children/adolescents)**
Borderline (Cluster B)	• Volatile emotional lives, swing wildly between idealizing and devaluing other people (**splitting** ego defense = people are very good or bad) • **Commonly asked on USMLE**, typical scenario is a highly disruptive hospitalized pt; on interview, he (but usually she) says some nurses are incompetent and cruel but wildly praises others (including you) • Exhibit self-destructive behavior (scratching or cutting themselves) • Ability to **disassociate:** they simply "forget" negative affects/experiences by covering them with overly exuberant, seemingly positive behavior

(continued)

Table 6.7 *Continued*	
Disorder	**Characteristics**
Histrionic (Cluster B)	• Require the attention of everyone, use sexuality and physical appearance to get it, exaggerate their thoughts with dramatic but vague language • Use disassociation and **repression** (block feelings unconsciously)—don't confuse with **suppression** (feelings put aside consciously)
Narcissistic (Cluster B)	• Feel entitled—strikingly so—because they are the best and everyone else is inferior, handle criticism very poorly
Dependent (Cluster C)	• Can do little on their own, nor can they be alone
Avoidant (Cluster C)	• Feel inadequate and are extremely sensitive to negative comments • Reluctant to try new things (e.g., make friends) for fear of embarrassment
Obsessive–compulsive (Cluster C)	• Preoccupied with detail: rules, regulations, neatness • Isolation is a common ego defense: putting up walls of self-restraint and detail orientation that keep away any sign of emotional affect

10. Rationalization: making the unreasonable seem acceptable (e.g., upon being fired, you say you wanted to quit anyway)

11. Reaction formation: set aside unconscious feelings and express exact opposite feelings (show extra affection for someone you hate)

12. Regression: resorting to childlike behavior (often seen in the hospital)

13. Sublimation: taking instinctual drives (sex) and funneling that energy into a socially acceptable action (studying) behavior or emotion

14. Suppression: the conscious process of pushing thoughts into the preconscious; the conscious decision to delay paying attention to an emotion or need in order to cope with the present reality

VI. Somatoform and Factitious Disorders

A. Definitions

1. Somatoform disorder = **lack of conscious manipulation of somatic Sx**

2. Factitious disorder = **consciously faking** or manipulating Sx for purpose of "assuming the sick role" **but not for material gain**

3. Malingering = consciously faking Sx **for purpose of material gain**

B. **Factitious Disorder**

1. Pt may mimic any Sx, physical or psychological, to assume the sick role

2. **Pt is not trying to avoid work or win a compensation claim**

3. Münchhausen syndrome = factitious disorder with predominantly physical (not psychologic) Sx

4. Münchhausen by proxy = pt claims nonexistent Sx in someone else under his/her care, e.g., parents bringing in their "sick" children

5. DDx = malingering

6. **HINT: The USMLE may present a scenario involving nurses or other health care workers as the pts (often involving an episode of apparent hypoglycemia), look for evidence of factitious disorder (e.g., low C-peptide levels suggesting insulin self-injection)**

7. Dx is by exclusion of real medical condition

8. Tx is nearly impossible; when confronted, pts often become angry, deny everything, tell you how horrible you are, and move on to someone else

C. **Somatoform Disorders**

1. Somatization Disorder

a. Often female pts with problems starting before age 30, with history of frequent visits to the doctor for countless procedures and operations (often exploratory) and often history of abusive/failed relationships

b. Sx = somatic complaints involving different systems, particularly GI (nausea, diarrhea), neurologic (weakness), and sexual (irregular menses), with no adequate medical explanation based on examination/lab findings

c. Dx = rule out medical condition and material or psychologic gain

d. Tx = **continuity of care**

(1) Schedule regular appointments so pt can express his/her Sx

(2) Perform physical examination but do not order labs

(3) As the therapeutic bond strengthens, strive to establish awareness in the pt that psychologic factors are involved, and, if successful in doing so, arrange a psychiatric consult—but if done too early or aggressively, pt may be reluctant or resentful

2. Conversion Disorder

   a. Sx are neurologic, not multisystem, and are not consciously faked

   b. Sensory deficits often fail to correspond to any known pathway, e.g., a stocking-and-glove sensory deficit that begins precisely at the wrist, studies will reveal intact neurologic pathways, and pts rarely get hurt, e.g., pts who are "blind" will not be colliding into the wall

   c. Dx requires identification of a stressor that precipitated the Sx as well as exclusion of any adequate medical illness

   d. Some of the pts who receive this Dx may eventually be found to have non-psychiatric causes of illness, e.g., brain tumors, multiple sclerosis

   e. Tx = supportive, Sx resolve within days (<1 mo), **do not tell pt that she/he is imagining the Sx, but suggest that psychotherapy may help with the distress**

   f. Px: the more abrupt the Sx, the more easily identified the stressor; the higher the premorbid function, the better the outcome

3. Hypochondriasis

   a. Sx = preoccupation with dz, pt does not complain of many Sx but misinterprets them as evidence of something serious

   b. Tx = regular visits to MD with every effort not to order labs or procedures, psychotherapy should be presented as a way of coping with stress, **again, do not tell pts that she/he is imagining the Sx**

4. Body Dysmorphic Disorder

   a. Sx = concern with body, **pt usually picks 1 feature, often on the face, and imagines deficits that other people do not see;** pt excessively exaggerates any slight imperfections, if present

   b. Look for a significant amount of emotional and functional impairment

   c. Tx = SSRIs may be helpful in some cases, surgery is not recommended

VII. Child and Adolescent Psychiatry

A. Psychological Testing

Psychological Tests

Intelligence	
Wechsler Adult Intelligence Scale—Revised (WAIS-R)	Tests ability to reason new situations, and assimilate, organize, and process this information. Tests cover verbal comprehension, performance at picture completion, block design, etc.
Wechsler Intelligence Scale for Children—Revised (WISC-R)	Tests children 6–16
Wechsler Preschool and Primary Scale of Intelligence (WPPSI)	Tests children 4–6
Personality	
Minnesota Multiphasic Personality Inventory (MMPI)	Most common objective personality test. Determines personality type
Rorschach	Most common projective test. Ink blot designs are interpreted, and defense mechanisms and thought disorders are evaluated
Achievement	
Wide-Range Achievement Test (WRAT)	Evaluates content-specific knowledge. Topics include spelling, reading, math, and science

B. Autism and Asperger's Syndrome

1. Autism is the prototypic **pervasive developmental disorder**, pervasive because the disorder encompasses so many areas of development: language, social interaction, emotional reactivity

2. The child is "living in his own world;" the autistic child fails to develop nml interactions with others and seems to be responding to internal stimuli

3. Si/Sx

   a. Becomes evident before the age of 3 yrs, often much earlier

   b. Baby does not seem to be concerned with the mother's presence or absence and makes no eye contact; as the baby becomes older, deficiencies in language (including repetitive phrases and made-up vocabulary) and abnormal behavior become more obvious

      c. Look for the behavioral aspects; the child often has a strange, persistent fascination with specific, seemingly mundane objects (vacuum cleaners, sprinklers) and may show stereotyped, ritualistic movements (e.g., spinning around)

      d. Impairment in social interactions, communication, and repetitive behaviors

      e. Autistic children have an inordinate need for constancy

  4. Think of Asperger's syndrome as autism **without** the language impairment

  5. **Contrary to older thought, poor parenting/bonding is not a cause of autism!—parents need reassurance about this**

  6. **Also, after dozens of large, scientific studies, not one has ever found evidence linking vaccines or vaccine preservatives (mercury or Thimerosal) to autism**

C. **Depression**

  1. Depression may present slightly differently depending on the age group

      a. Preschool children may be hyperactive and aggressive

      b. Adolescents show boredom, irritability, or openly antisocial behaviors

  2. Should look for the same Sx as described for adult depression: depressed mood, anhedonia, neurovegetative changes, etc.

  3. Tx

      a. Unlike adult depression, use of antidepressants is much more controversial with far fewer data supporting its effectiveness

      b. **Note:** children's mood disorders are especially sensitive to psychosocial stressors, so family Tx is a major consideration

D. **Separation Anxiety**

  1. Look for a child who seems a bit too attached to his parents or any other figures in his life; the child is worried that something will happen to these beloved figures or that some terrible event will separate them

  2. Si/Sx = sleep disturbances (nightmares, inability to fall asleep alone) and somatic Sx during times of separation (headaches, stomach upset at school)

  3. Tx = desensitizing Tx (gradually increasing the hours spent away from parents), in some cases imipramine is used

E. **Oppositional Defiant/Conduct Disorder**

  1. Differentiate the two by words and action (bark versus bite)

2. Oppositional defiant disorder Si/Sx ("bark")
    a. Pts are argumentative, temperamental, and defiant, more so with people they know well (they may seem harmless to you)
    b. They are often friendless and perform poorly in school
3. Conduct Disorder Si/Sx ("Bite")
    a. Pts bully others, start fights, may show physical cruelty to animals, violate/destroy other people's property (setting fires), steal things, stay out past curfews, or run away
    b. Pts do not feel guilty for any of these behaviors
    c. Glimpse into the child's family life often reveals pathology in the form of substance abuse or negligence
4. Oppositional defiant disorder may lead to conduct disorder, but the two are not synonymous
5. Tx = providing a setting with strict rules and expected consequences for violations of them

F. **Attention-deficit Hyperactivity Disorder (ADHD)**
    1. Si/Sx can be divided into the components suggested by their name
        a. Attention-deficit Sx = inability to focus on or perform tasks completely, easily distracted by random stimuli
        b. Hyperactivity Sx are more outwardly motor; child is unable to sit still, talks excessively, and can never "wait his turn" in group games
    2. Dx requires that Sx be present before age 7 yrs
    3. Tx = methylphenidate, an amphetamine (Ritalin, Concerta, Adderal)
        a. Parents and teachers notice improvement in the child's behavior if dx is correct.
        b. Because of concerns about impeding the child's growth, drug holidays are often taken (e.g., no meds over weekends or vacations)
        c. Children with ADHD do better with an extremely structured environment featuring consistent rules and punishments
        d. Px is variable, some children show remissions of hyperactivity, but quite a few continue to show Sx through adolescence and adulthood; children with ADHD have a higher likelihood of developing conduct disorders or antisocial personalities

G. **Tourette's Disorder**
    1. Tics are involuntary, stereotyped, repetitive movements, or vocalizations

2. **Tourette's Dx requires both a motor tic and a vocal tic present for ≥1 yr**

3. **Vocal tics often are obscene or socially unacceptable (coprolalia),** which is a cause of extreme embarrassment to the pt

4. **Tx = haloperidol is effective but not required in mild cases**

5. Psychotherapy is unhelpful in treating the tics per se but can be helpful in dealing with the emotional stress caused by the disorder

H. **Anorexia and Bulimia Nervosa**

1. Eating disorders are by no means limited to children, but because they often start in adolescence, they are mentioned here

2. Both disorders are associated with a profound disturbance in body image and its role in the person's sense of self-worth

3. Anorexia Si/Sx

   a. **By definition, anorexic pts are 85% below their expected body weight** because they do not eat enough, often creating elaborate rituals for disposing of food in meal settings, e.g., cutting meat into tiny pieces and rearranging them constantly on the plate

   b. **Amenorrhea occurs 2° to weight loss**

4. Bulimia Si/Sx

   a. More common than anorexia, **characterized by binge eating:** consuming huge amounts of food over a short period, with a perceived lack of control

   b. May be accompanied by active purging (vomiting, laxative use)

   c. **Unlike anorexics, who by definition have ↓ body weight,** bulimics often have a nml appearance

   d. **Abrasions over the knuckles** (from jamming the fingers into the mouth to induce vomiting) and **dental erosion** suggest the Dx

5. Tx

   a. Hospitalization may be required for anorexia to restore the pt's weight to a safe level, pt often resists hospitalization

   b. Monitoring serum electrolytes is essential because of vomiting; most worrisome consequence is cardiac dysfunction—as exemplified by singer Karen Carpenter, whose battle with anorexia led to her untimely death

   c. Psychotherapy is the mainstay of Tx for both dz

6. Overall, anorexia nervosa has a relatively poor Px with high morbidity and mortality, bulimics fare slightly better.

VIII. Abuse of Drugs

A. Introduction

1. Always consider drug abuse when a pt's life seems to be disintegrating, e.g., deteriorating family relations, work performance, financial stability

2. Generally (with many exceptions), withdrawal Sx are opposite those of intoxication, dysphoria is characteristic of all of them—**withdrawal is a sign of physiologic dependence**

3. Individual drugs (Table 6.8)

Table 6.8 Drug Intoxications and Withdrawal			
Drug	**Intoxication Si/Sx**	**Withdrawal**	**Tx**
Alcohol	Disinhibition, ↓ cognition Screen for alcoholism with **CAGE** • **C**—feeling the need to **cut** down • **A**—feeling **annoyed** when asked about drinking • **G**—feeling **guilty** for drinking • **E**—need a drink in the morning **(eye-opener)**	Tremor, seizures, delirium tremens (high mortality! Prevent with benzodiazepines)	• See Chapter 1. III.D.4.h
Cocaine/ amphetamine	Agitation, irritability, ↓ appetite, formication, ↑ or ↓ BP & HR, cardiac arrhythmia or infarction, stroke, seizure, nosebleeds	Hypersomnolence, dysphoria, ↑ appetite	• Benzodiazepine for seizures and for BP/HR • Ca⁺⁺ channel blockers for ischemia (β-blockers may worsen d/t unopposed α-agonism by the cocaine)

(continued)

Table 6.8 *Continued*

Drug	Intoxication Si/Sx	Withdrawal	Tx
Heroin (opioids)	Intense, fleeting euphoria, drowsy, slurred speech, ↓ memory, pupillary constriction, ↓ respiration **Triad of ↓ consciousness, pinpoint pupils, and respiratory depression should always lead to a suspicion of opioids**	Nausea/vomiting, pupillary dilation, and insomnia	• Naloxone to reverse acute intoxication • Withdrawal Tx with long methadone taper
Benzodiazepine and barbiturates	Respiratory and cardiac depression	Agitation, anxiety, delirium	• Intoxication → control airway, charcoal to reduce absorption, flumazenil can reverse benzos acutely, but can precipitate seizures so be cautious • Withdrawal Tx → taper doses
PCP	Intense psychosis, violence, rhabdomyolysis, hyperthermia	Similar, lasts for days to weeks	• Supportive, benzos or haloperidol for psychosis
LSD	Sensation is enhanced: colors are richer, music more profound, tastes heightened	Not withdrawal, but can have long-lasting psychosis	• Supportive

LSD, lysergic acid diethylamide; PCP, phencyclidine.

IX. Miscellaneous Disorders

A. Disorders of Sexuality and Gender Identity

1. Sexual identity is based on biology, e.g., men have testes
2. Gender identity is based on self-perception, e.g., biologic male perceives himself as a male

3. **Children have a firm conception of their gender identity very early (before age 3)**

4. Sexual orientation is who the person is attracted to; **homosexuality is not a psychiatric disorder**

B. **Dissociative Disorder (Multiple Personality Disorder)**

1. A pt seemingly possesses different personalities that can each take control at a given time

2. The pt's Hx may give some Hx of childhood trauma, e.g., abuse

3. Tx focuses on gradual integration of these personalities

4. Main differentials are **dissociative amnesia** and **dissociative fugue**

   a. Amnesia is a syndrome of forgetting a great deal of personal information

   b. Fugue refers to the syndrome of sudden travel to another place, with inability to remember the past and confusion of present identity

   c. **Neither case involves shifting between different identities**

C. **Adjustment Disorder**

1. Any behavioral or emotional Sx that occur in response to stressful life events in excess of what is nml

2. Obviously has a catch-all quality to it; **this will be a frequent answer option on the USMLE**

3. **Dx requires Sx within 3 mos of the stressor** (so Sx do not have to be immediate) and **must disappear within 6 mos of the disappearance of the stressor**

4. Bereavement may seem to be a type of adjustment disorder (stressor is death), but they are separate Dx

5. Depending on the setting, adjustment disorder may appear as depression or anxiety—but remember: **Axis I disorders such as major depression and generalized anxiety take precedence**

D. **Impulse-Control Disorders**

1. Pts are unable to resist the drive to perform certain actions **harmful to themselves or others**

2. Note the emotional response: these individuals **feel anxiety before the action and gratification afterward**

3. Intermittent explosive disorder

   a. Discrete episodes of aggressive behavior far in excess of any possible stressor

b. The key term is **episodic**; antisocial personalities also commit aggressive behaviors, but their aggression is present between outbursts of such behavior

4. Kleptomania
   a. Impulse to steal
   b. The object of theft is not needed for any reason (monetary or otherwise)
   c. The kleptomaniac often feels guilty after stealing

5. Pyromania
   a. Purposeful fire-setting
   b. Often a fascination with fire itself distinguishes this from the antisocial personality/conduct disorders, where the fire-setting is purposeful, e.g., revenge, and not the failure to resist an impulse

6. Trichotillomania = hair-pulling, resulting in observable hair loss

X. Sleep

A. **Nml sleep** consists of two different types:
1. Non–rapid eye movement (NREM) has four states (Table 6.9)
2. Rapid eye movement (REM)

B. **Sleep Stages** (see Table 6.9)

C. **Sleep Disorders**
1. Dyssomnias: difficulties with sleep
   a. Insomnia
      (1) Unable to fall asleep or stay asleep recurrently over a 1-mo period
      (2) Can be associated with stress, anxiety, drugs, and various medical and mental conditions

Table 6.9 Sleep Stages

Stages	Characteristics
Non-REM	Early slow-wave sleep
Stage 1	Alpha-waves (awake waves disappear) and theta-waves (time to sleep waves occur)
Stage 2	Sleep spindles
Stages 3 and 4	Delta-wave sleep (most difficult to awake from)
REM	Dreaming (suppressed by alcohol and drugs)

      (3) Tx = sleep routine, exercise, antihistamines, short course of benzodiazepines <2 wks to prevent rebound insomnia

  b. Hypersomnia

     (1) Narcolepsy: recurrent sleep attacks, associated with REM sleep and dreaming

       (a) Pts can suddenly collapse because of loss of all muscle tone (cataplexy)

       (b) Tx = stimulants such as methylphenidate or pemoline (Provigil)

     (2) Sleep apnea: periods of apnea occurring during sleep

       (a) Obstructive: ↑ inspiratory effort that fails to result in ↓ airflow

         (i) Most common; pts usually are obese heavy snorers who awake after a gasp for air, pts complain of excessive daytime sleepiness; spouse complains of loud snoring

         (ii) Can lead to pulmonary HTN, associated with hypothyroidism

         (iii) Tx = weight loss, continuous positive airway pressure (CPAP) at night to maintain patent airway, surgery if no relief and severely affecting lifestyle or danger to life

       (b) Mixed obstructive/central: periods of no inspiratory effort followed by inspiratory effect that is obstructed by collapse of oropharyngeal airway

       (c) Central: rare; loss of inspiratory effort

     (3) Pickwickian syndrome (central alveolar hypoventilation)

       (a) Triad of somnolence, obesity, and erythrocytosis

       (b) Gradual onset of hypercapnia, hypoxemia, and erythrocytosis

       (c) Weight of adipose on lungs and abdomen cause chronic alveolar hypoventilation

       (d) Tx = weight loss, CPAP

2. Parasomnias

  a. Night terror

     (1) Arises during NREM sleep

     (2) Child sits up suddenly in bed with diaphoresis, tachycardia, feeling frightened

     (3) Not full awake; pts usually fall back to sleep after the episode

    b. Nightmares
       (1) Occur during REM sleep
       (2) Usually occur after an emotional event, stress, or frightening movie
       (3) Pts are fully awake and have good recall of nightmare events
       (4) Also associated with drugs
    c. Sleepwalking (somnambulism)
       (1) Occurs during NREM sleep
       (2) Pts get out of bed and wander around; some pts can jump out of windows or open doors
       (3) Pts usually awaken with no memory of events
    d. Restless leg syndrome
       (1) Irresistible urge to move limbs
       (2) Most commonly causes limb-jerking movements during sleep that disrupts sleep stages
       (3) Can be primary with no known cause or secondary to iron deficiency, dopamine deficiency, or hypothyroidism
       (4) Dx = Lab studies to r/o underlying cause. Sleep study to evaluate severity
       (5) Tx = Dopamine agonist and treatment of underlying cause, i.e., thyroid replacement or iron

7. NEUROLOGY

I. Stroke

A. Terminology

1. Stroke = sudden, nonconvulsive focal neurologic deficit
2. Transient ischemic attack (TIA) = deficit lasting ≤24 hrs (usually <1 hr) but resolves completely
3. Emboli sources = **carotid atheroma (most common),** cardiac and fat emboli, endocarditis (metastasizing CA cells)
4. Lacunar infarct = small infarct in deep white mater, strongly associated with HTN and atherosclerosis
5. Watershed infarcts occur at border of areas supplied by different arteries (e.g., middle cerebral artery, anterior cerebral artery), often following prolonged hypotension

B. Presentation

1. Si/Sx depend on location of stroke (Table 7.1)
2. Wernicke's aphasia (temporal lobe lesion) = receptive, pt speaks fluently but words do not make sense: **Wernicke's is wordy**

Table 7.1 Presentation of Stroke

Si/Sx	Artery	Region (Lobe)
Amaurosis fugax (monocular blindness)	Carotid (emboli)	Ophthalmic artery
Drop attack/vertigo/CN palsy/coma	Vertebrobasilar (embolic)	Brainstem
Aphasia	Middle cerebral	Dominant frontal or temporal[a]
Sensory neglect and apraxia[b]	Middle cerebral	Nondominant frontal or temporal[a]
Hemiplegia	Middle or anterior cerebral	Parietal lobe on opposite side
Urinary incontinence and grasp reflex	Middle or anterior cerebral	Frontal
Homonymous hemianopia	Middle or posterior cerebral	Temporal or occipital

[a]Dominant = left in 99% of right-handers and >50% of left-handers.
[b]Apraxia = pt cannot follow command even if it is understood and the pt is physically capable of it.

3. Broca's aphasia (frontal lobe lesion) = expressive, pt is unable to verbalize: **Broca's is broken**
4. Edema occurs 2–4 days postinfarct, watch for this clinically (e.g., ↓ consciousness, projectile vomiting, pupillary changes) (Figure 7.1)
5. Decorticate (cortical lesion) posturing → flexion of arms
6. Decerebrate (midbrain or lower lesion) posturing → arm extension

C. **DDx**

1. Stroke, seizure (Sz), neoplasm, encephalitis, multiple sclerosis
2. Stroke causes = 35% atheroembolic, 30% cardiac, 15% lacunar, 10% parenchymal hemorrhage, 10% subarachnoid hemorrhage, ≤1% other (e.g., vasculitis, temporal arteritis, etc.)
3. Dx = CT (insensitive but rapid and readily available—if positive, Dx is made; if negative, still need MRI to rule out); MRI is gold standard (see Figure 7.1)
4. Rule out Sz → EEG, loss of bowel/bladder control and tongue injury

D. **Tx**

1. Tissue plasminogen activator (tPA) within 3–6 hrs of onset (preferably 1 hr) for occlusive dz **only** (i.e., not for hemorrhagic stroke)
2. **Intracranial bleeding is an absolute contraindication to tPA use!**
3. Correct underlying disorder, e.g., hyperlipidemia, hypertension, diabetes, valve abnormality, coagulopathy, atrial fibrillation
4. For embolic strokes give aspirin/warfarin anticoagulation for prophylaxis
5. If carotid is 70% occluded and pt has Sx → endarterectomy or endocarotid stent

E. **Px**

1. 20%–40% mortality at 30 days (20% atheroemboli, 40% bleed)
2. Less than one-third of pts achieve full recovery of lifestyle
3. Atheroembolic strokes recur at 10% per yr

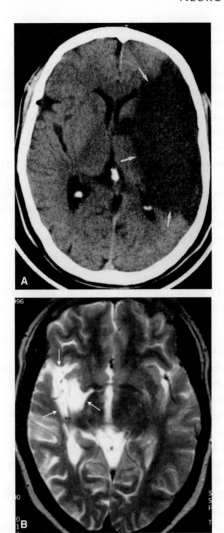

FIGURE 7.1

Cerebral infarction. **A.** Unenhanced CT scan showing a low-density region of the left cerebral hemisphere conforming to the distribution of the middle cerebral artery (*arrows*). **B.** MRI of another pt with a right middle cerebral artery territory infarct. The infarcted area (*arrows*) shows patchy high-signal intensity on this T2-weighted image. The *arrows* point to the anterior and posterior extents of the infarcted brain tissue. (From Armstrong P, Wastie M. *Diagnostic imaging*, 4th Ed. Oxford: Blackwell Science, 1998, with permission.)

II. Infection and Inflammation

A. **Meningitis**

1. 50% due to *Streptococcus pneumoniae,* 25% due to *Neisseria meningitidis; Haemophilus influenzae* rare now because of vaccination; *Listeria* seen in neonates, pregnant women, elderly, immunocompromised pts; Group B *Streptococcus (Streptococcus agalactiae)* and *Escherichia coli* are the #1 and #2 causes of neonatal meningitis

2. Si = **Meningismus** (pt cannot touch chin to chest), ⊕ **Kernig's sign** (pt is supine with hip and knees flexed at 90 degrees, examiner cannot extend knee), ⊕ **Brudzinski's sign** (pt is supine; when examiner flexes neck, pt involuntarily flexes hip and knees)

3. Cerebrospinal fluid (CSF) differential for meningitis (Table 7.2)

4. Presentations can be acute, subacute, chronic

5. Acute
   a. Send CSF for Gram stain, bacterial cultures; if patient has encephalitis or if HSV viral meningitis is suspected, send HSV PCR
   b. Treat all pts with suspected meningitis empirically by age until specific tests return (Table 7.3)
   c. Of viral causes, only HSV (acyclovir) and HIV (AZT) can be treated—otherwise Tx is supportive
   d. Bacterial meningitis (Table 7.4)

6. Subacute/Chronic Meningitis
   a. Si/Sx = per acute but evolves over wk → mo, ± fever
   b. DDx = fungal, mycobacterial, syphilis; noninfectious dzs include lymphoma/leukemia spread to CSF, or rarely carcinomatosis, SLE/vasculitis, sarcoid
   c. Send CSF for fungal Cx, cytology, India Ink, TB PCR
   d. Fungal meningitis
      (1) DDx = *Cryptococcus, Coccidioides,* other rarer dz

Table 7.2 Cerebrospinal Fluid Findings in Meningitis

	Cells	Protein	Glucose
Bacterial	↑↑ Neutrophils	↑	↓ (≤1/2 serum)
Viral	↑ Lymphocytes	↑/±	Nml
Fungal/TB	↑ Lymphocytes	↑↑↑↑	↓

Table 7.3	Empiric Therapy for Community Acquired Meningitis by Age	
Age	**Regimen**	**Common Etiologies**
Neonates (≤1 mo)	Ampicillin + ceftriaxone	S. agalactiae, Listeria, E. coli
Children to teens	Ceftriaxone + vancomycin[a]	S. pneumoniae, N. meningitidis
Adults <65 yrs or, immune competent	Ceftriaxone + vancomycin[a]	S. pneumoniae by far most common
Adults ≥65 yrs or with immune-compromise	Ceftriaxone + vancomycin[a] + ampicillin	As for adults above, but need to cover Listeria as well

[a]Due to increasing rate of β-lactam resistance in S. pneumoniae.

Table 7.4	Bacterial Meningitis		
Organism	**Epidemiology**	**Characteristics**	**Tx**
S. pneumoniae	#1 cause in adults; HIV, old age, asplenia, antibody deficiency, alcoholism all predispose	Can progress from otitis media, sinusitis, or bacteremia	Ceftriaxone or PCN G, vancomycin if resistant to β-lactams
N. meningitidis	Most commonly in teenagers and young adults in close populations (college dormitories, military barracks)	Petechiae on trunk, legs, conjunctivae—beware of Waterhouse–Friderichsen syndrome (adrenal infarct)	PCN G; rifampin or fluoroquinolone prophylaxis for close contacts
H. influenzae	Formerly #1 cause until conjugated HiB vaccine	Now rare	Ceftriaxone
S. agalactiae	#1 cause in neonates	Acquired at birth	Ampicillin
E. coli	Common in neonates	Acquired at birth	Ceftriaxone
L. monocytogenes	Elderly/neonates, HIV, pregnant, diabetes, steroids, eating unpasteurized cheese	Often negative CSF Gram stain; culture grows GPC with "tumbling motility"	Ampicillin
S. aureus	Trauma/neurosurgery	Wound infection from skin, or infected ventriculostomy	Vancomycin (MRSA) or oxacillin (MSSA)

NEUROLOGY

(2) *Cryptococcus* commonly seen in AIDS
  (a) India Ink stain will show *Cryptococcus* in CSF
  (b) Opening pressure is commonly very elevated
  (c) Cryptococcal antigen in CSF invariably ⊕
  (d) Tx = iv amphotericin +/− 5-fluorocytosine, followed by fluconazole; must perform serial LPs to lower the intracranial pressure, drawing off enough CSF to have a low closing pressure; and if the pressures repeatedly rise again on sequential days, eventually a shunt must be put in to control pressures
(3) *Coccidioides*
  (a) Suspect in Arizona, California
  (b) Higher risk in African-American, Hispanic, and Filipino pts
  (c) Diagnose by antibody ⊕ in serum or CSF
  (d) Tx = high-dose fluconazole
e. TB meningitis
  (1) Usually occurs in elderly by reactivation, grave Px
  (2) Dx is made by TB PCR of the CSF
  (3) Tx = **RIPE: R**ifampin, **I**NH, **P**yrazinamide, **E**thambutol plus corticosteroids (for meningeal TB)

B. **Encephalitis**

Si/Sx = altered mental status and focal neurological findings (Table 7.5)

C. **Abscess**

1. Si/Sx = headache, fever, ↑ intracranial pressure (ICP), focal neurologic findings
2. Risk factors = congenital right-to-left shunt (lung filtration bypassed), otitis, paranasal sinusitis, metastases, trauma, and immunosuppression
3. Anaerobes and aerobes, gram-positive cocci and gram-negative rods can be causes
4. Tx = antibiotics ⊕ surgical drainage
5. Brain abscesses are invariably fatal if untreated

III. Demyelinating Diseases

A. **Multiple Sclerosis (MS)**

1. Unknown etiology, but ⊕ genetic and environmental predispositions, ↑ common in pts who lived first decade of life in northern latitudes

Table 7.5 Encephalitis

Etiology	Si/Sx	Tx/Px
HSV	• Affects temporal lobe primarily • Altered mental status, personality changes, olfactory hallucinations • CSF often (but not always) has blood in it • EEG/MRI → temporal lobe dz • Dx confirmed by HSV PCR in CSF	• IV acyclovir
Other Viral Encephalitis	• Caused by a variety of viruses including enteroviruses, arboviruses (Eastern Equine, California, etc), West Nile, etc. • Presentations all overlap, with altered mental status and focal neurological findings • Dx by combination of antibody testing and PCR	• None
Toxoplasmosis	• In neonates it causes congenital hydrocephalus and mental retardation from transplacental infection • In adults, exposed via cat feces, disease reactivates in CNS when the pt becomes immunocompromised—#1 CNS lesion in AIDS • Presents with multiple ring-enhancing lesions on MRI (basal ganglia classically involved) → focal neurological deficits • Dx is by clinical syndrome in the right patient (AIDS) with multiple ring-enhancing lesions on MRI and response to therapy (shrinking lesions) 2 wks after starting empiric Toxo therapy	• Sulfadiazine + pyrimethamine • Primary prophylaxis with TMP-SMX for HIV patients with CD4 count <200/μL
Progressive Multifocal Leuko-encephalopathy (PML)	• Usually in AIDS, also increasingly seen in patients treated with antibodies against lymphocytes for cancer or autoimmunity • Caused by JC polyomavirus • Presents with diffuse white matter disease on brain MRI • Dx = clinical syndrome in the right host, plus CSF PCR for JC virus	• Treat the AIDS
Cysticercosis	• Caused by the helminth *Taenia solium* • Presents with seizures, typically in a Hispanic immigrant, or in someone with close contact with an Hispanic immigrant (e.g., live-in nanny) • MRI shows cysts in brain, old disease appears as calcified spots in brain • Patients may (but often don't) have blood or CSF eosinophils • Dx by clinical and imaging pictures, can send CSF antibody, which is specific	• Albendazole + steroids

2. Si/Sx = relapsing asymmetric limb weakness, ↑ deep tendon reflexes (DTRs), nystagmus, tremor, scanning speech, paresthesias, optic neuritis, ⊕ Babinski sign

3. Dx = Hx, MRI, lumbar puncture

4. MRI → periventricular plaques, multiple focal demyelination scattered in brain and spinal cord (**lesions disseminated in space and time**)

5. **Lumbar puncture → ↑ CSF immunoglobulins manifested as multiple oligoclonal bands on electrophoresis**

6. Tx = interferon-β or glatiramer acetate, may induce prolonged remissions in some pts

7. Px
   a. Variable disease course, with long remissions sometimes seen
   b. But can progressively decline → death in only a few years

B. **Guillain–Barré Syndrome**

1. Acute autoimmune demyelinating dz involving peripheral nerves

2. **Si/Sx = muscle weakness and paralysis ascending up from lower limbs, ↓ reflexes, can cause bilateral facial nerve palsy (Miller–Fischer variant of G–B)**

3. **May be proceeded by gastroenteritis** (classically *Campylobacter jejuni*), *Mycoplasma* or viral infxn, immunization, allergic reactions

4. **Dx = Hx of antecedent stimuli (discussed earlier), CSF → albumin-cytologic dissociation** (CSF protein ↑↑↑ without ↑ in cells seen)

5. Tx = plasmapheresis, IVIG, intubation for respiratory failure

6. Many, but not all, patients will eventually spontaneously recover after support through the acute illness—residual deficits are common even in those who recover

7. Respiratory failure and death can occur in remainder

C. **Central Pontine Myelinolysis**

1. Diamond-shaped region of demyelination in basis pontis

2. **Results from rapid correction of hyponatremia**

3. No Tx once condition has begun

4. Coma or death is common outcome

IV. Metabolic and Nutritional Disorders

A. **Carbon Monoxide Poisoning**

1. Seen in pts enclosed in burned areas or during the start of a cold winter (people are using their new gas heaters) → bilateral pallidal necrosis

2. Si/Sx = headache, nausea, vomiting, delirium, cherry-red color of lips

3. Dx = elevated carboxyhemoglobin levels

4. Tx = hyperbaric oxygen (first line) or 100% O_2

B. **Thiamine Deficiency**

1. Usually 2° to alcoholism

2. Beriberi peripheral neuropathy due to Wallerian degeneration

3. Wernicke's encephalopathy: **Wernicke's triad = confusion (confabulation), ophthalmoplegia, ataxia**

4. Wernicke's is related to lesions of mamillary bodies

5. Tx—supportive; but in alcoholics who are being given glucose, give thiamine prior to glucose (e.g., thiamine should be run in IV fluid without glucose) or can exacerbate mamillary body damage

C. **B_{12} Deficiency**

1. Subacute degeneration of posterior columns and lateral cortico-spinal tract

2. Si/Sx = weakness and ↓ vibration sense (both worse in legs), paresthesias, hyperreflexia, ataxia, personality change, dementia—**Note: neurologic deficits can occur even if no hematologic abnormalities are present!**

3. Dx is by high methylmalonic acid and homocysteine levels, which are more sensitive than B_{12} levels

4. Tx = B_{12} replacement

D. **Wilson's Dz (Hepatolenticular Degeneration)**

1. Defect in copper metabolism → lesions in basal ganglia

2. Si/Sx = in addition to hepatic disease, neurologically causes extrapyramidal tremors and rigidity, psychosis, manic-depression, typically in young people (teenagers, young adults)

3. **Pathognomonic → Kayser–Fleischer ring around the cornea** (Figure 7.2)

4. Dx = ↓ serum ceruloplasmin

5. Tx = penicillamine or liver transplant if drug fails

E. **Hepatic Encephalopathy**

1. Seen in cirrhosis, may result from brain toxicity 2° to excess ammonia and other toxins not degraded by malfunctioning liver

2. Sx = hyperreflexia, **asterixis** (flapping of extended wrists), dementia, Sz, obtundation/coma

3. Tx = lactulose, neomycin, and protein restriction to ↓ ammonia-related toxins

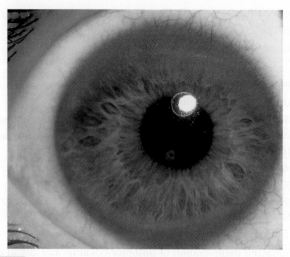

Kayser–Fleischer ring obscures peripheral iris details in a pt with Wilson's dz. (From Gold DH, Weingeist TA. *Color atlas of the eye in systemic disease.* Baltimore, MD: Lippincott Williams & Wilkins, 2001.)

F. **Tay–Sachs Dz**

1. Hexosaminidase A defect → ↑ ganglioside GM_2
2. Si/Sx = **cherry-red spot on macula**, retardation, paralysis, blind
3. Dx by Bx of rectum or by enzymatic assay, no Tx

V. Seizures

A. **Terminology**

1. Complex Sz → loss of consciousness (LOC); simple Sz → no LOC
2. Generalized Sz = entire brain involved; partial Sz = focal area
3. Tonic Sz → prolonged contraction; clonic Sz → twitches
4. Absence = complex generalized Sz → brief LOC
5. Grand mal = complex generalized tonic–clonic Sz

B. **Presentation**

1. Hx of prior head trauma, stroke, other CNS dz ↑ risk for Sz
2. Si/Sx = loss of bowel/bladder control, tongue maceration, postictal confusion/lethargy, focal findings indicate epileptogenic foci
3. If pt has Hx of Sz, always check blood level of medication

C. Tx

1. Tx Sz that recur or if pt has known epileptic focus (Tables 7.6 and 7.7)
2. Tx underlying cause: electrolyte, infxn, toxic ingestion, trauma, azotemia, stroke/bleed, delirium tremens, hypoglycemia, hypoxia
3. **Phenytoin causes gingival hyperplasia, hirsutism**
4. Carbamazepine causes leukopenia/aplastic anemia, hepatotoxic
5. Valproate causes neutropenia, thrombocytopenia, hepatotoxic
6. Stop Tx if no Sz for 2 yrs and nml EEG

Table 7.6 Seizure Therapy

Generalized Seizures	
Absence (petit mal)	
• Brief period of unresponsiveness (<30 seconds), pt stares blankly	
1st line	• ethosuximide, valproic acid
2nd line	• lamotrigine
Tonic-clonic (grand mal)	
• Dramatic convulsions with loss of consciousness, incontinence, post-ictal confusion	
1st line	• valproic acid, carbamazepine, phenytoin
2nd line	• lamotrigine, phenobarbital, primidone
Partial Seizures	
Simple partial	
• Sensory seizure or limited, focal motor seizure	
1st line	• carbamazepine, phenytoin
2nd line	• gabapentin, lamotrigine, phenobarbital, primidone, topiramate, valproic acid
Complex partial	
• Starts as simple partial but then generalizes	
1st line	• carbamazepine, phenytoin
2nd line	• gabapentin, lamotrigine, phenobarbital, primidone, topiramate, valproic acid
Status epilepticus	
• Unremitting seizure → respiratory compromise & rhabdomyolysis	
1st line	• lorazepam, diazepam
2nd line	• phenytoin
3rd line	• phenobarbital coma

NEUROLOGY

Table 7.7 Anti-Seizure Medications

Drug	Seizure Type	Characteristics
ethosuximide	• Absence (1st line)	• Non-sedating, causes mild GI side effects, rare idiosyncratic blood dyscrasias
valproic acid	• Absence (1st line) • Tonic-clonic (1st line) • Partial (2nd line)	• Can cause hepatotoxicity, blood dyscrasias • Also useful for bipolar syndrome
phenytoin	• Tonic-clonic (1st line) • Partial (1st line) • Status epilepticus (2nd line)	• Non-sedating, causes gingival hyperplasia, hirsutism, hypotension during IV load • Major inducer of cytochrome p450 enzymes • Can cause hepatic toxicity in patients with underlying liver disease
carbamazepine	• Partial (1st line) • Tonic-clonic (1st line)	• Causes blood dyscrasias, headaches, rashes • Also used to treat trigeminal neuralgia & bipolar syndrome • Contraindicated in absence seizures
phenobarbital	• Partial (2nd line) • Tonic-clonic (2nd line) • Status epilepticus (3rd line)	• Stimulates GABA signaling • Highly sedating, addictive • Marked cytochrome p450 enzyme induction • 3rd line for status by putting pt into a coma
primidone	• Partial (3rd line) • Tonic-clonic (3rd line)	• Metabolized to phenobarbital • Poorly tolerated, seldom used
gabapentin	• Partial (2nd line) • Tonic-clonic (2nd line)	• A GABA analog • An adjunctive therapy, not used by itself • Minor side effects include dizziness, ataxia • Also useful for neuropathic pain syndromes • Few drug interactions, ideal as adjunctive Tx
lamotrigine	• Partial (2nd line)	• May inhibit release of glutamate in the brain • Used as adjunct therapy, not by itself • Markedly alters levels of other anti-epileptics • Causes headache, GI upset, rash

Table 7.7	Continued	
Drug	**Seizure Type**	**Characteristics**
felbamate	• Partial (3rd line)	• Mechanism unclear, may relate to GABA • Used as monotherapy or adjunctive therapy • Blood dyscrasias & hepatotoxicity can be severe, reserve for refractory patients
topiramate	• Partial (2nd line) • Tonic-clonic (2nd line)	• Mechanism unclear, may relate to GABA • Causes cognitive slowing, tremor, GI upset • Used as adjunctive therapy in refractory pts
diazepam	• Status epilepticus (1st line) • Alcohol withdrawal seizure (1st line)	• Onset is faster than lorazepam, but remember redistribution of diazepam means that with a one-time dose its duration is shorter than lorazepam
lorazepam	• Status epilepticus (1st line) • Alcohol withdrawal seizure (1st line)	• Onset is slower than diazepam, but because of slower redistribution, with a one-time dose lorazepam effect lasts longer than diazepam

D. **Status Epilepticus**
 1. Continuous seizing lasting >5 min
 2. Tx = maintain and protect airway, IV benzodiazepines for immediate control, followed by phenytoin loading and phenobarbital for refractory cases
 3. **This is a medical emergency!**

VI. Degenerative Diseases

A. **Dementia versus Delirium Differential (Table 7.8)**
B. **Alzheimer's Dz (Senile Dementia of Alzheimer Type)**
 1. Most common cause of dementia—affects 5% of people age >70 yrs
 2. Si/Sx = dementia, anxiety, hallucination/delusion, tremor
 3. Occurs in Down's syndrome pts at younger ages (age 30–40 yrs)

Table 7.8 Dementia versus Delirium

	Dementia	Delirium
Definition	Both cause global decline in cognition, memory, personality, motor or sensory functions	
Course	Constant, progressive	Sudden onset, waxing/waning daily
Reversible?	Usually not	Almost always
Circadian?	Constant, no daily patter	Worse at night ("sundowning")
Consciousness	Normal	Altered (obtunded)
Hallucination	Usually not	Often, classically visual
Tremor	Often not	Often present (e.g., asterixis)
Causes	Alzheimer's, multi-infarct, Pick's dz, alcohol, brain infection/tumor, malnutrition (thiamine, B12, etc.)	Systemic infection, neoplasm, drugs (particularly narcotics and benzodiazepines), stroke, heart dz, alcoholism, uremia, electrolyte imbalance, hyper/hypoglycemia
Tx	Supportive (see later) for specifics, depending on the dz	Treat underlying cause; improve environment to increase familiarity of patient surroundings (particularly for older patients); if necessary, use drugs, do not use benzodiazepines which will worsen the problem; if necessary, use haloperidol or an atypical antipsychotic

4. Dx = clinical, with definitive Dx only possible at autopsy (neurofibrillary tangles)
5. Tx
   a. Cholinesterase inhibitors can slow dementia, but efficacy may only be present in early disease; there is no efficacy for late disease
   b. Antidepressants and antipsychotics can be used for psychosis
   c. Memantine is the first drug approved to treat moderate to severe stages of Alzheimer's; protects brain cells from damage caused by the chemical messenger glutamate, but efficacy is uncertain
6. Px = inevitable decline in function usually over approximately 10 yrs

C. **Multiinfarct Dementia**
1. Si/Sx = acute, stepwise ↓ in neurologic function, multiple focal deficits on exam, HTN, old infarcts by CT or MRI

    2. Dx = clinical, radiographic

    3. Tx = prevent future infarcts by ↓ cardiovascular risks

D. **Pick's Dz**

    1. Clinically resembles Alzheimer's, more in women, onset at younger age (50s)

    2. Predominates in frontal (more personality changes seen) and temporal lobes

    3. Dx = MRI → symmetric frontal or temporal atrophy, confirm by autopsy

    4. Tx/Px = as per Alzheimer's

E. **Parkinson's Dz**

    1. Parkinson's dz = idiopathic Parkinsonism, mid- to late-age onset

    2. Parkinsonism

        a. **Syndrome of tremor, cog-wheel rigidity, bradykinesia, classic shuffling gait, mask-like facies,** ± dementia from loss of dopaminergic neurons in substantia nigra

        b. DDx = Parkinson's dz, severe depression (bradykinesia and flat affect), intoxication (e.g., manganese, synthetic heroin), phenothiazine side effects, rare neurodegenerative dz

    3. Dx = clinical, rule out other causes

    4. Tx

        a. Sinemet (levodopa = carbidopa) best for bradykinesia

        b. Anticholinergics (benztropine/trihexyphenidyl) for tremor

        c. Amantadine → ↑ dopamine release, effective for mild dz

        d. Surgery—implanted deep brain electrical stimulation, or surgical pallidotomy for refractory cases

    5. Px = typically progresses over yrs despite Tx

F. **Huntington's Chorea**

    1. Si/Sx = progressive choreiform movements of all limbs, ataxic gait, grimacing → dementia, usually in 30s–50s (can be earlier or later)

    2. Autosomal CAG triplet repeat expansion in HD gene → atrophy of striatum (especially caudate nucleus), with neuronal loss and gliosis

    3. Dx = MRI → atrophy of caudate, ⊕ FHx

    4. Tx/Px = supportive, death inevitable

G. **Amyotrophic Lateral Sclerosis (Lou Gehrig's Dz, Motor Neuron Dz)**

1. Si/Sx = **upper and lower motor neuron dz** → muscle weakness with fasciculations (anterior motor neurons) progressing to denervation atrophy, hyperreflexia, spasticity, difficulty speaking/swallowing

2. Dx = clinical Hx, physical findings

3. Tx/Px = supportive, death inevitable, usually from respiratory failure

H. **Cerebral Palsy**

1. Dx = group of conditions that affect control of movement and posture. In approximately 70% of the cases, cerebral palsy results from the events occurring before birth that can disrupt nml development of the brain; in many cases, the cause of cerebral palsy is not known

2. Si/Sx = range from mild to severe, condition does not worsen as the child gets older

3. Types include

   a. **Spastic cerebral palsy:** most common form, individual's muscles are stiff, making movement difficult

   b. **Athetoid or dyskinetic cerebral palsy:** found in approximately 10%–20% of affected individuals, can affect the entire body, characterized by fluctuations in muscle tone, associated with uncontrolled movements

   c. **Ataxic cerebral palsy:** approximately 5%–10% of affected individuals have the ataxic form, which affects balance and coordination

4. Tx

   a. Botox injected into spastic muscles or baclofen to ↓ spasticity

   b. Selective dorsal rhizotomy may permanently reduce spasticity by cutting some of the nerve fibers that are contributing most to spasticity

5. Px = Some pts with Tx are able to work and study, depending on severity of condition

DERMATOLOGY

I. Terminology

1. Macule = flat discoloration, <1 cm in diameter (Figure 8.1)

2. Papule = elevated skin lesion, <1 cm in diameter (Figure 8.2)

3. Plaque = elevated skin lesion, >1 cm in diameter (Figure 8.3)

4. Vesicle = small fluid-containing lesion <0.5 cm in diameter (Figure 8.4)

5. Wheal = pruritic erythematous area that can enlarge to form urticaria (hives) (Figure 8.5)

6. Bulla = large fluid-containing lesion, >0.5 cm in diameter (Figure 8.6)

7. Lichenification = accentuated skin markings in thick epidermis as a result of scratching (Figure 8.7)

8. Keloid = irregular raised lesion resulting from scar tissue hypertrophy and extends beyond original scar. As opposed to hypertrophic scar which remains which stays within original scar (Figure 8.8)

9. Petechiae = flat, pinhead, nonblanching, red-purple lesion caused by hemorrhage into the skin: seen in any cause of thrombocytopenia

10. Purpura = larger than petechiae

11. Cyst = closed epithelium-lined cavity or sac containing liquid or semisolid material

12. Hyperkeratosis = ↑ thickness of stratum corneum (seen in chronic dermatitis)

13. Parakeratosis = hyperkeratosis with retention of nuclei in stratum corneum on histopathology and thinning of stratum granulosum (usually seen in psoriasis)

14. Acantholysis = loss of cohesion between epidermal cells (seen in pemphigus vulgaris)

15. Spongiosis = intercellular edema causing stretching and loss of desmosomal attachment, allowing formation of blisters within the epidermis (seen in acute and subacute dermatitis)

Text continues on page 396

FIGURE 8.1

This erythematous macule is the typical herald patch of pityriasis rosea.
(Courtesy of Dr. Steven Gammer.)

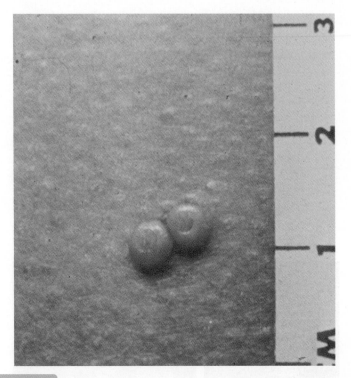

FIGURE 8.2
Papules of molluscum contagiosum. (Courtesy of Dr. Douglas Smith.)

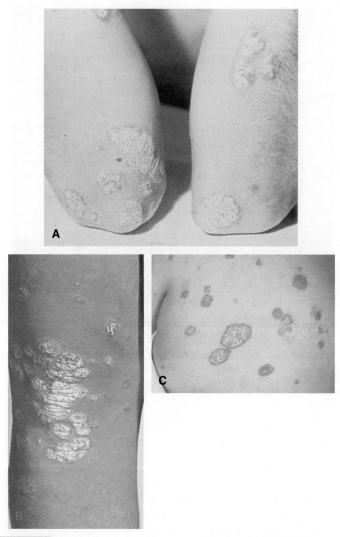

FIGURE 8.3
Erythematous plaques with silvery scales are typical of psoriasis and occur on the extensor surfaces, including the elbows **(A)** (Courtesy of Dr. Douglas Smith) and **(B)** knees (From Bickley LS. *Bate's guide to physical examination and history taking,* 8th Ed. Philadelphia, PA: Lippincott Williams & Wilkins, 2003, with permission), but can also occur on the body **(C).** (From Gold DH, Weingeist TA. *Color atlas of the eye in systemic disease.* Baltimore, MD: Lippincott Williams & Wilkins, 2001.)

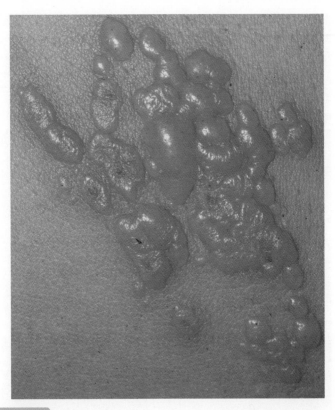

FIGURE 8.4

Vesicles of Herpes Simplex Virus (HSV) in the skin. (Courtesy of Dr. Steven Gammer.)

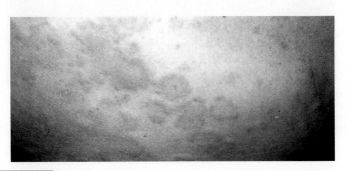

FIGURE 8.5

The ring-like wheals of urticaria. (From Axford JS. *Medicine.* Oxford: Blackwell Science, 1996, with permission.)

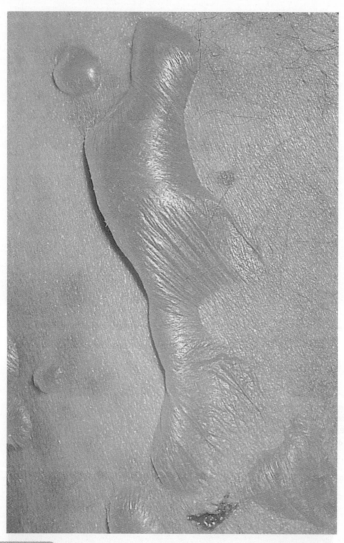

FIGURE 8.6

The large, tense bulla of bullous pemphigoid. (From Axford JS. *Medicine.* Oxford: Blackwell Science, 1996, with permission.)

FIGURE 8.7

Lichenification caused by repeated scratching in this pt with chronic eczematous dermatitis. (Courtesy of Dr. Steven Gammer.)

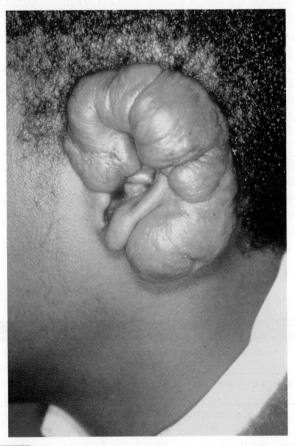

FIGURE 8.8

Keloid of the earlobe. (Courtesy of Dr. Douglas Smith.)

II. Topical Steroids (Table 8.1)

III. Infections

A. Acne

1. Inflammation of pilosebaceous unit caused by *Propionibacterium acnes* infection of blocked pore

2. Si/Sx = open comedones (blackheads) and closed comedones (whiteheads) on face, neck, chest, back, and buttocks; can become inflamed and pustular

3. Tx = topical antibiotics; Retin-A; benzoyl peroxide; systemic antibiotics; if acne is scarring, consider isoretinoin (Accutane), consider spironolactone in females.

B. Impetigo

1. Superficial skin infxn of epidermis

2. Si/Sx = honey-crusted lesions or vesicles occurring most often in children around the nose and mouth, can be bullous or nonbullous (Figure 8.9)

3. Common organisms include *Staphylococcus aureus* and *Streptococcus pyogenes*

4. Tx = topical or oral antibiotics against *S. aureus* and *Streptococcus* for 7–10 days

C. Folliculitis

1. Si/Sx = erythematous pustules around hair follicles, commonly noted around beard area

Table 8.1	Use of Topical Steroids	
Potency	**Drug**	**Use for Dz on**
Low	1% hydrocortisone	Face, genitals, skin folds (prevent atrophy/striae), also use in children for dz on body
Moderate	0.1% triamcinolone	Body/extremities, or ↑ dz on face, genitals, skin folds
High	Fluocinonide (Lidex)	Thick skin (palms/soles), or ↑ body dz, **do not use on face**
Very High	Diflorasone	Thick skin, or if very severe dz on body

Carrier substance: lotion = low potency; cream = mid potency; ointment = high potency.

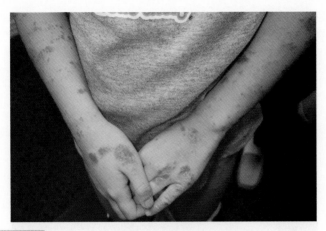

FIGURE 8.9

Crusted bullous impetigo. (Image provided by Stedman's.)

   2. *S. aureus* most common; *Pseudomonas aeruginosa* causes "hot tub" folliculitis (organism lives in warm water), also fungi and viruses

   3. Tx = local wound care, antibiotics only if severe

D. **Subcutaneous Infections**

   1. Cellulitis

     a. Si/Sx = spreading subQ infxn with classic signs of inflammation: *rubor* (red), *calor* (hot), *dolor* (pain), and *tumor* (swelling)

     b. *Staphylococcus* and *Streptococcus* most common etiologies

     c. Tx = vancomycin, cefazolin, or clindamycin

   2. Abscess (known as furuncle if small and localized, and carbuncle if extensive with deep pocket) (Figure 8-10)

     a. Local collection of pus, often with fever, ↑ white count

     b. Furuncle = pus collection in one hair follicle, often caused by *S. aureus*

     c. Carbuncle = pus collection involving many hair follicles

     d. Tx = incision and drainage (I&D), antibiotics targeting *S. aureus*, including MRSA (e.g., TMP-SMX, vancomycin, or clindamycin)

   3. Erysipelas

     a. Cellulitis in which infxn remains in the superficial dermal layer, leading to edema localized beneath the infxn

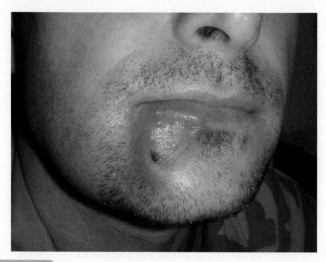

FIGURE 8.10

Subcutaneous abscess (furuncle). (Courtesy of Dr. Yang Xia)

  b. Presents with bright red skin with peau d'orange (orange peel-like) appearance, classically on cheeks but can be else-where

  c. *Streptococcus* is the cause (usually Group A Strep [GAS])

  d. Treat with penicillin

 4. Paronychia

  a. Infxn of skin surrounding nail margin that can extend into surrounding skin and into tendons within hand

  b. Commonly caused by *S. aureus,* also *Candida*

  c. Tx = warm compress, I&D if area is purulent, add antibiotics if severe

 5. Necrotizing Fasciitis

  a. Infxn from skin layers down to fascial planes with severe pain, fever, ↑ white count, local inflammation may be deceptively absent but pt will appear very ill (i.e., "pain out of proportion to exam findings")

  b. Caused by *S. pyogenes* (GAS), *Clostridium perfringens,* and now described with community acquired MRSA infxn

  c. **Tx = immediate, extensive surgical débridement, add penicillin or ceftriaxone (for *Streptococcus* and *Clostridium*) + vancomycin (for MRSA) + clindamycin**

(protein synthesis inhibitor; shuts down the production of toxins that mediate the tissue necrosis)

   d. Px = ↑↑↑ mortality unless débridement is rapid and extensive

E. **Scarlet Fever**

   1. *S. pyogenes* (GAS) is the cause

   2. Si/Sx

      a. **"Sunburn with goose bumps,"** rash, finely punctate, erythematous but blanches with pressure, initially on trunk, generalizes within hours

      b. Sandpaper rough skin, **strawberry tongue**, beefy-red pharynx, circumoral pallor

      c. **Pastia's lines = rash, most intense in creases of axillae and groin**

      d. Eventual desquamation of hands and feet as rash resolves

      e. Systemic Sx include fever, chills, delirium, sore throat, cervical adenopathy, all of which appear at same time as rash

   3. Complications include rheumatic fever and glomerulonephritis

   4. Tx = penicillin

F. **Hidradenitis Suppurativa**

   1. Si/Sx = plugged apocrine glands presenting as inflamed masses in groin/axilla, become secondarily infected

   2. Tx = surgical débridement, antibiotics and consider Retin A

G. **Erythrasma**

   1. Si/Sx = irregular erythematous rash found along major skin folds (axilla, groin, fingers, toes, and breasts) (Figure 8.11)

   2. Commonly seen in adult diabetics, caused by *Corynebacterium* spp.

   3. Dx = Wood's lamp of skin → **coral-red fluorescence, KOH prep negative**

   4. Tx = erythromycin

IV. Common Disorders

A. **Psoriasis**

   1. Si/Sx = pink plaques with silvery-white scaling **occurring on extensor surfaces such as elbows and knees** (see Figure 8.3B), scalp (classically with involvement behind the ears),

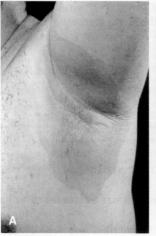
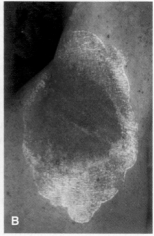

FIGURE 8.11

A. Erythrasma. **B.** Nml light. Coral-red axillary fluorescent as a result of coproporphyrin III, elaborated by *Corynebacterium minutissimum* under Wood's lamp. (From Axford JS. *Medicine.* Oxford: Blackwell Science, 1996, with permission.)

lumbosacral, glans penis, intergluteal cleft, and **fingernail pitting with onycholysis,** (Figure 8.12A), and can be associated with arthritis (Figure 8.12B)

2. Classic finding = **Auspitz sign** → removal of overlying scale causes pinpoint bleeding because of thin epidermis above dermal papillae

3. Classic finding = **Köbner's phenomenon** → psoriatic lesions appear at sites of cutaneous physical trauma (skin scratching, rubbing, or wound)

4. Psoriasis Variants

   a. Guttate psoriasis typically presents in a child or young adult, often after a streptococcal infxn, with acute eruption of small, drop-like, 1–10 mm diameter, salmon-pink papules, usually with a fine scale

   b. Pustular psoriasis is often localized to palms and soles, but can be generalized; presents with pustular lesions rather than classic psoriatic plaque (Figure 8.13)

   c. Inverse psoriasis presents with lesions in the intertriginous areas (e.g., axillae, groin, below the breasts) that are erythematous and appear like candidal infxns or tinea cruris

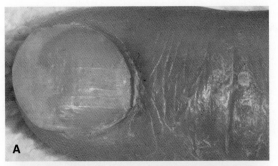

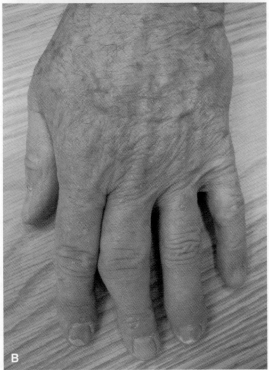

FIGURE 8.12

A. Involvement of the hands leads to pitting of the fingernails and onycholysis (lifting of the nail off the nailbed; Courtesy of Dr. Steven Gammer). **B.** Psoriatic arthritis. This pt has severe psoriatic arthritis with marked deformities. (Image provided by Stedman's.)

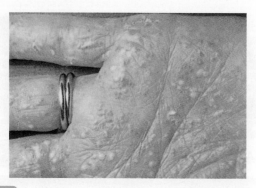

FIGURE 8.13

Pustular psoriasis.

5. Dx = clinical, Bx is criterion standard
6. Tx
   a. Localized lesions can be treated with topical steroids
   b. Narrow band UVB light and PUVA (**P**soralens + **UV A** light) effective for diffuse dz, but may ↑ risk of skin CA
   c. Methotrexate, cyclosporine, or TNF antagonists (e.g., infliximab, etanercept) are options for refractory, diffuse dz, especially if arthritis coexists

B. **Eczema (Eczematous Dermatitis)**
   1. Family of superficial, intensely pruritic, erythematous skin lesions
   2. Atopic Dermatitis
      a. Si/Sx = **an "itch that rashes,"** rash 2° to scratching chronic pruritus, commonly found on the face in infancy; later in childhood can present on the flexor surfaces such as antecubital and popliteal fossa
      b. Atopy
         (1) Inherited predisposition to asthma, allergies, and dermatitis
         (2) Dx is clinical
         (3) Tx = avoid irritants or triggers, keep skin moist with lotions, use steroids and antihistamines for Sx relief of itching and inflammation
   3. Contact Dermatitis
      a. Si/Sx = linear pruritic rash at site of contact
      b. Caused by delayed-type hypersensitivity reaction after exposure to poison ivy, poison oak, nickel, or chemicals
      c. Dx is clinical, Hx of exposure crucial
      d. Tx = oral steroid taper

4. Dyshidrotic eczema causes multiple pruritic papules and vesicles on the hand and sides of fingers

5. Seborrheic Dermatitis
   a. Chronic Inflammatory disorder affecting the areas of head and trunk where sebaceous glands are most prominent
   b. Can be caused by multiple factors, including fungal infection (*Malassezia*)
   c. Si/Sx = erythema, scaling, white flaking (dandruff) in the areas of sebaceous glands (face, especially around nasolabial folds, scalp, groin, axilla, and external ear), as shown in Figure 8.14

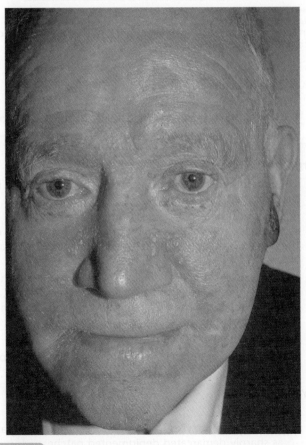

FIGURE 8.14

Seborrheic dermatitis.

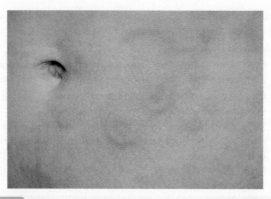

Urticarial wheals (acute urticaria). (From Axford JS. *Medicine.* Oxford: Blackwell Science, 1996, with permission.)

    d. Called "cradle cap" in infants

    e. Dx = clinical

    f. Tx = selenium shampoo (Selsun Blue) for scalp, 2% topical ketoconazole for face, topical or systemic steroids may be indicated

C. **Urticaria (Hives)**

    1. Common disorder caused by mast cell degranulation and histamine release

    2. Si/Sx = transient papular wheals, intensely pruritic, surrounded by erythema, **dermographism** (write word on the skin and it remains imprinted as erythematous wheals; Figure 8.15)

    3. Most lesions are immunoglobulin (Ig)E-mediated (Type I hypersensitivity), but exercise, certain chemicals in sensitive pts, and inhibitors of prostaglandin synthesis (e.g., aspirin) also can cause IgE-independent reactions

    4. Dx = skin testing or aspirin or exercise challenge

    5. Tx = avoidance of triggers, antihistamines, steroids, epinephrine

    6. Can cause respiratory emergency requiring intubation

D. **Hypopigmentation**

    1. Vitiligo

       a. **Loss of melanocytes** in discrete areas of skin, appearing as sharply demarcated depigmented patches (Figure 8.16)

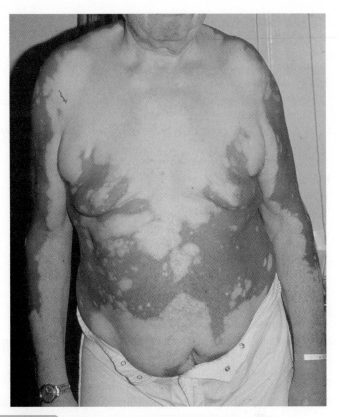

FIGURE 8.16

Extensive vitiligo. (Courtesy of Dr. Steven Gammer.)

b. Occurs in all races but most apparent in darkly pigmented pts
c. Chronic condition that may be autoimmune in nature
d. Associated with other systemic disorders, i.e., Hashimotos thyroiditis, Diabetes Mellitus, tuberous sclerosis, melanoma, etc.
e. Tx = minigrafting, total depigmentation, chronic UVA/UVB light Tx
f. Px = some pts remit over long term, others never do

2. Albinism
   a. **Melanocytes are present** but fail to produce pigment due to tyrosinase deficiency

  b. Si/Sx = white skin and eyelashes, nystagmus, iris translucency, ↓ visual acuity, ↓ retinal pigment, and strabismus

  c. Tx = avoid sun exposure, sunscreens

  d. Px = oculocutaneous form predisposes to skin CA

 3. Pityriasis Alba

  a. Nonpathologic areas of hypopigmentation on face or upper extremities

  b. Can be 2° to prior infxn or inflammation, often regress over time

  c. Differentiated from tinea versicolor by KOH prep

E. Hyperpigmentation

 1. Freckle (ephelis) is caused by nml melanocyte number but ↑ melanin within basal keratinocytes, darkens with sun exposure

 2. Lentigo is pigmented macules caused by melanocyte hyperplasia that, unlike freckles, does not darken with sun exposure

 3. Nevocellular Nevus

  a. Common mole, benign tumor derived from melanocytes

  b. Variations of nevi

   (1) Blue nevus = black-blue nodule present at birth, often mistaken for melanoma

   (2) Spitz nevus = red-pink nodule, often seen in children, confused with hemangioma or melanoma

   (3) Dysplastic nevus = atypical, irregularly pigmented lesion with ↑ risk of transformation into malignant melanoma, may be associated with an autosomal dominant inherited syndrome

  c. Dx = Bx; if Tx required, Tx is excision

 4. Mongolian Spot

  a. A benign, macular blue-gray birthmark usually on the sacral area of healthy infants

  b. Often seen in newborns of Asian, African, or Native American descent

  c. Usually present at birth or appears within the first weeks of life and typically disappears spontaneously within 4 yrs but can persist

  d. Lesions appear bruise-like and can be mistaken for child abuse, so good history of lesions is critical

  e. Dx = clinical, no Tx necessary

5. Melasma (Chloasma)
   a. Masklike hyperpigmentation on face seen in pregnancy
   b. Sunlight accentuates pigmentation, which typically fades postpartum
   c. Tx = minimize facial exposure to sun, hydroquinone cream, consider Q-switched Alexandrite laser.

6. Hemangioma
   a. Capillary hemangiomas present at birth
   b. Tx
      (1) Usually resolve on their own with time
      (2) Consider oral steroids or β-blockers if large
      (3) Surgical excision if affecting vision or airway
   c. Port-wine stains (purple-red on face or neck; Figure 8.17)
      (1) Can be associated with Sturge–Weber syndrome (see Table 8.3)
      (2) Must screen for glaucoma and CNS dz (CT scan)
      (3) Tx = laser Tx, will not regress spontaneously

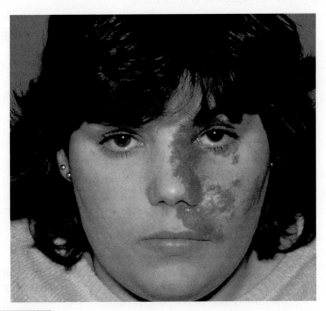

FIGURE 8.17

Port wine stain in a pt with Sturge–Weber syndrome. (From Gold DH, Weingeist TA. *Color atlas of the eye in systemic disease.* Baltimore, MD: Lippincott Williams & Wilkins, 2001.)

d. Strawberry hemangiomas (bright-red raised lesions) are benign, most disappear on their own

e. Cherry hemangiomas (benign small red papule); Tx = laser excision or electrodessication

7. Xanthoma

a. Yellowish papules, often accumulations of foamy histiocytes

b. Can be idiopathic or associated with familial hyperlipidemia (Figure 8.18)

c. If seen on eyelids, they are called "xanthelasma"

d. Tx = ↓ hyperlipidemia, surgically excise papules as needed

8. Pityriasis Rosea (Figure 8.19)

a. Erythematous maculopapular rash with scale apparent in center

b. Often preceded by a "herald patch" on trunk

c. **Can appear on back in a Christmas tree distribution**

d. Tx = sunlight, otherwise spontaneously remits in 6–12 wks. Can use topical steroids to expedite resolution

9. Erythema Nodosum (Figure 8.20)

a. Inflammation of subQ fat (panniculitis) and adjacent vessels

b. Characteristic lesions are **tender red nodules occurring on the lower legs** and sometimes forearms

c. Usually resolves in 6–8 wks; Tx directed at underlying cause

d. Common causes

(1) Infxns = *Mycoplasma, Chlamydia, Coccidioides immitis, Mycobacterium leprae,* and others

(2) Drugs = sulfonamides and contraceptive pills

(3) Inflammatory bowel dz, sarcoidosis, rheumatic fever

(4) Pregnancy

10. Dermatomyositis (see Internal Medicine VI.E.3)

11. Seborrheic Keratosis (Figure 8.21)

a. Black or brown benign plaques, appear to be stuck onto skin surface

b. Commonly seen in elderly, runs in families

c. Can be mistaken for melanoma

d. The sign of Lesser–Trélat is the association of multiple eruptive seborrheic keratoses with internal malignancy, most commonly adenoCA of the GI tract

12. Acanthosis Nigricans (Figure 8.22)

a. Black velvety plaques on flexor surfaces and intertriginous areas

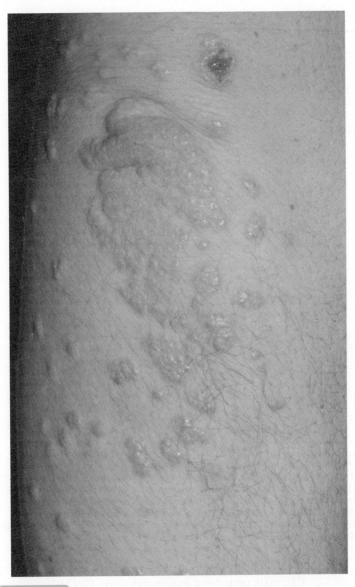

DERMATOLOGY

FIGURE 8.18

Multiple xanthoma (called eruptive xanthoma) in a pt with severe hypercho-lesterolemia. (Courtesy of Dr. Steven Gammer.)

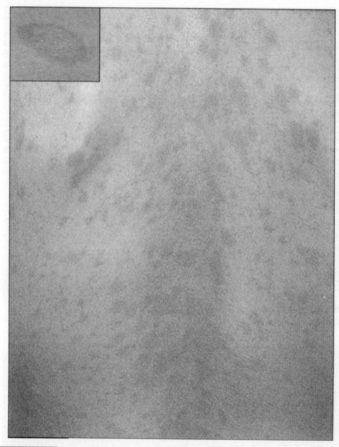

FIGURE 8.19

The herald patch (*inset*) of pityriasis rosea is typically found on the trunk and is much larger than the other papules (courtesy of Dr. Steven Gammer). Note the Christmas tree distribution of the lesions following the skin lines in a concave shape up vertically close to the spine and horizontally along the sides. (From Graham-Brown R, Burns T. *Lecture notes on dermatology*, 7th Ed. Oxford: Blackwell Science, 1996:211, with permission.)

   b. Seen in obesity and endocrine disorders (e.g., diabetes)

   c. Can mark underlying malignancy (e.g., GI/GU, lymphoma)

  13. Bronze Diabetes = 1° Hemochromatosis

   a. Familial defect causing intestinal hyperabsorption of iron

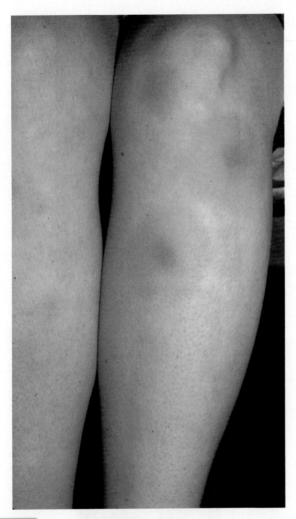

FIGURE 8.20

Erythema nodosum on the shins.

b. **Classic triad:** ↑ **skin pigmentation, cirrhosis, diabetes mellitus**
c. Other Sx = cardiomyopathy, pituitary failure, arthropathies
d. **Clinical pearl: hemochromatosis is the likely Dx in any pt with osteoarthritis involving the metacarpophalangeal joints**

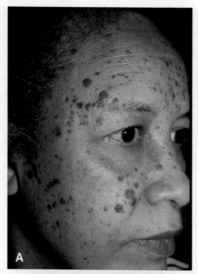

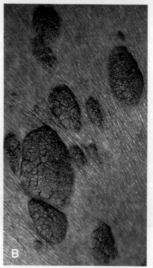

FIGURE 8.21

A. The black plaques of seborrheic keratosis appear to be "stuck-on." **B.** A close-up of their velvety/warty surface. (Both images courtesy of Dr. Steven Gammer.)

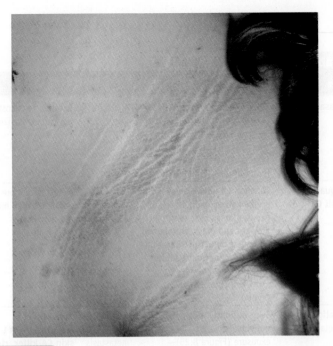

FIGURE 8.22

The fine, velvety plaque of acanthosis nigricans. (Courtesy of Dr. Steven Gammer.)

    e. Dx = transferrin saturation (iron/total iron-binding capacity) ≥50%

    f. Tx = phlebotomy, which improves survival if started early

F. **Verrucae (Warts)**

  1. Verruca vulgaris = hand wart

  2. Verruca plana (flat wart) smaller than vulgaris, seen on hands and face

  3. Human papilloma virus (HPV) Types 1–4 cause skin and plantar warts

  4. HPV-6 and HPV-11 cause anorectal and genital warts (condyloma acuminatum)

  5. HPV-16, HPV-18, HPV-31, HPV-33, HPV-35 cause cervical CA

  6. Condylomata lata are flat warts caused by *Treponema pallidum* (syphilis)

  7. Tx for skin Verrucae-salicylic acid, liquid nitrogen, topical imiquimod, intralesional candida

V. Cancer (Table 8.2)

Table 8.2	Skin Cancer		
Dz	**Si/Sx**	**Tx**	**Px**
Basal cell CA	Most common skin CA, classic **"rodent ulcer"** seen on face, with **pearly translucent borders and fine telangiectasias,** not usually found on lips (Figure 8.23)	Excision	Excellent—almost never metastasize
Squamous cell CA	Common in elderly, appears as erythematous nodules on sun-exposed areas that eventually ulcerate and crust, **frequently preceded by actinic keratosis = rough epidermal lesions on sun-exposed** areas such as lower lip, ears, and nose (Figure 8.24)	Excision, radiation	Metastasize more basal cell than but not as much as melanoma
Malignant melanoma	Seen in lightly pigmented individuals with ↑ sun exposure (Figure 8.25)— diagnose with **ABCDEs** <ul><li>**A**symmetry = malignant; symmetry = benign</li><li>**B**order = irregular; benign = smooth</li><li>**C**olor = multicolored; benign = one color</li><li>**D**iameter >6 mm; benign = <6 mm</li><li>**E**levation = raised above skin; benign = flat</li><li>**E**nlargement = growing; benign = not growing</li></ul>	Excision, chemo if metastasis likely	High rate of metastasis → **#1 skin CA killer, risk of mets ↑ with depth of invasion on Bx**

Text continues on page 418

Table 8.2 *Continued*			
Dz	**Si/Sx**	**Tx**	**Px**
Kaposi's sarcoma	Connective tissue CA caused by human herpes virus-8, appears as red-purple plaques or nodules on skin and mucosa, frequently affects lungs and GI viscera, seen in AIDS, elderly, or Mediterranean males (Figure 8.26)	HIV drugs, chemo	Benign unless damages internal organs
Cutaneous T-cell lymphoma	"Mycosis fungoides," presents with erythematous patches and plaques that may ultimately ulcerate, rash can precede malignancy by yrs, a leukemic phase of dz called "Sézary syndrome"	PUVA, topical chemo, radiation	Life expectancy 7–10 yrs without Tx

DERMATOLOGY

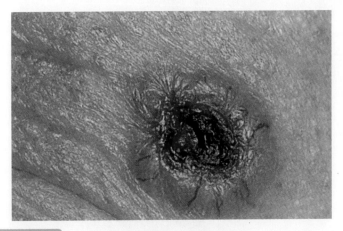

FIGURE 8.23

The rodent ulcer of basal cell CA. Note the telangiectasias as the borders.
(From Axford JS. *Medicine.* Oxford: Blackwell Science, 1996, with permission.)

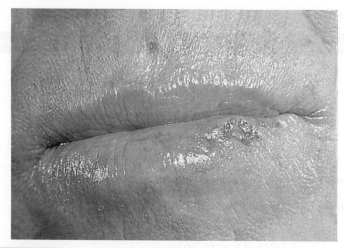

FIGURE 8.24

Squamous cell CA of the lip (early ulcer). (From Axford JS. *Medicine.* Oxford: Blackwell Science, 1996, with permission.)

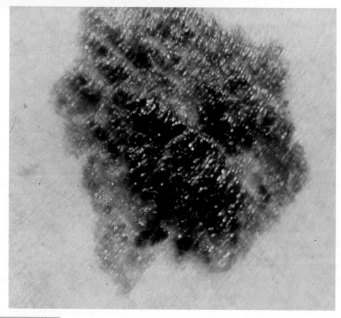

FIGURE 8.25

A melanoma with ABCDEs. The lesion is Asymmetric, with irregular Borders, is Multicolored, has a large Diameter, and is Elevated (plaque not macule). It was also Enlarging. (Courtesy of Dr. Douglas Smith.)

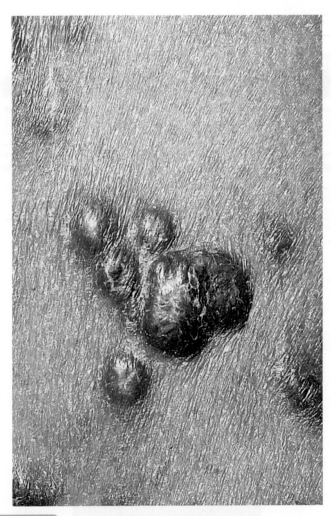

FIGURE 8.26

The red/purple nodules of Kaposi's sarcoma. (From Axford JS. *Medicine.* Oxford: Blackwell Science, 1996, with permission.)

VI. Neurocutaneous Syndromes (Phakomatoses; Table 8.3)

Table 8.3 Neurocutaneous Syndromes (Phakomatoses)

Dz[a]	Characteristics
Tuberous sclerosis (Figure 8.27)	Ash leaf patches (hypopigmented macules), Shagreen spots (leathery cutaneous thickening), adenoma sebaceum of the face, **sz, mental retardation**
Neurofibromatosis (NF) (Figure 8.28)	Si/Sx = **café-au-lait spots,** neurofibromas, meningiomas, acoustic neuromas, Kyphoscoliosis—NF-2 causes bilateral acoustic neuromas
Sturge–Weber syndrome (see Figure 8.17)	Si/Sx = **port-wine hemangioma of face** in CN V distribution, mental retardation, sz
Von Hippel–Lindau syndrome	Si/Sx = multiple hemangiomas in various organs, ↑ frequency of renal cell CA and polycythemia (↑ erythropoietin secretion)

[a]All are autosomal dominant except Sturge–Weber syndrome, which has no genetic pattern.

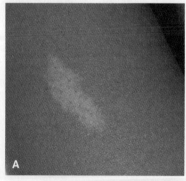

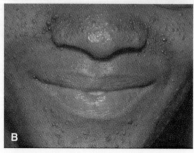

FIGURE 8.27

The ash leaf patch **(A)** and adenoma sebaceum **(B)** characteristic of tuberous sclerosis.

DERMATOLOGY

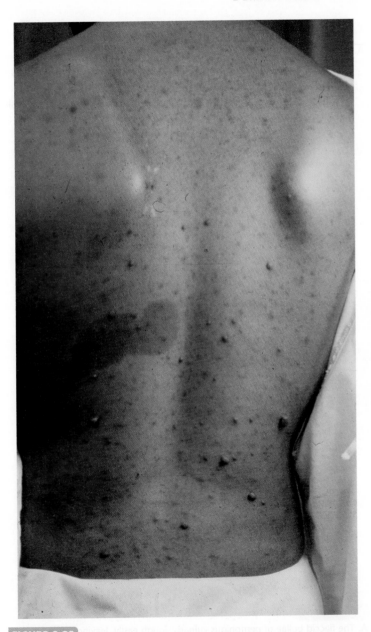

FIGURE 8.28

Several neurofibromas and a large café-au-lait spot. (Courtesy of Dr. Steven Gammer.)

VII. Blistering Disorders

A. Pemphigus Vulgaris (PG)

1. PG is a rare autoimmune disorder, **affecting 20- to 40-yr-olds**
2. Si/Sx = **flaccid epidermal bullae** that easily slough off leaving large denuded areas of skin (Nikolsky's sign; Figure 8.29), ↑ risk of 2° infxn

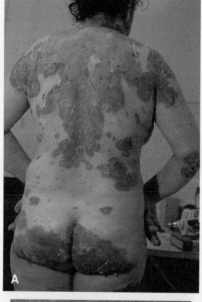

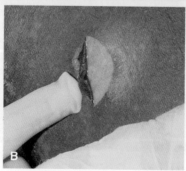

FIGURE 8.29

A. The flaccid bullae of pemphigus vulgaris slough easily, leaving inflamed, denuded areas of skin. **B.** Nikolsky's sign is present due to the weak attachment of the bullae to the underlying epidermis. (Courtesy of Dr. Steven Gammer.)

3. DDx = bullous pemphigoid
4. Dx = skin Bx → **immunofluorescence surrounding epidermal cells** showing "tombstone" fluorescent pattern
5. Tx = high-dose oral steroids, cyclosporine, Moflitel, antibiotics for infxn
6. Px = **often fatal if not treated**

B. **Bullous Pemphigoid**

1. Common autoimmune dz affecting **mostly the elderly**
2. Resembles PG but much less severe clinically
3. Si/Sx = **hard, tense bullae** that do not rupture easily and usually heal without scarring if uninfected (Figure 8.30)
4. Dx = skin Bx → immunofluorescence as a **linear band along the basement membrane, with** ↑ **eosinophils** in dermis
5. Tx = oral steroids
6. Px = much better than PG

C. **Erythema Multiforme**

1. Hypersensitivity reaction to drugs, infxns, or systemic disorders such as malignancy or collagen vascular dz
2. Si/Sx = **diffuse, erythematous target-like lesions** in many shapes (hence name "multiforme"), often accompanying a herpes eruption (Figure 8.31A)
3. **Stevens–Johnson syndrome = severe febrile form (sometimes fatal) → hemorrhagic crusting also affects lips and oral mucosa** (Figure 8.31B)
4. Dx = clinical, Hx of herpes infxn or drug exposure
5. Tx = stop offending drug, prevent eruption of herpes with acyclovir

D. **Porphyria Cutanea Tarda**

1. Autosomal dominant defect in heme synthesis (50% ↓ in uroporphyrinogen decarboxylase activity in RBC and liver)
2. Si/Sx = blisters on sun-exposed areas of face and hands, ↑ hair on temples and cheeks, **no abd pain** (differentiates from other porphyrias)
3. Dx = Wood's lamp of urine → **urine fluoresces with distinctive orange-pink color because of** ↑ **levels of uroporphyrins**
4. Tx = sunscreen, phlebotomy, chloroquine, no alcohol
5. Px = remitting/relapsing, exacerbations resulting from HIV, viral hepatitis, hepatoma, alcohol abuse, estrogen, sunlight

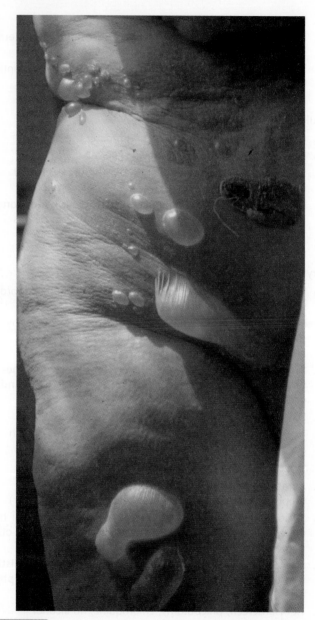

FIGURE 8.30

Multiple tense bullae of bullous pemphigold. (Courtesy of Dr. Steven Gammer.)

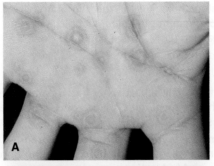

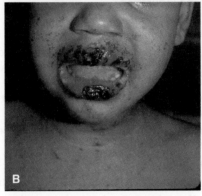

FIGURE 8.31

A. The target-like lesions of erythema multiforme. **B.** Stevens–Johnson syndrome is a more severe presentation of erythema multiforme in which mucosal surfaces are involved as well. (Courtesy of Dr. Steven Gammer.)

VIII. Vector–Borne Diseases

A. Bacillary Angiomatosis (Peliosis Hepatis)

1. Si/Sx = weight loss, abd pain, **rash with red or purple vascular lesions,** from papule to hemangioma size, located anywhere on skin and disseminated to any organ

2. DDx = Kaposi's sarcoma, cherry hemangioma

3. **Almost always seen in HIV⊕ pts or homeless population**

4. Caused by *Bartonella* spp., leading to dysregulated angiogenesis

5. **Cat-scratch dz caused by *Bartonella henselae* transmitted by kitten scratches; trench fever caused by *Bartonella quintana* spread by lice**

6. Dx = histopathology with Wharthin–Starry silver stain, visualization of organisms in lesion, blood culture, and polymerase chain reaction (PCR) can be done

7. Tx = erythromycin

B. **Lyme Dz**

1. Si/Sx = fever, chills, headaches, facial paralysis, lethargy, photophobia, meningitis, myocarditis, arthralgia, and myalgias

2. **Classic rash = erythema chronicum migrans → erythematous annular plaques with a red migrating border, central clearing, and induration**

3. Dx = PCR for *Borrelia burgdorferi* DNA, or skin Bx of migrating edge looking for causative spirochete

4. Prevent by spraying skin and clothes with DEET or permethrin; wear long pants in woods to prevent tick bite (*Ixodes dammini, Ixodes pacificus*)

5. Postexposure (i.e., after tick bite) prophylaxis with single-dose doxycycline

6. Once infected → high-dose penicillin, ceftriaxone, doxycycline or tetracycline for 2–4 wks

C. **Rocky Mountain Spotted Fever**

1. Si/Sx = acute-onset fever, headache, myalgias, classic rash

2. Rash = **erythematous maculopapular, starting on wrists and ankles then moving toward palms, soles, and trunk**

3. Rash may lead to cutaneous necrosis because of disseminated intravascular coagulation-induced occlusion of small cutaneous vessels with thrombi

4. Dx by Hx (exposure to outdoors or tick bite from *Dermacentor* spp.), serologies for *Rickettsia rickettsii,* skin Bx

5. Doxycycline or chloramphenicol

IX. Parasitic Infections

A. **Scabies**

1. Si/Sx = erythematous, **markedly pruritic papules and burrows located in intertriginous areas** (e.g., finger and toe webs, groin), lesions contagious (Figure 8.32)

2. Dx = microscopic identification of *Sarcoptes scabiei* mite in skin scrapings

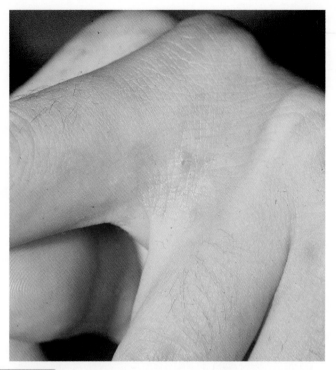

FIGURE 8.32

A papule located in the finger web is classic for scabies. (Courtesy of Dr. Steven Gammer.)

3. Tx = pt and all close contacts apply Permethrin 5% cream to entire body for 8–10 hrs, then repeat in 1 wk, wash all bedding in hot water the same day

4. Lindane cream is less effective, associated with neurotoxic adverse effects in kids

5. Symptomatic relief of hypersensitivity reaction to dead mites may be treated with antihistamines and topical steroids

B. **Pediculosis Capitis (Head Louse)**

1. Si/Sx = can be aSx, or pruritus and erythema of scalp may be noted, common in school-age children

2. Dx = microscope exam of hair shaft (Figure 8.33), nits may fluoresce with Wood's lamp

Text continues on page 428

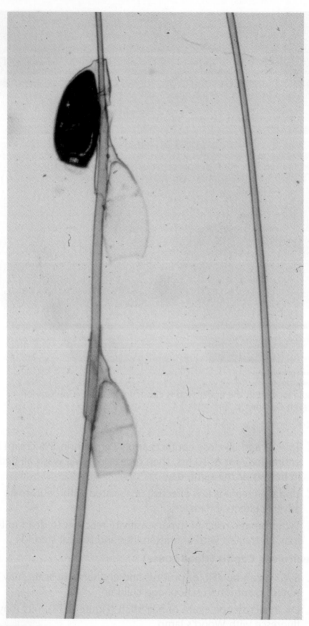

FIGURE 8.33

A louse and an empty casing attached to hair shaft. (Courtesy of Dr. Steven Gammer.)

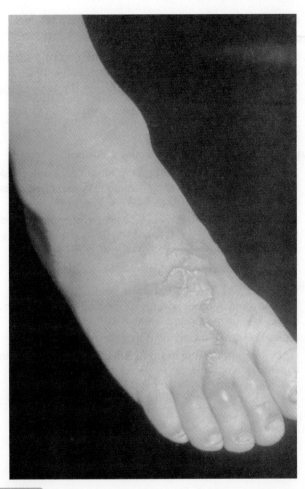

FIGURE 8.34

Cutaneous larva migrans. The skin shows a creeping eruption with the characteristic serpiginous, raised lesion. (From Sun T. *Parasitic disorders: pathology diagnosis, and management,* 2nd Ed. Baltimore, MD: Lippincott Williams & Wilkins, 1999.)

3. Permethrin shampoo or gel to scalp, may need to repeat

C. **Pediculosis Pubis ("Crabs")**

1. Si/Sx = very **pruritic papules in pubic area,** axilla, periumbilically in males, along eyelashes, eyebrows, and buttocks

2. Dx = microscopic identification of lice, rule out other sexually transmitted dz (STDs)

3. Tx = apply Permethrin 5% shampoo for 10 min, then repeat in 1 wk

D. **Cutaneous Larva Migrans (Creeping Eruption)**

1. Si/Sx = erythematous, pruritic, **serpiginous threadlike lesion** marking burrow of migrating nematode larvae, often on back, hands, feet, buttocks (Figure 8.34)

2. Organism = hookworms: *Ancylostoma, Necator, Strongyloides*

3. Dx = Hx of unprotected skin lying in moist soil or sand, Bx of lesion, lesion moves very slowly (e.g., 1–2 cm per day)

4. Tx = ivermectin orally or thiabendazole topically

E. Larva Currens

1. Si/Sx = rapidly moving linear, erythematous streaks in skin, moves 1–2 cm per hour

2. Caused by disseminated infxn by *Strongyloides*

3. Dx by ova and parasite exam (O&P) of stool or sputum (for hyperinfxn syndrome, in a very sick pt), or Bx

4. Tx = ivermectin

X. Fungal Cutaneous Disorders (Table 8.4)

Table 8.4 Fungal Cutaneous Disorders

Dz	Si/Sx	Dx	Tx
Tinea	• Erythematous, pruritic, scaly, well-demarcated plaques, typically annular (ring-like) with raised borders • Tinea cruris is intertriginous (typically groin) • Tinea corporis (i.e., ringworm) is on torso • Tinea capitis is on scalp, associated with hair loss and broken hair shafts • Tinea pedis is on foot (i.e., athlete's foot)	Clinical or KOH prep	Topical antifungal (oral needed for tinea capitis)
Onychomycosis	• Fingernails or toenails appear thickened, yellow, degenerating	Clinical or KOH prep	Lamisil, Itraconazole, fluconazole
Tinea versicolor	• Caused by *Pityrosporum ovale* (a.k.a. *Malassezia furfur*) • Multiple sharply marginated erythematous or hyperpigmented macules on face and trunk noticed in summer because macules will not tan—in a dark-skinned individual it can appear like vitiligo, but it is distinguished by multiple, individual circular lesions	KOH prep → yeast and hyphae with classic **spaghetti and meatball appearance**	Selenium sulfide shampoo Ketoconazole
Candida	• Erythematous scaling plaques, often in intertriginous areas (groin, breast, buttocks, web of hands)—distinguish from tinea cruris by the presence of satellite lesions beyond the edges of the main infxn (Figure 8.35A) • Oral thrush → cottage cheese-like white plaques on mucosal surface (Figure 8.35B) • Can extend to esophagus and cause dysphagia and odynophagia	KOH prep → budding yeast and pseudohyphae	Topical Nystatin or oral fluconazole

DERMATOLOGY

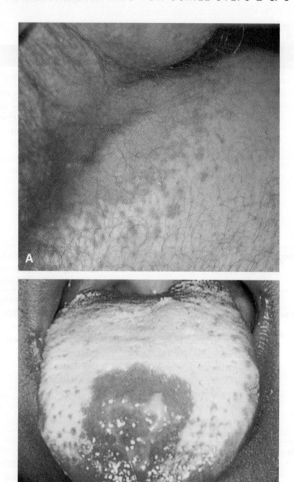

FIGURE 8.35

A. An erythematous intertriginous infxn is usually Candida if there are "satellite lesions" beyond the edges of the main infxn. (Courtesy of Dr. Steven Gammer.) **B.** Thrush on the tongue (From Weber J, Kelley J. *Health assessment in nursing,* 2nd Ed. Philadelphia, PA: Lippincott Williams & Wilkins, 2003.)

9. OPHTHALMOLOGY

I. Eyes

A. **Classic Syndromes or Sx**

1. Amblyopia
   a. ↓ vision 2° to failure of development of the pathway between the retina and visual cortex before ages 7–11
   b. Causes cataract, strabismus, or visual deprivation
   c. Si/Sx = Two-line difference in visual acuity between eyes, esotropia (inwardly rotated "crossed eyes") or exotropia (outwardly rotated "walled eyes"), diplopia, and refractive error not correctable with lenses
   d. Tx = early correction of cause of visual acuity disturbance

2. Bitemporal Hemianopsia (Figure 9.1)
   a. Unable to see in bilateral temporal fields
   b. Usually caused by a pituitary tumor

3. Internuclear ophthalmoplegia
   a. **Classically found in multiple sclerosis**
   b. Lesion of median longitudinal fasciculus
   c. Si/Sx = inability to adduct the ipsilateral eye past midline on lateral gaze (inability to perform conjugate gaze)
   d. Caused by lack of communication between contralateral CN VI nucleus and ipsilateral CN III nucleus

4. Parinaud's Syndrome
   a. Midbrain tectum lesion → bilateral paralysis of upward gaze
   b. Commonly associated with pineal tumor

5. Marcus Gunn Pupil (Afferent Pupillary Defect)
   a. Because of afferent defect of CN II, pupil will not react to direct light but will react consensually when light is directed at the nml contralateral eye
   b. **Characterized by swinging flashlight test**
      (1) Swing penlight quickly back and forth between eyes
      (2) Denervated pupil will not constrict to direct stimulation and **instead will actually appear to dilate when light is shone in it** because it is dilating back to baseline when consensual light is removed from other eye

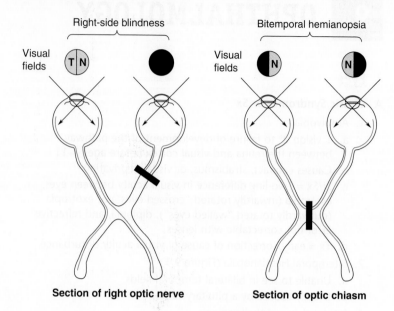

Section of right optic nerve

Section of optic chiasm

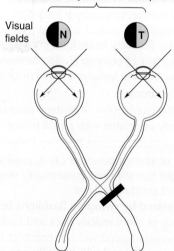

Section of right optic tract

FIGURE 9.1

Visual field defects. (From Moore KL, Dalley AF. *Clinical oriented anatomy*, 4th Ed. Baltimore, MD: Lippincott Williams & Wilkins, 1999.)

6. Argyll Robertson Pupil
   a. **Pathognomonic for 3° syphilis (neurosyphilis)**
   b. Pupils constrict with accommodation but do not constrict to direct light stimulation (pupils accommodate but do not react)
7. Lens Dislocation
   a. Occurs in homocystinuria, Marfan's and Alport's syndromes
   b. Lens dislocates superiorly in Marfan's (mnemonic: **Marfan's pts are tall, their lenses dislocate upward**), inferiorly in homocystinuria, and variably in Alport's syndrome
8. Kayser–Fleischer Ring
   a. **Pathognomonic for Wilson's dz**
   b. Finding is a ring of golden pigment around the iris (see Neurology, Figure 7.2)
9. Pterygium (Figure 9.2)
   a. Fleshy growth from conjunctiva onto nasal side of cornea
   b. Associated with exposure to wind, sand, sun, and dust

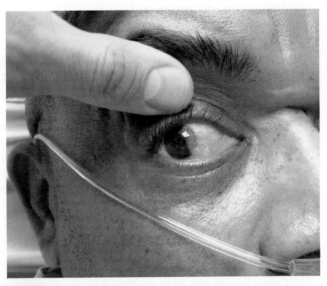

FIGURE 9.2

Right-sided pterygium. (Courtesy of Mark Silverberg, MD. From Greenberg MI, Hendrickson RG, Silverberg M, et al. *Greenberg's text-atlas of emergency medicine.* Philadelphia, PA: Lippincott Williams & Wilkins, 2004, with permission.)

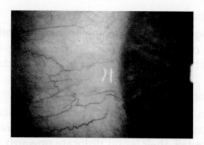

Clinical appearance of a pinguecula. (From James B, Chew C, Bron A. *Lecture notes on ophthalmology*, 8th Ed. Oxford: Blackwell Science, 1997, with permission.)

    c. Tx = cosmetic removal unless impairing vision; wear sunglasses and avoid dry eyes

10. Pinguecula (Figure 9.3)
    a. Benign yellowish nodules on either side of the cornea
    b. Commonly seen in pts >35
    c. Rarely grows and requires no Tx
    d. May have sensation of foreign body in eye

11. Subconjunctival Hemorrhage
    a. Spontaneous onset of a painless, bright-red patch on sclera
    b. Benign, self-limited condition usually seen after overexertion
    c. In the setting of trauma must r/o ruptured globe

12. Retrobulbar Neuritis
    a. Caused by inflammation of the optic nerve, usually unilateral
    b. **Seen in multiple sclerosis, often is the initial sign**
    c. Si/Sx = + afferent pupillary defect (APD), + pain, rapid loss of vision and pain upon moving eye, spontaneously remitting within 2–8 wks, each relapse damages the nerve more until blindness eventually results
    d. Funduscopic exam is nonrevealing; Dx by MRI of orbits
    e. Tx = corticosteroids

13. Optic Neuritis
    a. Inflammation of optic nerve within the eye
    b. Causes include viral infxn, multiple sclerosis, vasculitis, methanol, meningitis, syphilis, tumor metastases
    c. Si/Sx = variable vision loss and ↓ pupillary light reflex, + APD if unilateral

Table 9.1 Palpebral Inflammation

Dz	Si/Sx	Tx
Chalazion	• Inflammation of internal meibomian sebaceous gland • Presents with swelling on conjunctival surface of eyelid	Warm compresses, steroid ointment
Hordeolum (stye)	• Infxn of external sebaceous glands of Zeiss or Mol • Presents with tender red swelling at lid margin (Figure 9.4)	Hot compress, can add antibiotics
Blepharitis	• Inflammation of eyelids and eyelashes resulting from infxn (*S. aureus*) or 2° to seborrhea • Presents with red, swollen eyelid margins, with dry flakes noted on lashes • **Without Tx can extend along eyelid (cellulitis)**	Wash lid margins daily with baby shampoo, control scalp seborrhea with shampoo
Orbital cellulitis	• Marked swelling and erythema of eye, often with proptosis, ↓ vision, limited eye movement (Figure 9.5) • Distinguished from pre-septal (outside the orbit) cellulitis by change in vision and limited eye movement, which are not seen in preseptal cellulitis • **Can spread to cavernous sinus, leading to deadly thrombosis and meningitis**	Treat emergently with IV vancomycin + 3rd generation cephalosporin, CT scan to r/o abscess

    d. **Funduscopic exam reveals disk hyperemia**

    e. If pt is >60 yrs, Bx temporal artery to rule out temporal arteritis

    f. Tx = corticosteroids

B. **Palpebral Inflammation (Table 9.1)**

C. **Red Eye**

    1. **Assess pain, visual acuity, type of eye discharge, and pupillary abnormalities in all pts**

    2. DDx (Table 9.2)

D. **Dacryocystitis (Tear Duct Inflammation)**

    1. Infxn of lacrimal sac, usually caused by *Staphylococcus aureus*, *Streptococcus pneumoniae*, *Haemophilus influenzae*, or *Streptococcus pyogenes*

Text continues on page 440

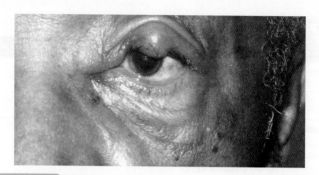

FIGURE 9.4

Stye (hordeolum).

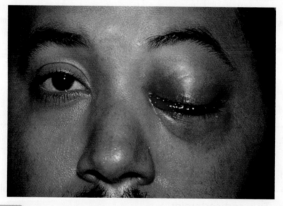

FIGURE 9.5

Orbital cellulitis presenting with massive swelling, chemosis, erythema, and poor ocular motility. (From Tasman W, Jaeger E. *The Wills eye hospital atlas of clinical ophthalmology,* 2nd Ed. Baltimore, MD: Lippincott Williams & Wilkins, 2001.)

Table 9.2 Red Eye

Dz	Si/Sx	Cause	Tx
Bacterial conjunctivitis	• Minimal pain, no vision changes • **Purulent** discharge • No pupillary changes • **Rarely** preauricular adenopathy (only *Neisseria gonorrhoeae*)	*S. pneumoniae*, *Staphylococcus* spp., *N. gonorrhoeae*, *Chlamydia trachomatis* (in neonates, sexually active adults)	Topical fluoroquinolone or erythromycin
Viral conjunctivitis	• Minimal pain, no vision changes • **Watery** discharge • No pupillary changes • **Often preauricular adenopathy** • **Often pharyngitis** (adenovirus)	Adenovirus most common, others = HSV, varicella, EBV, influenza, echovirus, coxsackie virus	No Tx required, self-limiting dz
Allergic conjunctivitis	• No pain, vision, or pupil changes • **Marked pruritus** • **Bilateral** watery eyes	Allergy/hay fever	Antihistamine or steroid drops
Hyphema	• **Blood in anterior chamber of eye, fluid level noted** (Figure 9.6) • Pain, no vision changes • No discharge, no pupil changes	Blunt ocular trauma	Check intraocular pressure (IOP): **<25mm Hg if sickle cell dz; <30 mm Hg if no Sickle cell dz**
Xerophthalmia	• Minimal pain, vision blurry, no pupillary changes, no discharge • **Bitot's spots** visible on exam (desquamated, conjunctival cells) • **Keratoconjunctivitis sicca** (Sjögren's dz) **Dx by Schirmer test** (place filter paper over eyelid; if not wet in 15 min → Dx)	Sjögren's dz or vitamin A deficiency	Artificial tears, vitamin A

OPHTHALMOLOGY

(continued)

Table 9.2 *Continued*

Dz	Si/Sx	Cause	Tx
Corneal abrasion	• **Painful, with photophobia** • No pupil changes • Watery discharge • Dx by fluorescein stain to detect areas of corneal defect	Direct trauma to eye (finger, stick, etc.)	Antibiotics, eye patch, examine daily
Keratitis	• **Pain,** photophobia, tearing • **↓ vision** • Can be caused by herpes zoster of CN V, 1st branch (Figure 9.7) • **Herpes simplex shows classic dendritic branching on fluorescein stain** (Figure 9.8) • **Pus in anterior chamber (hypopyon) is a grave sign** (Figure 9.9C)	Adenovirus, HSV, *Pseudomonas, S. pneumoniae, Staphylococcus* spp., *Moraxella* (often in lens wearers)	**Emergency, immediate Ophthalmology consult** Tx = topical vidarabine
Uveitis	• Inflammation of the iris, ciliary body, and/or choroid • **Pain, miosis,** photophobia • **Flare and cells** seen in aqueous humor **on slit-lamp examination** (Figure 9.9)	Seen in seronegative spondylo-arthro-pathy, IBD sarcoidosis, or infxn (CMV, syphilis, TB)	Tx underlying dz
Angle-closure glaucoma	• **Severe pain** • **↓ vision,** halos around lights • **Fixed mid-dilated pupil** • Eyeball firm to pressure • Vomiting	↓ Aqueous humor outflow via canal of Schlemm—mydriatics can also cause	**Emergency,** IV mannitol and glaucoma acetazolamide, laser iridotomy timolol, brimonidine
Subconjunctival hemorrhage (Figure 9.8)	Spontaneous onset of painless bright red patch caused by rupture of episcleral vessel	Overexertion, valsalva, or trauma. Can also be seen in pts with uncontrolled HTN	• Self-limited • Check blood pressure

CMV, cytomegalovirus; EBV, Ebstein-Barr virus; HSV, herpes simplex virus.

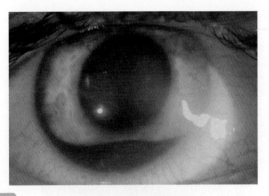

FIGURE 9.6

Hyphema. (From Moore KL, Dalley AF. *Clinical oriented anatomy*, 4th Ed. Baltimore, MD: Lippincott Williams & Wilkins, 1999.)

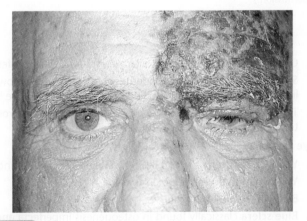

FIGURE 9.7

Herpes zoster ophthalmicus. (From Tasman W, Jaeger E. *The Wills eye hospital atlas of clinical ophthalmology*, 2nd Ed. Baltimore, MD: Lippincott Williams & Wilkins, 2001.)

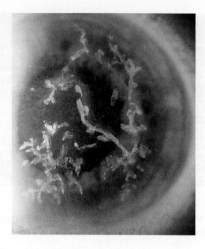

FIGURE 9.8

Classic zoster pseudo-dendrites are elevated mucous plaques with tapered ends. (From Tasman W, Jaeger EA, eds. *The Wills eye hospital atlas of clinical ophthalmology,* 2nd Ed. Philadelphia, PA: Lippincott Williams & Wilkins, 2001, with permission.)

2. Can be secondary to chronic allergies, trauma, or skin infection
3. Si/Sx = inflammation and tenderness of nasal aspect of lower lid, purulent discharge may be noted or expressed (Figure 9.10)
4. Tx = Keflex, I&D if an abscess has formed, will need dacrocystorhinstomy (DCR) in the future to prevent recurrence

E. **Eye Colors**

1. **Yellow eye** (icterus) from bilirubin staining of sclera (jaundice)
2. **Yellow vision** seen in digoxin toxicity
3. Blue Vision due to Viagra use
4. **Blue sclera** classically found in osteogenesis imperfecta and Marfan's dz
5. **Opaque eye;** can be cataract, tumor, or glaucoma and other causes
   a. Opacity of lens severe enough to interfere with vision
   b. Causes = congenital, diabetes (sorbitol precipitation in lens), galactosemia (galactitol precipitation in lens), Hurler's dz (see Appendix)
   c. R/o Retinoblastoma in kids

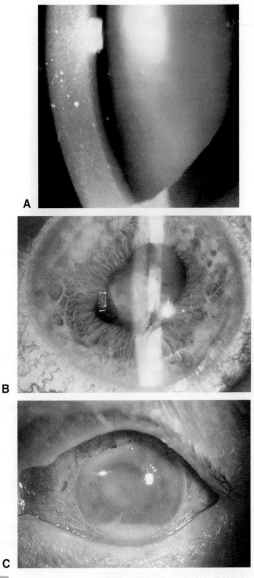

FIGURE 9.9

Signs of anterior uveitis. **A.** Keratic precipitates on the corneal endothelium. **B.** Posterior synechiae (adhesions between the lens and iris) give the pupil an irregular appearance. **C.** Hypopyon, white cells have collected as a mass in the inferior anterior chamber. (From Tasman W, Jaeger E. *The Wills eye hospital atlas of clinical ophthalmology,* 2nd Ed. Baltimore, MD: Lippincott Williams & Wilkins, 2001.)

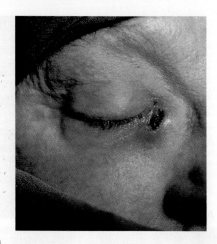

Dacryocystitis that, unusually, points through the skin. (From James B, Chew C, Bron A. *Lecture notes on ophthalmology,* 8th Ed. Oxford: Blackwell Science, 1997, with permission.)

F. **Retina**

1. Diabetic Retinopathy

    a. Occurs after approximately 10 yrs of diabetes

    b. Direct correlation with levels of HgA1c, i.e., the higher the levels, the higher the incidence

        (1) Background type

            (a) Flame hemorrhages, microaneurysms, and hard or soft exudates (cotton-wool spots) on retina (Figure 9.11A and B)

            (b) Tx is strict glucose and HTN control

        (2) Proliferative type

            (a) More advanced dz, with neovascularization easily visible around fundus (hyperemia) and hard exudates (Figure 9.11C)

            (b) Tx is photocoagulation (laser ablation of blood vessels in the retina), which slows dz progression but is not curative

2. Age-related Macular Degeneration

    a. Causes painless loss of visual acuity

    b. Dx by altered pigmentation in macula

    c. Pts often retain adequate peripheral vision

    d. Tx = antioxidants and Anti-VEGF

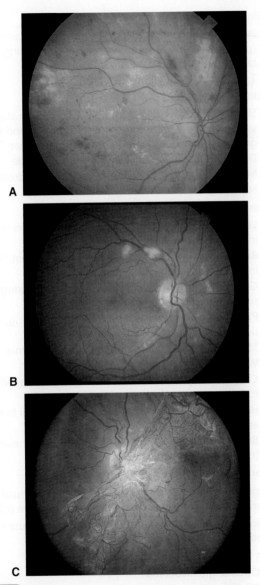

FIGURE 9.11

A. Sign of retinal vascular dz: hemorrhage and exudate. **B.** Sign of retinal vascular dz: cotton-wool spots. **C.** Sign of retinal vascular dz: new vessels, here particularly florid arising at the disk. (From Tasman W, Jaeger E. *The Wills eye hospital atlas of clinical ophthalmology,* 2nd Ed. Baltimore, MD: Lippincott Williams & Wilkins, 2001.)

3. Retinal Detachment
   a. Presents with painless, dark vitreous floaters, flashes of light (photopsias), blurry vision, eventually progressing to a curtain of blindness as detachment worsens
   b. Tx = urgent Ophthalmology consult

4. Retinitis Pigmentosa
   a. Slowly progressive defect in night vision (often starts in young children) with ring-shaped scotoma (blind spot) that gradually increases in size to obscure more vision
   b. Dz is hereditary with unclear transmission mode
   c. May be part of the Laurence–Moon–Biedl syndrome
   d. No Tx

5. Classic Physical Findings of Retina
   a. **Leukocoria** = absent red reflex, actually appears white, seen in retinoblastoma
   b. **Roth spots** = small hemorrhagic spots with central clearing in retina associated with endocarditis
   c. **Copper wiring, flame hemorrhages, A-V nicking** seen in subacute HTN and/or atherosclerosis
   d. **Papilledema** appears as disk hyperemia, blurring, and elevation, associated with ↑ intracranial pressure
   e. **"Sea fan"** neovascularization in sickle cell anemia
   f. **Wrinkles** on retina seen in retinal detachment
   g. **Cherry-red spot on macula** seen in Tay–Sachs, Niemann–Pick dz, central retinal artery occlusion
   h. Hollenhorst plaque = yellow cholesterol emboli in retinal artery
   i. **Brown** raised macule on retina = **malignant melanoma** (most common intraocular tumor in adults)

G. **Glaucoma**

1. Progressive optic neuropathy with characteristic visual field loss often (not always) related to ↑ intraocular pressure (IOP)

2. Major cause of blindness in the aging (leading cause of blindness in African-Americans)

3. Can be open or closed type
   a. Open-angle glaucoma
      (1) Causation unknown, mechanical versus vascular versus toxic (glutamate) theory
      (2) Rarely causes pain or corneal edema

(3) Constriction of visual field in later stages

(4) Incidence ↑ with age

(5) On funduscopic examination, classic finding ↑ in size of optic cup with thinning of neural rim

(6) Tx

    (a) Medical = cholinergics, α-agonists, β-blockers, carbonic anhydrase inhibitors, prostaglandin analog

    (b) Laser surgery to stretch trabecular meshwork and facilitate outflow

    (c) Surgery to facilitate alternate drainage pathway for aqueous

  b. Angle-closure glaucoma

    (1) Can be chronic or acute, the latter is an emergency

    (2) Typically idiopathic, can be drug induced (mydriatics)

    (3) Mydriatics cause the peripheral iris to move forward and occlude the aqueous fluid outflow tract

    (4) Prodromal Sx = sudden pain in eye and head, halos around lights, blurry vision, nausea and vomiting

    (5) Acute attack causes severe throbbing pain in eye, radiating to CN V distribution, blurry vision, nausea/vomiting, fixed, mid-dilated pupil, redness

    (6) This is considered an emergency because blindness can occur, must decrease IOP before nerve damage

    (7) Tx

        (a) IV or oral acetazolamide, topical timolol, pilocarpine (stretches and pulls the iris away from the angle)

        (b) Mydriatics **not** recommended (can exacerbate condition)—laser iridotomy follows to establish alternate pathway for aqueous to flow allowing iris to bow back into position

        (c) Laser iridotomy indicated in aSx eye to prevent future occurrence of angle closure

H. **Orbital Tumors**

  1. Adult

    a. Cavernous hemangioma

      (1) Most common adult tumor

      (2) Large well-circumscribed vascular tumor (proptosis of eye)

b. Metastases
  (1) Breast, lung, prostate most common
  (2) 10% of orbital tumors
c. Lymphoid tumors
  (1) Older pts
  (2) Spectrum from benign reactive lymphoid hyperplasia to lymphoma
  (3) Orbital involvement—radiotherapy; if systemic, radiation and chemotherapy
d. Fibrous histiocytoma—mesenchymal tumor
e. Mucocele—cystic mass of sinuses caused by duct obstruction, frontal and ethmoid sinuses most commonly involved
f. Fibrous dysplasia—bony tumor
g. Schwannoma
  (1) Tumor of peripheral nerve
  (2) Seen in neurofibromatosis

2. Pediatric
  a. Capillary hemangioma
    (1) Most common orbital tumor in children
    (2) Vascular tumor
    (3) Tx = β-blockers
  b. Dermoid cyst—benign cystic mass with connective tissue and skin appendages (hair, sebaceous glands)
  c. Leukemia
    (1) Myelogenous leukemia—chloroma
    (2) Lymphocytic leukemia—can also produce orbital infiltration
  d. Rhabdomyosarcoma
    (1) Most common primary orbital malignancy in children
    (2) Px, botryoid
  e. Lymphangioma
    (1) Tumor of early childhood with large lymph channels
    (2) Often have hemorrhage
  f. Neuroblastoma
    (1) Most common metastatic tumor in children
    (2) Ecchymosis with proptosis

I. **Orbital trauma (Table 9.3)**
J. **Ophthalmic Medications (Table 9.4)**

Table 9.3 Eye-related Trauma

Dz	Si/Sx	Tx
Chemical burns	• Alkali burns most damaging. Severe pain, erythema, conjunctival injection or blanching/necrosis; complete opacification of cornea in severe cases	• Immediate irrigation of eye with nml saline and removal of particulate debris • Check vision and pH • Immediate ophthalmology consult • Complete history of events surrounding exposure and exam of eye, face, and airway
Eyelid laceration	• May be superficial or involve deeper structures such as levator muscle, tarsal plate, and orbital septem. Medial lacerations can include lacrimal system (canaliculus) • Penetrating foreign bodies must be ruled out as a cause of laceration	• Ophthalmology consult for repair of lid/lacrimal system
Foreign body	• Pencils, glass, metal, wood, bullet • May cause corneal abrasion if hidden beneath eyelids • May be intraocular or intraorbital • CT scan is gold standard for imaging (never MRI. the magnet moves metallic object and may cause further damage) • Teardrop or odd-shaped pupil occasionally seen with penetrating foreign bodies	• Ophthalmology consult • External examination of eyelids, orbital walls, conjunctive, visual acuity, pupils, and extraocular movements • Slit-lamp examination of cornea with fluorescein dye • Eye shield prior to transport • Stabilize any objects protruding from orbit • Give IV broad spectrum antibiotics • Give antiemetics to control nausea and vomiting and prevent ↑ IOP • Tetanus prophylaxis • Glass and some metals are inert and are well tolerated • Wood must be removed immediately to prevent endophthalmitis

(continued)

OPHTHALMOLOGY

Table 9.3 *Continued*

Dz	Si/Sx	Tx
Ruptured globe (open globe injury)	• Full thickness corneal/corneoscleral/scleral laceration 2° to blunt or penetrating trauma	• Urgent surgical repair to close eye and IV antibiotics • Orbital imaging to look for intraocular foreign bodies; **beware** of sympathetic ophthalmia—a rare auto-immune uveitis that can affect the injured eye and then progress to uninjured eye • Tx—enucleate any irreversibly injured globes within 2 wks to prevent exposure to retinal antigens
Retinal detachment	• Commonly associated with blunt trauma to eye • Presents with painless, dark vitreous floaters, flashes of light (photopsias), and blurry vision • Progresses to a curtain of blindness in vision as detachment worsens • Retinal tear or hole visualized in periphery • Wrinkles on retina seen in retinal detachment	• Ophthalmology consult for urgent surgical reattachment
Hyphema	• Pain, blurriness blunt ocular trauma • Irregular pupil • Blood in anterior chamber of eye, fluid level noted	• Ophthalmology consult
Blowout fracture	• Thin bones of orbit "blow out" from ↑ intraorbital pressure • Most commonly orbital floor and medial wall • Enophthalmos, diplopia, and occasionally extraocular muscle entrapment, usually inferior rectus	• CT scan of orbit • Ophthalmology • Otolaryngology consult
Traumatic optic neuropathy	• Caused by indirect trauma to optic nerve, direct trauma from compression by hematoma or bone fragments • Afferent pupillary defect (Marcus Gunn pupil) • Vision loss	• Ophthalmology consult • Tx controversial—observation versus IV high-dose steroids (recent large study showed no benefit of steroids or decompression)

(continued)

Table 9.3 *Continued*

Dz	Si/Sx	Tx
Retrobulbar hemorrhage	• Can be seen with blunt trauma to eye and postoperatively after sinus surgery and blepharoplasty • Proptosis, resistance to retropulsion, ↑ IOP, ↓ extraocular motility, and afferent pupillary defect	• Ophthalmology consult • Surgical lateral canthotomy and lateral tendon cantholysis to relieve pressure may be necessary
Ocular melanoma	• Rare tumor commonly associated with dysplastic nevus syndrome	

Table 9.4 Opthalmic Medications

Drug Class	Examples	Use	Side Effects
Anesthetics	• Proparacaine hydrochloride • Tetracaine	• ↓ corneal sensation • Inhibiting corneal blink reflex and ↓ pain • Removal of foreign bodies and examination of injured cornea	• Repeated long-term use can lead to corneal ulceration, perforation • Can cause ocular allergic reaction
Steroids (topical)	• Prednisolone • Loteprednol • Rimexolone	• Iritis	• May potentiate a herpes simplex keratitis, bacterial, or fungal infxn if misdiagnosed • Cataracts and ↑ IOP seen in long-term use of steroid eye drops (steroid-induced glaucoma) • Ophthalmologist-directed use only

(continued)

Table 9.4 *Continued*

Drug Class	Examples	Use	Side Effects
Anticholinergics	• Short acting—Tropicamide, Cyclopentolate hydrochloride • Long acting—Scopolamine hydrobromide, Atropine sulfate	• Mydriatic and cycloplegic agents use to fully examine retina and facilitate refraction	• Rarely nausea, vomiting, and syncope • Acute angle closure glaucoma
Adrenergics	• Phenylephrine hydrochloride	• Mydriatic only, no cycloplegic effects	• HTN and tachycardia at higher concentrations
Decongestants	• Naphazoline hydrochloride • Phenylephrine hydrochloride • Tetrahydrozoline hydrochloride	• Used to relieve red eye • Cause vasoconstriction of conjunctival vessels	• Rebound vasodilation and worsening red eye
Antibacterials	• Tobramycin • Ciprofloxacin • Sulfacetamide • Erythromycin	• Prophylactic or organism specific bacterial Tx • Under the direction of an ophthalmologist	• Allergic reactions • Tobramycin toxic to corneal epithelium
Antiviral	• Vidarabine • Trifluridine	• Herpes Simplex Virus	• Allergic reactions • Punctuate keratopathy
NSAID	• Diclofenac • Ketorolac	• Ocular allergy	• Allergic reaction • Tachyphylaxis

Table 9.4 *Continued*

Drug Class	Examples	Use	Side Effects
Glaucoma	• β-blockers; e.g., Timolol (nonselective), betaxolol (β-1 selective)	• ↓ aqueous humor formation	• Systemic absorption can cause bronchospasm, bradycardia, and hypotension
	• Parasympatho-mimetics; i.e., pilocarpine	• ↑ outflow	• Lacrimation, salivation, nausea, vomiting, and headache
	• Sympathomimetic epinephrine (β-agonist), iopidine (α-agonist)	• ↑ outflow (β agonist), ↓ aqueous production (α-agonist)	• HTN, headache, cardiac arrhythmias (iopidine causes allergic reaction)
	• Carbonic anhydrase inhibitors (acetazolamide)	• ↓ aqueous formation	• Allergic reactions (sulfa base), nausea, vomiting, tingling of hands/feet. Avoid in pts with sickle cell trait or anemia, causes acidosis which ↑ sickling
Dry eye	Artificial tears	Ophthalmic lubricant	Allergic reaction to preservatives

10. RADIOLOGY

I. Helpful Terms and Concepts

A. **Lucent versus Sclerotic Lesions**

1. On plain film, a "lucency" is a focal area of bone or tissue that has a ↓ density, usually resulting from a pathologic process

2. On X-ray, a lucent bone lesion may appear like a dark, punched-out hole in the surrounding nml bone

3. In contrast, sclerotic bone lesions appear denser than the surrounding bone, and thus on X-ray appears whiter and more intense than its surroundings

B. **Hypodense versus Hyperdense**

1. Tissue density on CT can be characterized by how light or dark it appears relative to surrounding nml parenchyma

2. Hypodense lesions appear darker than nml tissue, whereas hyperdense lesions are brighter

3. Air- or fluid-filled lesions, such as cysts and abscesses, are common hypodense lesions

C. **Ring Enhancement**

1. Ring enhancement refers to a bright intensity that can be observed surrounding many lesions on both CT and MRI

2. This usually indicates local edema around a mass lesion, and in the brain it can indicate breakdown of the blood–brain barrier

D. **Radiopaque versus Radiolucent**

1. The more radiopaque an object is, the brighter it appears on plain film

2. Dental fillings, bullets, and metal prostheses are very radiopaque, so they appear white on plain film

3. The more radiolucent an object is, the darker it appears on plain film

Table 10.1	Common Radiologic Studies
Study	**Indications**
CT versus MRI	• CT → faster, less expensive, greater sensitivity for acute head trauma, better for detection of spinal cord compression • MRI → better visualization of soft tissue, allows multiplanar imaging (axial, coronal, sagittal, and oblique), no ionizing radiation
Endoscopic retrograde cholangiopancreatography (ERCP)	Pancreatitis 2° to choledocholithiasis, cholestatic jaundice
Utz[a]	Abd aortic aneurysm, gallbladder dz, renal and adrenal masses, ectopic pregnancy, kidney stones
Carotid Doppler Utz	Carotid artery stenosis, assessing flow dynamics
Intravenous pyelogram (IVP)	Genito-urinary obstruction
Kidney, ureter, bladder (KUB) X-ray[a]	Kidney stones, solid abd masses, abd free air
Lateral decubitus chest plain film	For determination of whether a suspected pleural effusion will layer

[a]Note: 80/20 rule: Gallstones diagnosed 80% of the time and kidney stones 20% of the time by Utz. Kidney stones diagnosed 80% of the time and gallstones only 20% of the time by X-ray.

II. Common Radiologic Studies (Table 10.1)

III. An Approach to a Chest X-Ray (Figure 10.1)

A = Airway—is trachea midline? and Alignment—symmetry of clavicles

B = Bones—look for fractures, lytic lesions, or defects

C = Cardiac silhouette—normally occupies <1/2 chest width

D = Diaphragms—flattened (e.g., chronic obstructive pulmonary dz)? Blunted angles (effusion)? Elevated (airspace consolidation)?

E = External soft tissues—lymph nodes (especially axilla), subQ emphysema, other lesions

F = Fields of the lung—opacities, nodules, vascularity, bronchial cuffing, etc.

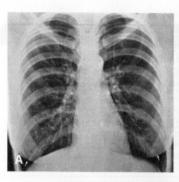

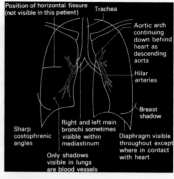

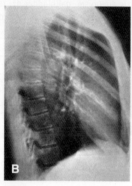

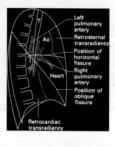

FIGURE 10.1

Nml chest. **A.** PA view. The *arrows* point to the breast shadows of this female pt. **B.** Lateral view. Note that the upper retrosternal area is of the same density as the retrocardiac areas and the same as over the upper thoracic vertebrae. The vertebrae are more transradiant (i.e., blacker) as the eye travels down the spine, until the diaphragm is reached. *Ao, aorta; T, trachea.* (From Armstrong P, Wastie M. *Diagnostic imaging,* 4th Ed. Oxford: Blackwell Science, 1998, with permission.)

IV. Common Radiologic Findings (Table 10.2)

Table 10.2 Common Radiologic Findings

Finding/Description	DDx

Multiple contrast-enhancing lesions on CT or MRI	**Neoplastic:**
	• Metastases (see Figure 10.2)
	  ◊ Breast CA and bronchogenic lung CA most common
	  ◊ Also malignant melanoma, prostate, lymphoma
	Infectious:
	• Bacterial abscess
	• Toxoplasmosis
	• Cysticercosis
	Vascular:
	• Infarct
	Degenerative:
	• Demyelinating dz

Nonsclerotic skull lucency	**Infectious:** • TB • Syphilis • Osteomyelitis **Neoplastic:** • Multiple myeloma • Metastases **Trauma:** • Burr hole **Endocrine:** • Hyperparathyroidism
Sclerotic bone lesions (Figure 10.3)	**Infectious:** • Osteomyelitis (presents with periosteal reaction) • Syphilis **Congenital:** • Fibrous dysplasia • Tuberous sclerosis **Neoplastic:** • Metastases—primarily prostate and breast • Lymphoma • Multiple myeloma—usually presents with multiple lesions (see Figure 1.15) • Osteosarcoma **Vascular:** • Healing fracture callus

(continued)

Table 10.2 *Continued*

Finding/Description	DDx
"Bone within bone" sign	**Endocrine:** • Growth arrest and recovery • Paget's dz • Osteopetrosis **Intoxication:** • Heavy metal poisoning
Inferior surface rib notching	**Vascular:** • Coarctation of the aorta—**classic finding** • Superior vena cava obstruction **Congenital:** • Chest wall A-V malformation
Ivory vertebral body Sclerotic change in single vertebra	**Neoplastic:** • Sclerotic metastases • Lymphoma **Endocrine:** • Paget's dz
Honeycomb lung Fibrotic replacement of lung parenchyma with thick-walled cysts	**Idiopathic:** • Idiopathic interstitial fibrosis • Histiocytosis X • Sarcoidosis **Congenital:** • Cystic fibrosis • Tuberous sclerosis • Neurofibromatosis **Autoimmune:** • Scleroderma • Rheumatoid arthritis **Intoxication:** • Allergic alveolitis • Asbestosis • Bleomycin • Nitrofurantoin • Cyclophosphamide
Ground glass opacities on lung CT Hazy, granular ↑ in density of lung parenchyma that usually implies an acute inflammatory process	**Inflammation:** • Interstitial pneumonia • Hypersensitivity pneumonitis • *Pneumocystic carinii* pneumonia • Alveolar proteinosis
Water-bottle-shaped heart on PA plain film	Pericardial effusions with >250 mL of fluid

Table 10.2 *Continued*

Finding/Description	DDx
Pulmonary edema Classically, severe pulmonary edema appears as **a bat's wing shadow**	**Vascular:** • Congestive heart failure **Inflammatory:** • Adult respiratory distress syndrome • Mendelson's syndrome **Intoxication:** • Smoke inhalation **Trauma:** • Near drowning
Blunting of costophrenic angles 300–500 mL of fluid is needed before blunting of the lateral costophrenic angles becomes apparent (see Figures 10.4 and 10.5)	Pleural effusion
Kerley B lines Interlobar septa on the peripheral aspects of the lungs that become thickened by dz or fluid accumulation (see Figure 10.6)	**Vascular:** • Left ventricular failure • Lymphatic obstruction **Inflammatory:** • Sarcoidosis • Lymphangitis carcinomatosa
Multiple lung small soft tissue Densities <2 mm	**Inflammatory:** • Sarcoidosis • Miliary TB • Fungal infxn • Parasites • Extrinsic allergic alveolitis **Neoplastic:** • Metastases **Endocrine:** • Hemosiderosis

(continued)

Table 10.2 *Continued*

Finding/Description	DDx
Lung nodules >2 cm Ghon complex—calcified granuloma classic for TB, found at lung base along hilum (see Figure 10.7)	**Neoplastic:** • Metastases • 1° lung CA • Benign hamartoma **Intoxication:** • Silicosis **Idiopathic:** • Histiocytosis X **Inflammatory:** • Sarcoidosis • TB • Wegener's • Fungal infxns • Abscess
Hilar adenopathy	**Inflammatory:** • Sarcoidosis (bilateral, eggshell calcification) • Amyloidosis **Intoxication:** • Silicosis **Neoplastic:** • Bronchogenic CA (unilateral) • Lymphoma
Cavity Annular opacity with central lucency (see Figure 10.8)	**Infectious:** • TB (apex) • Lung abscess • Fungal • Amebiasis **Neoplastic:** • Bronchogenic CA • Metastases • Lymphoma **Autoimmune:** • Rheumatoid lung dz
Unilaterally elevated diaphragm (see Figure 10.9)	**Trauma:** • Phrenic nerve palsy **Congenital:** • Pulmonary hypoplasia scoliosis **Vascular:** • Pulmonary embolism

Table 10.2 *Continued*

Finding/Description	DDx
Bilaterally elevated diaphragm	• Obesity • Pregnancy • Fibrotic lung dz
Steeple sign Narrowed area of subglottic trachea **Thumb sign**	Parainfluenza virus (croup) Epiglottitis classically caused by Haemophilus influenzae

Pneumoperitoneum
Free air under the diaphragm on an
upright chest film or upright abdomen
Double-wall sign on abd plain film
Appearance of the outer and
inner walls of bowel is almost
pathognomonic for pneumoperitoneum
	Inflammatory:
	• Perforation
	  ◊ Ulcer
	  ◊ Diverticulitis
	  ◊ Appendicitis
	  ◊ Toxic megacolon
	  ◊ Infarcted bowel
	Also can be:
	• Peritoneal dialysis
	• Pneumomediastinum that has tracked
	  inferiorly
	• Diaphragmatic rupture

Gasless abdomen on abd plain film (see Figure 10.10)	• Obstruction • Severe ascites • Pancreatitis
Filling defects in stomach on upper GI series	• Gastric ulcer • Gastric CA
Dilated small bowel (see Figures 10.10 and 10.11)	**Mechanical obstruction:** • Postsurgical • Incarcerated hernia • Intussusception • Paralytic ileus **Inflammatory:** • Celiac sprue • Scleroderma
Coffee bean sigmoid volvulus (see Figure 10.12)	• Large-bowel obstruction • Paralytic ileus
String sign on barium swallow Narrowing of the terminal ileum caused by thickening of the bowel wall	• Crohn's dz

(continued)

RADIOLOGY

Table 10.2 *Continued*

Finding/Description	DDx
Lead pipe sign on barium enema Smooth, narrowed colon without haustra	• Inflammatory bowel dz (see Figure 10.13)
Apple core lesion Circumferential growth in the bowel lumen	• Colon CA
Liver calcifications	**Inflammatory:** • Granuloma • Hydatid cyst **Neoplastic:** • Hepatoma
Gas in portal vein Linear lucencies that reach within 2 cm of liver capsule	**Vascular (seen in adults):** • Mesenteric infarct • Air embolism **Inflammatory (children):** • Necrotizing enterocolitis
Unilateral cystic renal mass Hypodensities with thin walls	**Inflammatory:** • Renal abscess • Hemodialysis-induced cyst • Hydatid cyst **Congenital:** • Bilateral renal cysts • Polycystic kidney dz **Neoplastic:** • Renal cell CA
String of beads on renal arteriogram Multiple dilatations alternating with strictures of both renal arteries	• Fibromuscular dysplasia

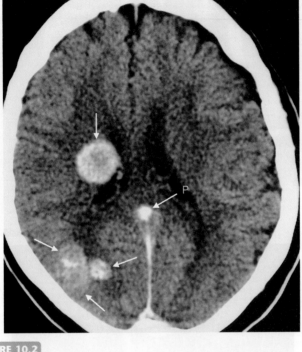

FIGURE 10.2

Metastases (*arrows*). *P, pineal.* (From Armstrong P, Wastie M. *Diagnostic imaging,* 4th Ed. Oxford: Blackwell Science, 1998, with permission.)

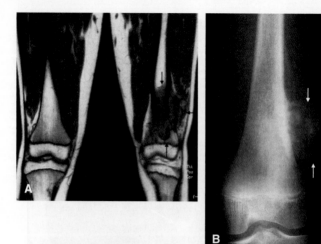

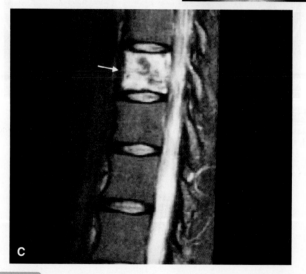

FIGURE 10.3

MRI of bone tumors. **A.** T1-weighted scan of osteosarcoma in the lower shaft and metaphysis of the left femur. The extent of tumor (*arrows*) within the bone and the soft-tissue extension are both very well shown. This information is not available from the plain film. **B.** However, the plain film provides a more specific diagnosis because the bone formation within the soft-tissue extension (*arrows*) is obvious. **C.** T2-weighted scan of lymphoma in the T10 vertebral body (*arrow*). The very high signal of the neoplastic tissue is highly evident even though there is no deformity of shape of the vertebral body. (From Armstrong P, Wastie M. *Diagnostic imaging,* 4th Ed. Oxford: Blackwell Science, 1998, with permission.)

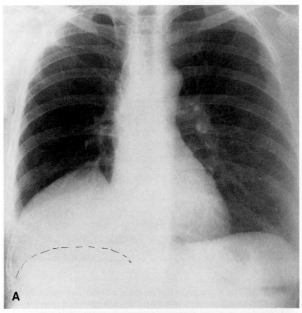

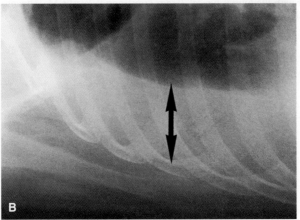

FIGURE 10.4

Large right subpulmonary effusion (pt has had right mastectomy). Almost all the fluid is between the lung and the diaphragm. The right hemidiaphragm cannot be seen. **A.** Estimated position is penciled in. **B.** In the lateral decubitus view, the fluid moves to lie between the lateral chest wall and the lung edge (*arrows*). (From Armstrong P, Wastie M. *Diagnostic imaging,* 4th Ed. Oxford: Blackwell Science, 1998, with permission.)

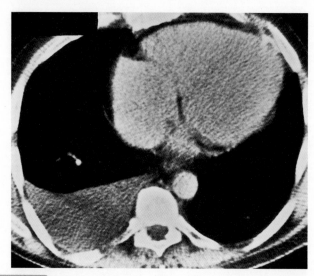

FIGURE 10.5

CT of pleural fluid. The right pleural effusion is of homogeneous density, with a CT number between zero and soft tissue. Its well-defined, meniscus-shaped border with the lung is typical. (From Armstrong P, Wastie M. *Diagnostic imaging,* 4th Ed. Oxford: Blackwell Science, 1998, with permission.)

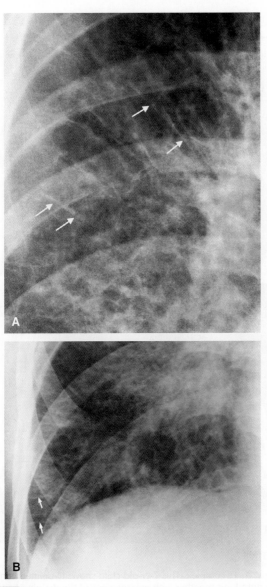

FIGURE 10.6

Septal lines. **A.** Kerley A lines (*arrows*) in a pt with lymphangitis carcinomatosa. **B.** Kerley B lines in a pt with pulmonary edema. The septal lines (*arrows*) are thinner than the adjacent blood vessels. The B lines are seen in the outer cm of lung where blood vessels are invisible or very difficult to identify. (From Armstrong P, Wastie M. *Diagnostic imaging,* 4th Ed. Oxford: Blackwell Science, 1998, with permission.)

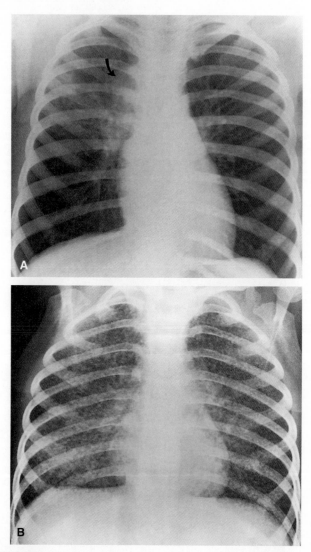

FIGURE 10.7
Tuberculosis. **A.** 1° complex. This 7-yr-old child shows ill-defined consolidation in the right lung together with enlargement of the draining lymph nodes (*arrow*). **B.** Miliary TB. The innumerable small nodular shadows uniformly distributed throughout the lungs in this young child are typical of miliary TB. In this instance, no 1° focus of infxn is visible. (From Armstrong P, Wastie M. *Diagnostic imaging*, 4th Ed. Oxford: Blackwell Science, 1998, with permission.)

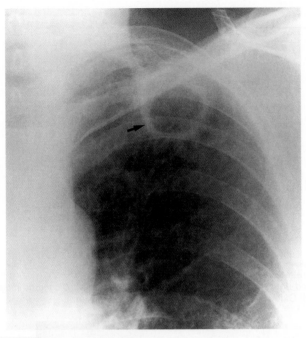

FIGURE 10.8

Fungus infxn. The cavity (*arrow*) in this pt from the southeastern US was the result of North American blastomycosis. Note the similarity to TB. Other fungi, e.g., histoplasmosis, can give an identical appearance. (From Armstrong P, Wastie M. *Diagnostic imaging*, 4th Ed. Oxford: Blackwell Science, 1998, with permission.)

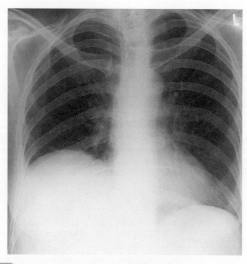

FIGURE 10.9

Elevated right diaphragm. (From Armstrong P, Wastie M. *Diagnostic imaging,*
4th Ed. Oxford: Blackwell Science, 1998, with permission.)

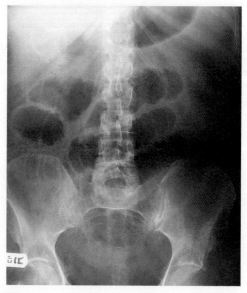

FIGURE 10.10

Small-bowel obstruction: distended small bowel and absence of gas shadows in the colon. (From Armstrong P, Wastie M. *Diagnostic imaging,* 4th Ed.
Oxford: Blackwell Science, 1998, with permission.)

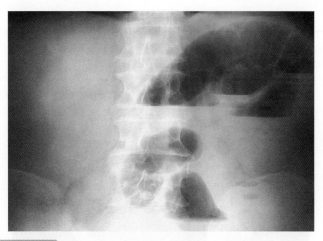

FIGURE 10.11

Erect film demonstrating multiple small-bowel air–fluid levels. (From Armstrong P, Wastie M. *Diagnostic imaging,* 4th Ed. Oxford: Blackwell Science, 1998, with permission.)

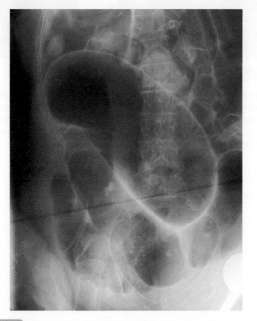

FIGURE 10.12

Sigmoid volvulus with a grossly distended sigmoid. (From Armstrong P, Wastie M. *Diagnostic imaging,* 4th Ed. Oxford: Blackwell Science, 1998, with permission.)

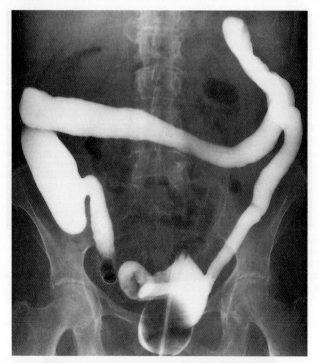

FIGURE 10.13

Ulcerative colitis. With long-standing dz, the haustra are lost and the colon becomes narrowed and shortened, coming to resemble a rigid tube. Reflux into the ileum through an incompetent ileocecal valve has occurred. (From Armstrong P, Wastie M. *Diagnostic imaging,* 4th Ed. Oxford: Blackwell Science, 1998, with permission.)

11. EMERGENCY MEDICINE

I. Toxicology

Toxin	Si/Sx	Dx	Antidote
Acetaminophen	Nausea/vomiting within 6 hrs, ↑ liver enzymes, ↑ prothrombin time (PT) at 24–48 hrs	Blood level	*N*-acetylcysteine within 8 hrs
Alkali agents	Derived from batteries, dish washer detergent, drain cleaners, ingestion causes mucosal burns → dysphagia and drooling	Clinical	NPO
Anticholinergic	**Dry as a bone, mad as a hatter, blind as a bat, hot as a hare, full as a flask** (no sweat, delirium, mydriasis, fever, urinary retention)	Clinical	Physostigmine
Arsenic	**Mees lines** (white horizontal stripes on fingernails [late sign]), **nausea/vomiting/Diarrhea**, seizures, shock	Blood level	Dimercaprol
Aspirin	Tinnitus, respiratory alkalosis, **anion gap metabolic acidosis with nml S_{osm}**	Blood level	Bicarbonate, dialysis
Benzodiazepine	Slurred speech, ataxia, drowsiness	Clinical	Flumazenil if iatrogenic overdose
β-Blockers	Bradycardia, heart block, obtundation, **hyperkalemia**	Clinical	Glucagon, IV calcium
Carbon monoxide	**Headache, nausea/vomiting**, confusion, coma, **cherry-red skin**	Carboxy-hemoglobin	100% O_2 or hyperbaric O_2

(continued)

Toxin	Si/Sx	Dx	Antidote
Cyanide	In sec to min → **almond-scented breath**, coma	Clinical	Sodium nitrite, sodium thiosulfate, **Hydroxocobalamine**
Digoxin	Yellow halos, **bradycardia, heart block, hyperkalemia**	Blood level[a]	Antidigoxin, **Fab antibodies**
Ethylene glycol	**Calcium oxalate crystals in urine, anion gap, metabolic acidosis with high S_{Osm}**	Bicarb level, **Osm gap**	**Fomepizole**[a]
Heparin	Bleeding, thrombocytopenia	Clinical (↑ partial thrombo-plastin time [PTT] level)	Protamine
Iron	Vomiting, bloody diarrhea, acidosis, CXR → radiopaque tablets	Blood level	Deferoxamine
Isoniazid	Confusion, peripheral neuropathy (seizure)	Clinical	Pyridoxine
Lead	**Microcytic anemia with basophilic stippling,** ataxia, retardation, peripheral neuropathy	Blood level	EDTA, Dimercaprol
Mercury	**"Erethism" = ↓ memory, insomnia, timidity, delirium (mad as a hatter)**	Blood level	Dimercaprol
Methanol	**Anion gap metabolic acidosis with high S_{Osm},** blindness, **optic disk, hyperemia**	Blood level	Bicarbonate, **Fomepizole**
Opioids	CNS/respiratory depression, miosis	Clinical	Naloxone
Organophosphate	Incontinence, cough, bronchospasm, miosis, bradycardia, heart block, tremor	Clinical	Atropine, pralidoxime
Phenobarbital	CNS depression, hypothermia, miosis, hypotension	Clinical	Supportive

Toxin	Si/Sx	Dx	Antidote
Quinidine	Torsade de pointes (ventricular tachycardia), tinnitus, vertigo widens QRS complex and prolongs QT interval	Blood level[b]	IV magnesium
Theophylline	First Sx = hematemesis, then CNS → seizures or coma, cardiac → arrhythmias, hypotension	Blood level	Charcoal, cardiac monitor
Tricyclics	Anticholinergic Sx, QRS >100 ms, tachy, coma	Clinical	Bicarbonate bolus
Warfarin	Bleeding	↑ PT	Vitamin K

[a]See *N Engl J Med* 1999;340:832–838.
[b]Correlates in acute but not chronic toxicity.
S_{Osm}, serum osmolality.

II. Fish and Shellfish Toxins[a]

Ciguatera

1. Most common fish-borne illness worldwide and the most common type of nonbacterial food poisoning reported in the US

2. Species of fish include barracuda, grouper, snapper, and sea bass (reef fish)

3. The bigger the fish, the higher the concentration of ciguatoxin

4. Ciguatoxin has anticholinesterase and cholinergic properties; its toxicity is related to the competitive inhibition of calcium-regulated cell membrane sodium channels

5. Sx: Begin within 6 hrs of eating a Ciguatoxic fish
   a. GI complaints: vomiting, watery diarrhea, abd cramps, lasts 24–48 hrs
   b. Neurologic symptoms: paresthesias of lips and extremities, reversal of hot–cold sensation, vertigo, blurred vision, tremor, ataxia, feeling of loose painful teeth. May persist for months and are aggravated by alcohol consumption or stress
   c. Shock: hypotension, respiratory failure

6. Tx: prevention, supportive measures, IV mannitol can be given for severe cases, and amitriptyline for paresthesias

Scombroid

1. A histamine-like reaction associated with marine tuna, mackerel, jacks, dolphin (mahi-mahi), and bluefish

2. Scombrotoxin formed when surface bacteria Proteus and Klebsiella on the fish secrete the enzyme histidine decarboxylase and convert histidine in the fish flesh to histamine. This and other histamine-like substances act to produce the clinical effects

(continued)

Scombroid *(Continued)*

3. Sx: flushing hot sensation of face and neck, pruritus, urticaria, headache, dizziness, burning sensation in mouth and throat, bronchospasm, angioedema, and hypotension can occur

4. Tx: supportive, antihistamines, cimetidine, and bronchodilators

Paralytic Shellfish

1. Caused by ingestion of mollusks (mussels, clams, oysters, and scallops) that have concentrated the *Saxitoxin*

2. Sx: paresthesias of mouth and extremities, sensation of floating, vomiting, diarrhea, ataxia, vertigo, and muscle paralysis (generalized peripheral nerve dysfunction)

3. Fatality rate of 8%–9%, with deaths occurring in 1–12 hrs 2° to respiratory failure

4. *Saxitoxin* acts by inhibiting sodium channels in nerve terminals blocking nerve and muscle action potential propagation

5. Tx: supportive, no known antidote, protect airway, and consider mechanical ventilation

Neurotoxic Shellfish

1. Caused by ingestion of mollusks that have concentrated the *Brevitoxin*

2. Sx: not as bad as paralytic shellfish; paresthesias like those seen in ciguatera poisoning (hot/cold reversal), vomiting, diarrhea, no paralysis or respiratory failure. Self-limited

3. Aerosolized *Brevetoxin* during a red tide at the beach can cause rhinorrhea, conjunctivitis, bronchospasm, and cough

4. *Brevetoxin* acts by opening sodium channels of postganglionic cholinergic nerve fibers and depolarize skeletal muscle

5. Tx: supportive and symptomatic

Tetrodotoxin

1. Rare in US. Caused by eating Japanese puffer fish (*Fugu*), blue ringed octopus, newts, and salamander

2. Sxs: begin within minutes of ingestion, paresthesias of face and extremities, salivation, hyperemesis, weakness, ataxia, dysphagia, ascending paralysis, respiratory failure, hypotension, bradycardia, fixed dilated pupils

3. Tetrodotoxin is chemically related to saxitoxin, causing a similar blockade of sodium channels in nerve terminals. There are also direct effects of the toxin on the medulla, and reversible competitive blockade at the motor end plate

4. Tx: Supportive, airway and ventilatory support, anticholinesterase inhibitors; i.e., edrophonium. Px is good if pt survives first 24 hrs

[a]Eastaugh J, Shepherd S. Infectious and toxic syndromes from fish and shellfish consumption: a review. *Arch Intern Med.* 1989 Aug;149(8);1735–1740.

III. Bites and Stings

Bite or Sting	Sx	Tx
Bee/wasp	Local inflammation or anaphylactic reaction possible	• Scrape out stinger if present, wash with soap and water • **Airway,** IV fluids, O_2, Cardiac monitoring for systemic effects • **Epinephrine** (1:1000) 0.3–0.5 mL SQ in adults, 0.01 mL/kg in children, may be given a second time in 10–15 min • **Diphenhydramine** 25–50 mg IV/IM, and **methylprednisolone:** 80–120 mg IV, followed by prednisone taper upon stabilization
Black Widow ("red hourglass" on abdomen)	Sharp pain at site, with deep burning, aching pain along extremity, and vomiting, headache, chest tightness, HTN, rigid abd muscles, back spasms	• **Airway,** IV fluids, O_2, cardiac monitoring for systemic effects • Antivenin is curative. Wound care, tetanus prophylaxis, pain relief
Brown Recluse Spider ("brown-yellow violin" on thorax)	Painless bite, nausea, myalgias and arthralgias, fever, chills, rash, necrosis at bite site	Wound care, dapsone, plastic surgery consult for significant necrosis
Snake (depends on geographical region)	Fang puncture marks, vomiting, diarrhea, restlessness, dysphagia, muscle weakness, fasciculations, generalized bleeding	• Advanced cardiac life support (ACLS) resuscitation as needed • Type specific antivenin. Tetanus prophylaxis, coagulopathy, compartment syndrome of affected extremity
Cats	Tender regional lymphadenopathy can occur, with local edema, erythema, decreased range of motion (tenosynovitis), commonly caused by *Pasteurella*	Copious irrigation and wound care, administer amoxicillin-clavulonate (or iv ampicillin-sulbactam), tetanus prophylaxis

(continued)

Bite or Sting	Sx	Tx
Dogs	Local edema and erythema, assess nature of bite, unprovoked worrisome for rabies, provoked → unlikely rabies	Copious irrigation and wound care, tetanus prophylaxis, rule out fractures, amoxillin-clavulonate (or iv ampicillin-sulbactam)
Human	Treat all knuckle injuries in a fight as a human bite, can present with erythema, edema, purulence, pain, fever, and chills	Copious irrigation, tetanus prophylaxis, augmentin PO, IV antibiotics for severe unresolving infxn or in immunocompromised, rule out fractures

IV. ENT Trauma*

Dx	Si/Sx	Tx

Foreign body	1. Ear—insect or object in ear
	2. Nose—persistent unilateral nasal drainage
	3. Airway—persistent pneumonia
	4. Esophageal—three most common areas of narrowing and lodging of foreign bodies
	  a. Cervical esophagus 16 cm from dental incisors
	  b. Cardioesophageal level 23 cm from incisors
	  c. Gastroesophageal 40 cm from incisors
		1. ENT consult for extraction. Mineral oil in ear to kill insects while you wait. Don't irrigate vegetable matter or it will swell
		2. ENT consult for extraction
		3. CXR PA and lateral, and pulmonary or ENT consult for bronchoscopy and extraction
		4. CT scan of neck

TM perforation	• Commonly occurs after a slap in the face or cotton swab in ear	• PO antibiotics and ear gtts • Water precautions

Dx	Si/Sx	Tx
Auricular hematoma	• Commonly seen in wrestlers with repeated trauma to ears • Ecchymotic fluctuant • If left untreated, necrosis of auricular perichondrium can occur and pts develop a cauliflower ear	1. ENT consult fluid collection 2. Incision and drainage of hematoma with drain left in place and Bolster dressing sutured in 3. PO antibiotics and careful followup
Blunt laryngeal trauma	• Hoarseness, stridor, voice changes, airway obstruction, subcutaneous emphysema, and hemoptysis	• ENT consult. CXR, fiberoptic scope, and CT to evaluate injury and possible fracture • Airway observation in monitored setting. May need to secure airway (tracheostomy) • Humidified oxygen and steroids. Surgery may be needed in severe trauma
Nasal Fx	• There may be external and/or internal structural deviation • Must rule out septal hematoma/septal abscess to prevent ischemic compression of perichondrium and septal cartilage necrosis leading to saddle nose deformity • Evaluate for CSF leak • Repair any superficial lacerations	• Any nosebleed should be stopped as described in Epistaxis • X-rays are not very helpful. Physical exam is all you need • ENT consult • Septal hematoma/abscess must be drained with a rubber train left in place • Neurosurgery should be informed of potential CSF leak • Because of edema and severe pain, most fracture (open or closed) reductions occur within 7–10 days in the OR under anesthesia if cosmesis or nasal airway is a concern • Antistaphylococcal antibiotic prophylaxis given

(continued)

Dx	Si/Sx	Tx

Facial fracture	• LeFort fractures are the classic facial trauma fractures
	• Look for mobile palate (fractures always involve the pterygoid plates)
	1. Types of LeFort fractures
	  a. LeFort 1 = maxilla fracture
	  b. LeFort 2 = pyramidal fracture on nasofrontal suture line
	  c. LeFort 3 = total craniofacial dysjunction
		• ENT/plastics/or maxillofacial consult
		• Open versus closed reduction with fixation devices (wiring versus plating)

Mandible Fx	1. Most commonly affects the condyle, body, and angle of mandible in that order 2. Multiple sites usually affected simultaneously 3. Sx: pain, malocclusion, trismus, crepitance, mucosal lacerations 4. Classified as favorable if fracture fragments pull in the direction of splinting fracture. Unfavorable if forces on fracture line pull fragments apart	1. CT and panorex views are usually diagnostic 2. Antibiotics and pain meds needed 3. Open or closed reduction of fracture is needed and can be performed by oral surgery, plastics, or ENT

*Note: All of the above conditions should be stabilized and evaluated by an Otorhinolaryngologist.

12. ETHICS/LAW/ CLINICAL STUDIES

I. Biostatistics

A. **Table of Definitions** (Table 12.1)

B. **Study Types**
1. Prospective is less prone to bias than retrospective
2. Interventional is less prone to bias than observational
3. Clinical trial
   a. Prospective interventional trial in which pts are randomized into an intervention group and a control group
   b. Randomization blunts the effect of confounding factors
   c. Blinding both clinician and pt (double-blind) further decreases bias

Table 12.1	Biostatistics
Term	**Definition**
Sensitivity	Probability that test results will be positive in pts with disease
Specificity	Probability that test results will be negative in pts without disease
False positive	Pt without disease who has a positive test result
False negative	Pt with disease who has a negative test result
PPV	Positive predictive value: probability pt with positive test actually has disease
NPV	Negative predictive value: probability pt with negative test actually has no disease
Positive Likelihood Ratio	Sensitivity/(1 − specificity)
Negative Likelihood Ratio	Specificity/(1 − sensitivity)
Incidence	# of newly reported cases of disease divided by total population
Prevalence	# of existing cases of disease divided by total population at a given time

(continued)

Table 12.1 *Continued*

Term	Definition
Relative risk	From cohort study (prospective)—risk of developing dz for people with known exposure divided by the risk of developing dz without exposure
Odds ratio	From case-control study (retrospective)—approximates relative risk by calculating an odds ratio, which is comparing the proportion of people with disease who had a specific risk factor divided by the proportion of people without disease who had the same risk factor (if dz is rare, odds ratio approaches true relative risk)
Variance	Estimate of the variability of each individual data point from the mean
Std deviation	Square root of the variance
Type I error (α-error)	Null hypothesis is rejected even though it is true—e.g., the study says the intervention works, but it only appears to work because of random chance
Type II error (β-error)	Null hypothesis is not rejected even though it is false—e.g., the study fails to detect a true effect of the intervention
Power ($1 - \beta$)	Estimate of the probability a study will be able to detect a true effect of the intervention—e.g., power of 80% means that if the intervention works, the study has an 80% chance of detecting this but a 20% chance of randomly missing it

4. **Cohort study**
   a. Population is divided by exposure status
   b. Requires large population (cannot study rare disease)
   c. Can study multiple effects by exposure
   d. **Gives relative risk if prospective**
   e. Can be prospective or retrospective
5. **Case-control study**
   a. Pts divided into those with dz (cases) and those without dz (controls)
   b. Fewer pts are needed (good for rare disease)
   c. Can study correlation of multiple exposures
   d. Gives odds ratio

II. Calculation of Statistical Values (Table 12.2)

A. Two-by-Two table
   1. The first column shows the patients who have disease and the second column shows the patients who do not have disease

Table 12.2 Sample Calculation of Statistical Values

	Pt has Dz	Pt does not have Dz	
Positive test	a = True positive	b = False positive	PPV = a/(a + b)
Negative test	c = False negative	d = True negative	NPV = d/(c + d)

PPV = a/(a + b)
NPV = d/(c + d)
Sensitivity = a/(a + c)
Specificity = d/(b + d)

2. The top row indicates the patients the test says have disease, and the bottom row indicates the patients the test says do not have disease
3. A = True Positives, B = False Positives, C = False Negatives, D = True Negatives

B. Test Accuracy
   1. There are 2 major measurements of test accuracy: sensitivity and specificity
      a. Sensitivity
         (1) Defined as the ability of the test to detect disease in a patient when the disease is really present
         (2) Sensitivity = # people the test says have disease/total # people who really have disease
         (3) By the 2 × 2 table, sensitivity = (true positives/true positives + false negatives) = a/(a + c)
         (4) **A test with high sensitivity is used to rule OUT disease**
         (5) Thus, tests with high sensitivity are useful when they are NEGATIVE, e.g. anti-nuclear antibody (ANA) to r/o systemic lupus erythematosis (SLE)
      b. Specificity
         (1) Defined as the ability of the test to accurately say that disease is not present when it is really not present
         (2) Specificity = the # people without disease who the test says do not have disease/total # people who really do not have disease
         (3) By the 2 × 2 table, specificity = true negatives/false positives + true negatives = d/(b + d)
         (4) **A test with high specificity is used to rule IN disease**
         (5) Thus, tests with high specificity are useful when they are POSITIVE, e.g., anti-ds-DNA for SLE
   2. **Sensitivity and specificity do not take into consideration the pre-test probability of disease, so they cannot be used as measurements of post-test probability of disease**

3. Post-test Probability of Disease
   a. Positive Predictive Value (PPV)
      (1) PPV = the probability that a person really has disease when the test says they have disease
      (2) PPV = (true positives/true positives + false positives) = a/(a + b)
      (3) PPV is used to rule IN disease
      (4) A test with a high PPV is useful if it is positive, but if it is negative, it cannot be used to rule out disease
      (5) **Tests with high specificities (rarely false positive) tend to have high PPVs**
   b. Negative Predictive Value (NPV)
      (1) NPV = the probability that a person does not have disease when the test says he does not have disease
      (2) NPV = (true negatives/false negatives + true negatives) = d/(c + d)
      (3) NPV is used to rule OUT disease
      (4) A test with a high NPV is useful if it is negative, but if it is positive, it cannot be used to rule in disease
      (5) **Tests with high sensitivities (rarely false negative) tend to have high NPVs**
   c. Effect of pre-test probability on post-test probability
      (1) As pre-test probability of disease increases, PPV increases and NPV decreases for the same test with the same sensitivity and specificity
      (2) As pre-test probability of disease decreases, PPV decreases and NPV increases for the same test with the same sensitivity and specificity
      (3) **Because PPV and NPV vary dramatically by pre-test probability, the PPV and NPV published in one study cannot be extrapolated to your patients unless the pre-test probability is the same both in the study and in your patient**
C. Likelihood Ratios (LRs)
   1. **LRs are calculated strictly based upon sensitivity and specificity; they do not take into account pre-test probability of disease and therefore are more portable between studies than are predictive values**
   2. $\oplus$LR = sensitivity/(1 − specificity)
   3. −LR = specificity/(1 − sensitivity)

4. Use ⊕LR when a test is positive, and use –LR when a test is negative
5. How to use LRs to calculate post-test probabilities of disease
   a. Step 1 = estimate the pre-test probability of disease
   b. Step 2 = convert the pre-test probability of disease from a percentage to a ratio called the pre-test odds
      (1) Examples
          (a) If pre-test prob = 10%, pre-test odds = 1:9
          (b) If pre-test prob = 25%, pre-test odds = 1:3
          (c) If pre-test prob = 50%, pre-test odds = 1:1
          (d) If pre-test prob = 75%, pre-test odds = 3:1
          (e) If pre-test prob = 90%, pre-test odds = 9:1
   c. Step 3 = multiply the pre-test odds by the LR
      (1) If the test you have used on the patient is positive, you multiply the first number in the pre-test odds ratio by the ⊕LR: assume ⊕LR = 5 and odds ratio is 1:9 → (5 × 1) :9 = 5:9
      (2) If the test you have used on the patient is negative, you multiply the second number in the pre-test odds ratio by the –LR: assume –LR = 5 and ratio is 1:9 → 1:(9 × 5) = 1:45
   d. Step 4 = Once you have calculated your post-test odds, convert it back into a percentage: this is now your post-test probability of disease
      (1) Post-test probability = numerator/(numerator + denominator)
      (2) Example: assume post-test odds are 6:3, post-test probability = 6/(6 + 3) = 6/9 = 67%
   e. Overall example
      (1) Assume a test has a sensitivity of 80% and a specificity of 90%
      (2) You estimate your patient's pre-test probability of disease to be only 10%
      (3) If you run the test on the patient and it comes back positive, the post-test probability of disease is as follows:
          (a) Pre-test odds = 1:9
          (b) ⊕LR of test = 0.8/(1 − 0.9) = 0.8/0.1 = 8
          (c) Post-test odds = 8 × (1:9) = 8:9
          (d) Post-test probability = 8/(8 + 9) = 8/17 = 47%

(4) If you run the test on the patient and it comes back negative, the post-test probability of disease is as follows:
   (a) Pre-test odds = 1:9 (same odds since same pre-test probability)
   (b) −LR of test = 0.9/(1 − 0.8) = 0.9/0.2 = 4.5
   (c) Post-test odds = (1:9) × 4.5 = 1:40.5
   (d) Post-test probability = 1/(1 + 40.5) = 1/41.5 = 2.4%

6. What is a good LR?
   a. As a general rule of thumb, LRs of 1–4 indicate the test will not be very useful at changing pre-test probabilities, and, therefore, these tests are not very good
   b. LRs of 5–10 indicate a good test, which will significantly change your pre-test probability of disease
   c. LRs of >10 are very good

D. Tips on Using Two-by-Two Tables

Always fill the table in assuming 100 pts—it is easier to do the math this way. The prevalence of the disease (50%) tells you that 50 pts should be in the first column because 50% of 100 pts have the disease. Therefore, 50 pts should also be in the second column (if 50 of 100 pts have the disease, 50 pts also do NOT have the disease). The sensitivity tells you that 45 of the pts in the first column should be in the top row because the test will find 90% of the 50 pts who have the disease. The specificity tells you that 40 of the pts in the second column should be in the bottom row because the test will correctly describe 80% of the 50 people who truly do not have the disease (and incorrectly claim that 20% of the 50 pts who truly do not have the disease do have the disease).

Now the disease prevalence tells you that 10 pts should be in the first column (10% of 100 pts have the disease). Therefore, 90 pts should be in the second column (if 10 of 100 pts have the disease, 90 pts do NOT have the disease). The sensitivity tells you that 9 of the pts in the first column should be in the top row because the test will find 90% of the 10 pts who have the disease. The specificity tells you that 72 of the pts in the second column should be in the bottom row because the test will correctly describe 80% of the 90 people who truly do not have the disease (and incorrectly claim that 20% of the 90 pts who do not have the disease do have the disease).

Example 1	For Disease X, a theoretical screening test is **90% sensitive and 80% specific**. In Africa where the disease has a **prevalence of 50%**, the test's **PPV** = 82% (a/[a + b] = 45/55) and the **NPV is 89%** (d/[c + d] = 40/45).

	Pt has Dz	Pt does not have Dz
Positive test	45	10
Negative test	5	40

Example 2	Now study the **same test for the same disease (X)** in America where the **prevalence of the disease is 10%**. The test characteristics remain the same: **90% sensitive and 80% specific**. The test's **PPV = 33%** (a/[a + b] = 9/27) and the **NPV = 99%** (d/[c + d] = 72/73). **The same test has drastically different predictive values depending on the disease prevalence!!!**

	Pt has Dz	Pt does not have Dz
Positive test	9	18
Negative test	1	72

III. Law and Ethics (Table 12.3)

A. Legal and Ethical Issues

1. Malpractice
   a. A civil wrongdoing (tort), not a crime
   b. Must satisfy the four "Ds"
      (1) Dereliction: deviation from the applicable standard of care
      (2) Duty: a physician–pt relationship was established with a duty to treat
      (3) Damages: injury or measurable damages occur
      (4) Directly: injury or damages directly result from physicians actions or inactions
   c. May be required to pay compensatory damages (money) for pt's suffering
   d. Studies have shown physicians with poor communication skills and interactions with pts are most likely to be sued for malpractice

2. Informed Consent
   a. Must be obtained from pt by a physician knowledgeable in the Dx and Tx in question before any procedure

Table 12.3 Ethical/Legal Terms

Abandonment = Termination of the physician–pt relationship by the physician without reasonable notice to the pt and without the opportunity to make arrangements for appropriate continuation and follow-up care

Assault = Intentional and unauthorized act of placing another in apprehension of immediate bodily harm

Battery = Intentional and unauthorized touching of a person, directly or indirectly, without consent. A surgical procedure performed upon a person without expressed or implied consent can constitute battery unless it is done to save life in an emergency situation and consent is therefore implied

Causation = The causal connection between the act or omission of the defendant and the injury suffered by the plaintiff. The plaintiff must show causation of an injury by the defendant in order to prove negligence

Common Good = (1) respect for persons; (2) social welfare; and (3) peace and security. All three of these elements dictate the common good of healthcare provision

Comparative Negligence = The principle adopted by most states that reduces a plaintiff's recovery proportional to the plaintiff's degree of fault in causing the damage

Consent = Voluntary act by which one person agrees to allow another person to do something. "Expressed consent" is directly and unequivocally given, either orally or in writing. "Implied consent" is shown by signs, actions, facts, or by inaction and silence, which raise a presumption that consent has been given. It may be implied from conduct (implied-in-fact), e.g., when someone rolls up his or her sleeve and extends his or her arm for vein puncture, or by the circumstance (implied-in-law), e.g., an unconscious person in an emergency situation

Damages = Money received through judicial order by a plaintiff sustaining harm, impairment, or loss to his or her person or property as the result of the accidental, intentional, or negligent act of another

Disproportionate Means = Any Tx that, in the given circumstances, either offers no reasonable hope of benefit (taking into account the well-being of the whole person) or is too burdensome for the pt or others, i.e., the burdens or risks are disproportionate or outweigh the expected benefits of the Tx

Deposition = Sworn, officially transcribed out-of-court testimony of a witness or party taken before a trial

Due Care = The degree of care that a prudent and competent person engaged in the same profession would exercise under similar circumstances. A test for liability for negligence. Also called reasonable care

Duty = An obligation recognized by the law. When the pt–physician relationship exists, the pt has a right to be attended and treated by the physician according to the required standard of care and the physician has a correlative duty to provide such care

Table 12.3 *Continued*

Fiduciary = Person in a position of confidence or trust who undertakes a duty to act for the benefit of another under a given set of circumstances

Futility = Efforts to achieve a result that is unreasonable or impossible. Covers Tx that: (1) will not serve any useful purpose; (2) causes needless pain and suffering; and (3) does not achieve the goal of restoring the pt to an acceptable quality of life

Good Samaritan Law = A statute, some form of which has been enacted in all 50 states and the District of Columbia, which exempts from liability a person, such as a physician passer-by, who voluntarily renders aid to an injured person but who negligently, but not unreasonably negligently, causes injury while rendering the aid

Human Dignity = Intrinsic worth that is inherent in every human being

Informed Consent = Requires a physician to obtain a pt's voluntary agreement to accept Tx based upon the pt's awareness of the nature of his or her dz, the material risks and benefits of the proposed Tx, the alternative Tx and risks, or the choice of no Tx at all

Privilege = Physician–pt privilege is the right to exclude from evidence in a legal proceeding any confidential communication that a pt makes to a physician for the purpose of Dx or Tx, unless the pt consents to the disclosure

Settlement = Agreement usually involving an exchange of money for a release of the right to sue made between opposing parties in a lawsuit which resolves their legal dispute

Wrongful death = Lawsuit brought on behalf of a deceased person's survivors that alleges that death was attributable to the willful or negligent act of another

b. Pts must be presented with their Dx, potential Tx, and the risks and benefits of each Tx

c. A competent adult or emancipated minor must then voluntarily consent or not consent to the Tx prior to starting

d. Considered *Battery* or *Negligence* if not obtained

e. Emergency waiver of consent

   (1) **There is no such thing as a 2-physician consent from a legal standpoint**

   (2) In an emergency, if pt is unable to consent, the physician must document justification for why the procedures must be performed as an emergency exception to informed consent

f. Ethics committee involvement may be required in the cases in which patient's wishes are unknown or caregiver or family members are unable to agree on plan of care.

3. Confidentiality
   a. Fosters trust in doctor–pt relationship and respects pt's privacy
   b. Can be overridden if there is a potential harm to a third party and there is no less invasive way for warning or protecting those at risk
4. *Primum Non Nocer,* Nonmaleficence
   a. "Above all, do no harm"
   b. A balance must exist in the care of pts, and risks and benefits of all interventions must be considered
   c. If a physician cannot act to benefit the pt, then at least do no harm
5. Beneficence
   a. Fiduciary relationship exists between the doctor and pt
   b. Physicians are trusted to act on behalf of the well-being of their pts
6. Death
   a. With the advent of cardiopulmonary life support systems, the definition of death is no longer simply a cessation of breathing or circulation
   b. Death is now also defined as complete irreversible loss of entire brain function to include cortical and brain stem function
   c. Pts must be "warm and dead" to be considered dead, there are many stories of people revived from freezing cold temperatures who were thought to be dead
   d. Persistent Vegetative State (PVS): have brain stem function but no cortical function
   e. Organ donation wishes of patient and family should be discussed
7. Advance Directives
   a. Allows competent pts to indicate their health-related preferences or a surrogate decision-maker prior to becoming incapacitated
   b. Living Will: Written instructions related to health-related preferences in the event the pt becomes incapacitated and is unable to communicate his or her wishes otherwise
   c. Durable Power of Attorney: A surrogate is designated to make health care decisions on behalf of the incapacitated pt
   d. Various states have limitations on Advance Directives; an attorney should be consulted if there are any questions regarding your particular state

8. Do Not Resuscitate (DNR) Orders
   a. Initiated by the attending staff physician after receiving informed consent from appropriate health care decision-maker
   b. Cardiopulmonary Resuscitation (CPR) is withheld
   c. Limited DNR orders may also be seen such as Do not Intubate (DNI) and chest compressions only
   d. These should all be clearly visible to all staff so that pt's requests can be followed in an emergency

IV. Doctoring

A. Introduction

1. Pt–Doctor (physician) relationship is based on trust, confidence, mutual understanding, and communication
2. Pt interviews and interactions must be conducted in a humanistic, culturally sensitive manner
3. In cooperation with other health care professionals, such as interpreters, an appreciation for racial and cultural diversity must always be conveyed
4. Nonbiased health care delivery to the pt and their family must be conveyed at all times
5. Tx plans must be realistic, mutually understood, and mutually agreed upon to achieve compliance

B. Interview

1. Introduce self to pt; assure an interpreter is present if a foreign language is spoken
2. Face pt, and always speak to pt and their family directly and not to the interpreter
3. Try not to interrupt pt when speaking
4. Interviewing techniques (Table 12.4)
5. Pt history: chief complaint, history of present illness (HPI), past medical history (PMH), past surgical history (PSH), family history (FH), social history (SH), and allergies
6. Helpful Interviewing Mnemonic (**HEADSSS**)
   a. Originally developed to interview adolescents but can be used for all ages as a way to break the ice of an initial interview and to cover major areas
   b. **HEADSSS** assessment allows physicians to evaluate critical areas in each pt's life that may be detrimental to their health
      (1) **H**ome environment: Who does pt live with? Any recent changes? Quality of family interaction (if applicable)?

Table 12.4 Interviewing Techniques

Technique	Description	Example
Empathy	Communicating an understanding of pt's feelings	"I can tell you must really be upset about this situation."
Paraphrasing	Communicates an understanding of content	"So, you have been waiting 3 hrs for your appointment."
Silence	A pause in a conversation is worth a thousand words. Doctor and pt can use this time to watch each other's nonverbal posturing and to take an inventory of how interview is going	"........................"
Open-ended questions	Allows pt and family to express themselves fully regarding the topic in question	"Why have you come to the hospital today?"
Questions for the doctor	Allows pt to express their concerns and to assure themselves of what has been discussed during the interview and what still has not been addressed	"Do you have any questions for me?"
Direct questioning	Allows the interviewer to focus on an important topic	"Now, tell me more about how you got that bruise on your arm."
Identifying/validation	Allows pt's concerns to appear acceptable and worth discussing	"I am also afraid of doctors and hospitals; please tell me more about why you are here."

(2) **H**ealth risks: Exposure to TB, Hepatitis, asbestos, ciga-rette smoke, radiation

(3) **E**mployment and **E**ducation: Is pt in school? Favorite subjects? Academic performance? Are friends in school? Any recent changes? Does pt have a job? Future plans?

(4) **A**ctivities: What does pt like to do in spare time? Who does pt spend time with? Involved in any sports/exercise? Hobbies? Attends parties or clubs?

(5) **D**rugs: Has pt ever used tobacco? Alcohol? Marijuana? Other illicit drugs? If so, when was the last use? How often? Do friends or family members use drugs? Who does the pt use these substances with?

    (6) **S**exual activity: Sexual orientation? Is pt sexually active? Number of sexual partners? Does the pt use condoms or other forms of contraception? Any history of STDs or pregnancy?

    (7) **S**uicide: Does the pt ever feel sad, tired, or unmotivated? Has the pt ever felt that life was not worth living? Any feelings of wanting to harm self? If so, does the pt have a plan? Has the pt ever tried to harm self in the past? Does the pt know anyone who has attempted suicide?

    (8) **S**afety: Does the pt use a seat belt or bike helmet? Does the pt enter into high-risk situations? Does the pt have access to a firearm? Is the pt's home environment safe?

C. Identifying Abuse

1. Not necessarily physical in nature, can be physical assault, sexual assault, psychological abuse, economic control, and/or progressive social isolation

2. Depending on state laws, certain potential abuse situations mandate reporting—failure to report subjects practitioner to disciplinary action, fines, and/or liability

3. Department of Social Services should be made aware of suspected child abuse and elder abuse cases

4. Cameras and rape kits should be made available in all emergency departments to property handle potential evidence

5. Must know and understand cultural demographics of community served. Certain cultural medicine rituals may be misinterpreted by health practitioners:

    a. Cupping: Cupping, pinching, or rubbing (also known as coining). Thought to restore balance by releasing excessive "air"

        (1) Small cups are used, i.e., small shot glasses. A small amount of alcohol is put into the cup and ignited, and the cup is immediately pressed tight against the skin (forehead, abdomen, chest, or back). A vacuum is produced by the combustion of the alcohol and the evacuation of oxygen from the cup. The developing vacuum then sucks out noxious materials or excess energy into the cup from the body. A circular ecchymotic area is left on the skin

        (2) Pinching: Pressure is applied by pinching the skin between the thumb and index finger to the point of producing a contusion. Done at the base of the nose, between the eyes, on the neck, chest, or back

(3) Rubbing is usually in the same areas as pinching and involves firmly rubbing lubricated skin with a spoon or a coin in order to bring toxic "air" to the body surface

b. Female genital mutilation carried out today in more than 30 countries across Africa and the Middle East

D. **Cultural Medicine**

1. Hot and Cold Theory: Seen in Latin American cultures; illness is caused by an imbalance of hot and cold. Eating appropriately hot or cold type foods as needed can restore balance

2. Prominent among Mexican-American folk healers is the curandero, a type of shaman who uses white magic and herbs to effect cures

E. **Interpreter**

1. In order to provide best available pt services, all efforts should be made to facilitate communications with pt in their language, using an interpreter whenever possible

2. Physician must always face pt and speak directly to pt while discussion is translated

3. Have pt repeat instructions to you through interpreter to assure understanding

4. Whenever possible use a trained interpreter, and avoid using family members to prevent embarrassment and miscommunication of discussion

V. Health Care Delivery

A. **Hospitals**

1. Tertiary Medical Center: Receives referrals from community, has latest technologies, including organ transplantation, Level 1 trauma, etc. Most academic medical centers

2. Intermediate Hospital: No organ transplantation, much of the same technology as a major medical center

3. Community Hospital: Provides basic services, lacks major staffing and technology of larger medical centers

B. **Health Maintenance Organizations (HMOs)**

1. Provide health care to people who have prepaid enrollment

2. Various Models Exist: Staff Model, Preferred Provider Organization (PPO), and Independent Practice Association (IPA)

a. Staff Model: Physicians are salaried employees or contracted to provide medical services to members. All pts must be seen by a primary care physician prior to referral to most specialists

b. PPOs: Occurs when an insurance company has established contracts with certain independent providers, allowing pts to choose physicians not normally on their list of providers for a surcharge

c. IPAs: Physicians paid on an agreed-upon fee-for-service whenever a member of the HMO uses their services

3. Capitation: Physicians are paid a certain amount per pt, per year, regardless of the amount of services provided to each of the pts assigned

C. **Extended Care Facilities**

1. Nursing Homes/Skilled Nursing Facilities (SNFs)

   a. Provide IV fluids, nutrition, and medications

   b. Nursing staff available 24 hr

2. Intermediate Care Facilities (ICF)

   a. Provide assistance mainly with activities of daily living

   b. Nursing not necessarily available 24 hr

D. **Hospice**

1. Specializes in providing terminal care to pts in their final moments of life

E. **Medicare/Medicaid**

1. Medicare: Authorized under the Social Security Act

   a. Provides health insurance to people >65 yrs old or who are disabled and receive social security, does not cover prescription medications

2. Medicaid: Also authorized under the Social Security Act

   a. Unlike Medicare, it is provided to the very poor who usually receive other types of public assistance—qualifications vary by state, does cover prescription medications

F. **Accountable Care Organizations (ACOs)**

1. New type of health care organization created under the Patient Protection and Affordable Care Act

2. An ACO is comprised of a group of coordinated healthcare providers in which payments are linked to quality of care delivered

3. As per the Center for Medicare and Medicaid Services, an ACO is "an organization of health care providers that agrees to be accountable for the quality, cost, and overall care of Medicare beneficiaries who are enrolled in the traditional fee-for-service program who are assigned to it"

G. **Hospital Personnel**

1. Nurses: Many levels of training
   a. Nurse's Aid: Basic medical vocational training
   b. Licensed Practical Nurse/Licensed Vocational Nurse (LPN/LVN): undergo a 1-yr program of nursing vocational training followed by a state licensing exam
   c. Registered Nurse: May have a Bachelors degree or Associates degree, have passed state nursing board exams and have a registered state license
   d. Clinical Nurse Specialist: Usually Masters degree prepared nurse, has advanced training in a specific medical area, i.e., intensive care, cardiac care, enterostomal care, etc.
   e. Nurse Practitioner: Usually Masters degree prepared nurse, practice as a family nurse practitioner, pediatric nurse practitioner, nursing midwife
   f. Doctoral Nurses: Hold Doctorate degree in various areas, mainly work in academic nursing schools as professors and researchers

2. Physician Assistant: Usually Bachelors degree level of education; many states now are requiring a Masters Degree and a state licensing exam. Function as independent practitioners under the supervision of a physician

H. Hospital Safety

1. In an attempt to decrease hospital readmission and improve patient safety, the Patient Safety and Quality improvement Act of 2005 was enacted.

2. Patient Safety Act requires hospitals to track the following:
   a. Incidents—patient safety events that reached the patient, whether or not there was harm
   b. Near misses or close calls—patient safety events that did not reach the patient

3. Joint Commission on Accreditation of Healthcare Organizations (JCAHO) requires reporting of the following:
   a. Sentinel Events are defined as any unanticipated event in a healthcare setting resulting in death, physical or psychological injury to a patient, not related to the natural course of the patient's illness.
   b. Root Cause Analysis must be preformed to identify the root causes of problem or events and to prevent future similar events from occurring

APPENDIX

A. ZEBRAS AND SYNDROMES

Dz	Description/Sx
Achondroplasia	Autosomal dominant dwarfism due to early epiphyseal closure → shortening and thickening of bones
	Si/Sx = leg bowing, hearing loss, sciatica, infantile hydrocephalus. Pts can have nml lifespan
Adie syndrome	Adie syndrome is a neurological disorder affecting the pupil of the eye and the <u>autonomic nervous system</u>. It is characterized by one eye with a pupil that is larger than normal and constricts slowly in bright light (tonic pupil), along with the absence of deep tendon reflexes, usually in the <u>Achilles tendon</u>. Adie syndrome may be the result of a viral or bacterial infection that causes inflammation and damage to neurons in the *ciliary ganglion*, an area of the brain that controls eye movements, and the *spinal ganglion*, an area of the brain involved in the response of the autonomic nervous system. Most cases of Adie syndrome are not progressive, life threatening, or disabling.
Adrenoleukodystrophy	X-linked recessive defect in long-chain fatty acid metabolism due to a peroxisomal enzyme deficiency. Causes rapidly progressing central demyelination, adrenal insufficiency, hyperpigmentation of skin, spasticity, seizures, death by age 12
Albers-Schönberg dz (osteopetrosis)	↑↑ Skeletal density because of osteoclastic failure → multiple fractures due to ↓ perfusion of thick bone, also causes anemia due to ↓ marrow space blindness, deafness, and cranial nerve dysfunction because of narrowing, impingement of neural foramina
Alkaptonuria	Defect of phenylalanine metabolism causing accumulation of homogentisic acid. Presents with black urine, ochronosis (blue-black pigmentation of ear, nose, cheeks), arthropathy due to cartilage-binding homogentisic acid
Alport's syndrome	X-linked hereditary collagen defect causing sensorineural hearing loss, lens dislocation, hematuria (glomerulonephritis)
Argyria	Dermal deposits of silver bound to albumin. Related to prolonged exposure or ingestion of silver-containing products. Dx = slate-gray skin color, including mucosa and sclera. Tx = psychosocial support, discoloration is irreversible (see Figure A.1)

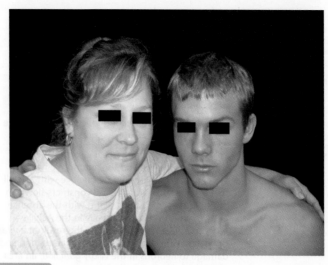

FIGURE A.1   Argyria.

Note the slate-gray skin discoloration of the young man on the **right**, in contrast to the nml skin color of the woman on the **left**. (Courtesy of Scott C. Wickless, Tor Shwayder, Davide Iacobelli, and Susan Smolinske. From Greenberg MI, Hendrickson RG, Silverberg M, et al. *Greenberg's text-atlas of emergency medicine*. Philadelphia, PA: Lippincott Williams & Wilkins, 2004, with permission.)

Dz	Description/Sx
Ataxia-telangiectasia	DNA repair defect affects B and T lymphocytes. Autosomal recessive dz usually appears by age 2. Physical signs include ataxia of gait, telangiectasias of skin and conjunctiva, recurrent sinus infxns
Banti's syndrome	"Idiopathic portal HTN." Splenomegaly and portal HTN following subclinical portal vein occlusion. Insidious onset, occurring yrs after initial occlusive event
Bartter's syndrome	Kidney dz that causes Na, K, and Cl wasting. Despite ↑ levels of renin, BP remains low
Beckwith–Wiedemann syndrome	Autosomal dominant fetal overgrowth syndrome of macrosomia, microcephaly, macroglossia, organomegaly, omphalocele, distinctive lateral earlobe fissures, hypoglycemia associated with hyperinsulinemia, ↑ incidence of Wilms' tumor
Bernard–Soulier syndrome	Autosomal recessive defect of platelet GPIb receptor (binds to von Willebrand factor), presents with chronic, severe mucosal bleeds and giant platelets on blood smear

Binswanger's dz	Subacute subcortical dementia caused by small artery infarcts in periventricular white matter. Usually seen in long-standing HTN but is rare
Brugada syndrome	Brugada syndrome causes a disruption of the heart's normal rhythm. Signs and symptoms usually develop in adulthood and include ventricular arrhythmia that can cause fainting, seizures, difficulty breathing, or sudden death. These complications typically occur when an affected person is resting or asleep. The underlying cause of Brugada syndrome can not always be identified. In some cases it is due to mutations in the _SCN5A_ gene. Other cases are not genetic (are not due to a gene mutation), but acquired due to adverse reactions to drugs or associated with very low or high levels of potassium, or high levels of calcium.
Bruton's agammaglobulinemia	X-linked block of B-cell maturation, causing ↓ B-cell levels and immunoglobulin G (IgG) levels. Presents with recurrent bacterial infxns in infants aged >6 mos
CADASIL (Cerebral Autosomal Dominant Arteriopathy with Sub-cortical Infarcts and Leukoencephalopathy)	CADASIL (Cerebral Autosomal Dominant Arteriopathy with Sub-cortical Infarcts and Leukoencephalopathy) is an inherited disease of the blood vessels that occurs when the thickening of blood vessel walls blocks the flow of blood to the brain. The disease primarily affects the small blood vessels in the white matter of the brain. CADASIL is characterized by migraine headaches and multiple strokes, which progresses to dementia. Other symptoms include white matter lesions throughout the brain, cognitive deterioration, seizures, vision problems, and psychiatric problems such as severe depression and changes in behavior and personality. Individuals may also be at higher risk of heart attack. Symptoms and disease onset vary widely, with signs typically appearing in the mid-30s. Some individuals may not show signs of the disease until later in life. CADASIL is caused by a change (or mutation) in a gene called _NOTCH3_ and is inherited in an autosomal dominant manner.
Caisson's dz	Decompression sickness ("the bends") caused by rapid ascent from deep-sea diving. Sx occur from 30 min–1 hr = joint pain, cough, skin burning/mottling
Caroli's dz	Segmental cystic dilation of intrahepatic bile ducts complicated by stones and cholangitis, can be CA precursor

Dz	Description/Sx
Charcot–Marie–Tooth dz	Autosomal dominant peroneal muscular atrophy causing foot drop and stocking-glove ↓ in vibration/pain/temperature sense and deep tendon reflex (DTR) in lower extremities. Histologically → repeated demyelination and remyelination of segmental areas of the nerve. Pts may present as children (Type 1) or adults (Type 2)
Chédiask-Higashi syndrome	Autosomal recessive defect of microtubule function of neutrophils, leads to ↓ lysosomal fusion to phagosomes. Presents with recurrent *Staphylococcus* and *Streptococcus* infxns, albinism, peripheral and cranial neuropathies
Cheyne–Stokes respirations	Central apnea seen in congestive heart failure, ↑ intracranial pressure, or cerebral infxn/inflammation/trauma: cycles of central apnea followed by regular crescendo-decrescendo breathing (amplitude first waxes and then wanes back to apnea); Biot's is an uncommon variant seen in meningitis in which the cycles consist of central apnea followed by stead amplitude breathing that then shuts back off to apnea
Chronic granulomatous Dz (CGD)	Phagocytes lack respiratory burst or NADPH oxidase, so can engulf bacteria but are unable to kill them. Presents with recurrent infxns with *Aspergillus* and *Staphylococcus aureus* infxns. Tx = recombinant interferon-g
Cystinuria	Autosomal recessive failure of tubular resorption of cystine and dibasic amino acids (lysine, ornithine, arginine), clinically see cystine stones. Tx = hydration to ↑ urine volume, alkalinization of urine with bicarbonate and acetazolamide
Danon disease	Danon disease is a type of lysosomal storage disorder. Lysosomes are compartments within the cell that use enzymes to break down large molecules into smaller ones that the cell can use. In Danon disease there is a defect in the wall (membrane) of the lysosome. The defect is caused by mutations in the *LAMP2* gene. Danon disease is chiefly characterized by <u>cardiomyopathy</u> (heart disease), although other signs and symptoms may occur as well. Danon disease is inherited in an <u>X-linked fashion</u>, as a result males tend to be more severely affected than females. Females who carry the <u>*LAMP2*</u> gene mutation may or may not develop signs and symptoms.

de Quervain's tenosynovitis	Tenosynovitis causing pain on flexion of thumb (motion of abductor pollicis longus)
Diamond–Blackfan syndrome	"Pure red cell aplasia," a congenital or acquired deficiency in the RBC stem cell. Congenital disorder is sometimes associated with abnormal facies, cardiac, and renal abnormalities. Tx = steroids
DiGeorge's syndrome	Embryologic defect in development of pharyngeal pouches 3 and 4 → thymic aplasia that causes T-cell deficiency and parathyroid aplasia. Most commonly presents with tetany due to hypocalcemia 2° to hypoparathyroidism and recurrent severe viral, fungal, or protozoal infxns
Dressler's syndrome	Acute pericarditis, develops within 2–4 wks after acute MI or heart surgery, may be due to autoimmune reaction to myocardial antigens
Eagle syndrome	Eagle syndrome is a collection of symptoms that includes recurrent throat and ear pain, foreign body sensation (or the feeling that something is stuck in one's throat), dysphagia (difficulty swallowing), and/or facial pain. This condition is a direct result of an elongated styloid process of the temporal bone or calcified stylohyoid ligament. The actual cause of the elongation is a poorly understood process. Diagnosis is made both radiographically and by physical examination. Treatment of Eagle syndrome is both surgical and nonsurgical.
Ehlers–Danlos syndrome	Autosomal dominant defect in collagen synthesis, variable expressivity. Si/Sx = loose joints, pathognomonic ↑ skin elasticity, mitral regurgitation, genu recurvatum of knee (fixed in hyperextension), aortic dilation
Ehlers–Danlos syndrome vascular type	Ehlers–Danlos syndrome vascular type is a connective tissue disease. Symptoms include thin, translucent skin, easy bruising, characteristic facial appearance, and fragile arteries, intestine, and/or uterus. It is inherited in an autosomal dominant manner and is caused by mutations in the COL3A1 gene. (see Figure A.2)
Ellis–van Creveld	Syndrome of polydactyly + single atrium
Erb's paralysis	Waiter's tip—upper-brachial plexopathy (C5–6)
Evan's syndrome	IgG autoantibody-mediated hemolytic anemia and thrombocytopenia, associated with collagen-vascular dz, thrombotic thrombocytopenic purpura, hepatic cirrhosis, leukemia, sarcoidosis, Hashimoto's thyroiditis. Tx = prednisone and IVIG

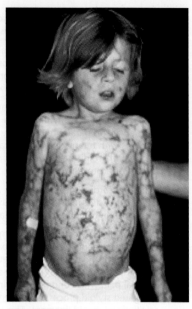

FIGURE A.2
Ehlers–Danlos syndrome vascular type.

Dz	Description/Sx
Fabry's dz	X-linked defect in galactosidase, Sx = lower-trunk skin lesions, corneal opacity, renal/cardiac/cerebral dz that are invariably lethal in infancy or childhood
Fanconi's anemia	Autosomal recessive disorder of DNA repair. Presents with pancytopenia, ↑ risk of malignancy, short stature, birdlike facies, café-au-lait spots, congenital urogenital defects, retardation, absent thumb
Fanconi syndrome	Dysfunction of proximal renal tubules, congenital or acquired (drugs, multiple myeloma, toxic metals), presenting with ↓ reabsorption of glucose, amino acids, phosphate, and bicarbonate. Associated with renal tubular acidosis Type II, clinically see glycosuria, hyperphosphaturia, hypophosphatemia (Vitamin D-resistant rickets), aminoaciduria (generalized, not cystine specific), systemic acidosis, polyuria, polydipsia
Farber's dz	Auto-recessive defect in ceramidase, causing ceramide accumulation in nerves, onset within the month of birth, death occurs by age 2

Felty's syndrome	Rheumatoid arthritis plus splenomegaly and neutropenia, often with thrombocytopenia
Fibrolamellar CA	Variant of hepatocellular CA. Occurs in young people (20–40 yrs), is not associated with viral hepatitis or cirrhosis. Has a good Px. Histologically shows nests and cords of malignant hepatocytes separated by dense collagen bundles
Fitz-Hugh–Curtis syndrome	Chlamydia or gonorrhea perihepatitis as a complication of pelvic inflammatory dz. Presents with right upper quadrant pain and sepsis
Galactosemia	Deficient galactose-1-phosphate uridyltransferase blocks galactose conversion to glucose for further metabolism, leading to accumulation of galactose in many tissues. Sx = failure to thrive, infantile cataracts, mental retardation, cirrhosis. Rarely due to galactokinase deficiency, blocking the same path at a different step
Gardner's syndrome	Familial polyposis syndrome with classic triad of desmoid tumors, osteomas of mandible or skull and sebaceous cysts
Gaucher's dz	Most frequent cause of lysosomal enzyme deficiency in Ashkenazi Jews. Autosomal recessive deficiency in β-glucocerebrosidase. Accumulation of sphingolipids in liver, spleen, and bone marrow. Can be fatal if very expensive enzyme substitute (alglucerase) not administered
Glanzmann's thrombasthenia	Autosomal recessive defect in GPIIb-IIIa platelet receptor that binds fibrinogen, inhibiting platelet aggregation, presents with chronic, severe mucosal bleeds
Glycogenoses	Genetic defects in metabolic enzymes causing glycogen accumulation. Si/Sx = hepatosplenomegaly, general organomegaly, exertional fatigue, hypoglycemia. Type I = von Gierke's dz; Type II = Pompe's dz; Type III = Cori's dz; Type V = McArdle's dz
Hartnup's dz	Autosomal recessive defect in tryptophan absorption at renal tubule. Sx mimic pellagra = the 3 Ds: Dermatitis, Dementia, Diarrhea (tryptophan is niacin precursor). Rash is on sun-exposed areas, can see cerebellar ataxia, mental retardation, psychosis. Tx = niacin supplements
Hepatorenal syndrome	Renal failure without intrinsic renal dz, occurring during fulminant hepatitis or cirrhosis, presents with acute oliguria and azotemia, typically progressive and fatal

Dz	Description/Sx
Hepatopulmonary syndrome	Development of intrapulmonary arteriovenous malformations (AVMs) in the setting of cirrhosis that causes pulmonary shunting with severe refractory hypoxia; pts present with platypnea, which is dyspnea when standing that improves with lying down; pathophysiology of AVM formation in the setting of cirrhosis is not understood, and the only Tx is liver transplantation, which may cause regression of AVMs
Holt–Oram syndrome	Autosomal dominant atrial septal defect in association with fingerlike thumb or absent thumb, cardiac conduction abnormalities, other skeletal defects
Homocystinuria	Deficiency in cystine metabolism. Sx mimic Marfan's = lens dislocation (downward in homocystinuria as opposed to upward in Marfan's), thin bones, mental retardation, hypercoagulability, premature atherosclerosis → strokes and MIs
Hunter's dz	X-linked lysosomal iduronidase deficiency, less severe than Hurler's syndrome. Sx = mild mental retardation, cardiac problems, micrognathia, etc.
Hurler's dz	Defect in iduronidase, causing multiorgan mucopolysaccharide accumulation, dwarfism, hepatosplenomegaly, corneal clouding, progressive mental retardation, death by age 10
Incontinentia pigmenti	Rare X-linked, dominant defect of the NEMO gene (Nuclear factor κ B Essential Modulator = IKBKG-IKK γ), resulting in excessive deposits of melanin in the body. Presents with neonatal erythematous skin rash, with spiral lines of small fluid-filled blisters transforming into rough, warty skin growths. Eventually, areas of hyperpigmentation develop which later become atrophied and hypopigmented. Dental problems, alopecia with scarring, and seizures and muscle weakness can occur, and can be associated with a variety of anatomical defects (e.g., dwarfism, club foot, skull deformities). Extremely wooly or kinky hair and severe immune system dysfunction may also appear

IRAK-4 deficiency	IRAK-4 deficiency is a rare inherited <u>primary immunodeficiency</u> that is characterized by severe recurrent <u>pyogenic</u> bacterial infections. Individuals with IRAK-4 deficiency seem to be particularly susceptible to infections caused by bacteria called *Streptococcus pneumoniae*. The deficiency is caused by <u>mutations</u> in a <u>gene</u> called *IRAK4* (interleukin 1 receptor-associated kinase 4).[1] The *IRAK4* gene provides instructions for making an enzyme that is crucial for protective immunity against specific bacterial infections.[2]
Isovalinic acidemia	"Sweaty-foot odor" dz. Caused by a defect in leucine metabolism, leads to buildup of isovaline in the bloodstream, producing characteristic odor
Jervell and Lange-Nielsen syndrome	Jervell and Lange-Nielsen syndrome is a form of <u>long QT syndrome</u>. Symptoms include deafness from birth, <u>arrhythmia</u>, fainting, and sudden death. There are two different types, Jervell and Lange-Nielsen syndrome type 1 and type 2. It is inherited in an <u>autosomal recessive</u> fashion.[1]
Job's syndrome	B-cell defect causing hyper-IgE levels, but defects in other IgG and immune functions. Presents with recurrent pulmonary infxns, dermatitis, excess teeth (pts unable to shed their baby teeth), frequent bone fractures, classic "gargoyle facies," IgE levels 10- to 100-fold higher than nml
Kasabach–Merritt	Expanding hemangioma trapping platelets, leading to systemic thrombocytopenia
Keshan's dz	Childhood cardiomyopathy 2° to selenium deficiency, very common in China
Klippel–Trénaunay–Weber syndrome	Autosomal dominant chromosomal translocation → prematurity, hydrops fetalis, hypertrophic hemangioma of leg, Kasabach–Merritt thrombocytopenia
Klumpke's paralysis	Clawed hand—lower brachial plexopathy (C8, T1) affecting ulnar nerve distributions, often presents with Horner's syndrome as well
Leber's congenital amaurosis (LCA)	Autosomal recessive disorder of photoreceptors appearing at birth or in infancy causing blindness, lack of papillary response, and nystagmus
Leigh's dz	Mitochondrially inherited dz → absent or ↓↓ thiamine pyrophosphate. Infants or children present with seizures, ataxia, optic atrophy, ophthalmoplegia, tremor

Dz	Description/Sx
Lesch–Nyhan syndrome	Congenital defect in Hypoxanthine-Guanine Phosphoribosyl Transferase (HPRT) → gout, urate nephrolithiasis, retardation, choreiform spasticity, self-mutilation (pts bite off their own fingers and lips). Mild deficiency → Kelley–Seegmiller syndrome = gout without nervous system Si/Sx
Leukocyte adhesion deficiency	Type I due to lack of β_2-integrins (LFA-1), Type II due to lack of fucosylated glycoproteins (selectin receptors). Both have plenty of neutrophils in blood but cannot enter tissues due to problems with adhesion and transmigration. Both present with recurrent bacterial infxns, **gingivitis, poor wound healing, delayed umbilical cord separation**
Lhermitte sign	Tingling down the back during neck flexion, occurs in any craniocervical disorder
Liddle's dz	Dz mimics hyperaldosteronism. Defect in the renal epithelial transporters. Si/Sx = HTN, hypokalemic metabolic alkalosis
Li–Fraumeni's syndrome	Autosomal dominant inherited defect of p53 leading to 1° CA of a variety of organ systems presenting at an early age
Maple syrup urine dz	Disorder of branched-chain amino acid metabolism (valine, leucine, isoleucine). Sx include vomiting, and pathognomonic maplelike odor of urine
Marchiafava–Bignami syndrome	Overconsumption of red wine → demyelination of corpus callosum, anterior commissure, middle cerebellar peduncles. Possibly anoxic/ischemic phenomenon
Marfan's dz	Genetic collagen defect → tall, thin body habitus, long and slender digits, pectus excavatum, scoliosis, aortic valve dilation → regurgitation, aortic dissection, mitral valve prolapse, joint laxity, optic lens dislocations, blue sclera. Think about Abe Lincoln when considering this disease: tall and thin
Melanosis coli	Overzealous use of laxatives causing darkening of colon but no significant dz

MELAS and MERRF syndrome	Mitochondrial Encephalopathy and Lactic Acidosis (MELAS) syndrome and Myoclonic Epilepsy associated with Ragged Red Fibers (MERRF) syndrome are genetic, mitochondrial disorders (therefore maternally inherited) in which electron transport is disrupted, usually due to a mutation in the mitochondrial leucine–transfer RNA gene. Presentation and severity is variable, depending on the cellular distribution of defective mitochondria throughout the body. MELAS can involve Type 2 diabetes, seizures, psychosis, stroke, renal failure, heart failure, hearing loss. MERRF Sx include seizures, myopathy with ragged-red fibers on Bx, including ptosis and ophthalmoparesis, cerebellar ataxia, dementia, or deafness. Screen with serum lactate/ pyruvate ratio ($\geq$20:1 suggests Dx), confirm with muscle Bx or genetic test
Mendelson's syndrome	Chemical pneumonitis following aspiration of acidic gastric juice pt presents with acute dyspnea, tachy- pnea, and tachycardia, with pink and frothy sputum
Meralgia paresthetica	Condition common to truckers, hikers, and overweight individuals who wear heavy backpacks or very tight- fitting belts compressing inguinal area. This causes pts to have a diffuse unilateral pain and paresthesias along anterior portion of upper thigh, corresponding to lateral femoral cutaneous nerve. Typically self-limiting but can treat with steroids for refractory dz
Minamata dz	Toxic encephalopathy from mercury poisoning, classically described from fish eaten near Japanese mercury dumping site
Mönckeberg's arteriosclerosis	Calcific sclerosis of the media of medium-size arteries, usually radial and ulnar. Occurs in people >50 yrs, but it does **not** obstruct arterial flow because intima is not involved. Unrelated to other atherosclerosis and does not cause dz
Münchhausen's syndrome	Factitious disorder in which the pt derives gratification from feigning a serious or dramatic illness. In Münchhausen's by proxy, the pt derives gratification from making someone else ill (often a mother injures her child for attention)

Dz	Description/Sx
Nevoid basal cell carcinoma syndrome	Nevoid basal cell carcinoma syndrome is a type of genetic tumor syndrome. Signs and symptoms include an increased risk for certain types of noncancerous and cancerous tumors, skin pits in the palms and soles of the feet, large head size, and bone abnormalities involving the spine, ribs, or skull. Nevoid basal cell carcinoma syndrome is caused by a mutation in the gene _PTCH1_. It is inherited in an <u>autosomal dominant</u> fashion (see Figure A.3).
Niemann–Pick's dz	Autosomal recessive defect in sphingomyelinase with variable age at onset (↑ severe dz in younger pt) → demyelination/neurologic Sx, hepatosplenomegaly, xanthoma, pancytopenia
Noonan's syndrome	Autosomal dominant with Sx similar to Turner's syndrome → hyperelastic skin, neck webbing, ptosis, low-set ears, short stature, pulmonary stenosis, atrial-septal (AS) defect, coarctation of aorta, small testes. Presents in males, X and Y are both present

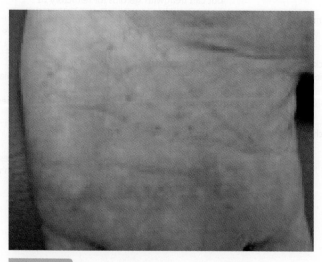

FIGURE A.3

Nevoid basal cell carcinoma syndrome.

Ochoa syndrome	Ochoa syndrome is a congenital (present from birth) disorder characterized by an unusual facial expression and obstructive disease of the urinary tract. When affected infants smile, their facial musculature turns upside down or "inverts" so that they appear to be crying. The urinary abnormality is an obstructive uropathy involving failure of nerve signals between the bladder and the spinal cord resulting in incomplete emptying of the bladder.[1] Other urinary symptoms may include incontinence, urinary tract infections, and hydronephrosis. The syndrome, which has been linked to mutations in the HPSE2 gene on the long arm (q) of chromosome 10 (10q23-q24), is inherited in an autosomal recessive fashion. Treatment, which involves bladder re-education, prophylactic antibiotics, anticholinergic therapy (to decrease bladder hyperactivity), and alpha-blockers, is important in the prevention of upper urinary tract deterioration and renal failure.
Ortner's syndrome	Impingement of recurrent laryngeal nerve by the enlarging atrium in mitral regurgitation, leading to hoarseness
Osteogenesis imperfecta	Genetic disorder of diffuse bone weakness due to mutations resulting in defective collagen synthesis. Multiple fractures 2° to minimal trauma = brittle bone dz. Classic sign = blue sclera due to translucent connective tissue over choroid
Peliosis hepatis	Rare 1° dilation of hepatic sinusoids. Associated with exposure to anabolic steroids, oral contraceptives, danazol. Irregular cystic spaces filled with blood develop in the liver. Cessation of drug intake causes reversal of the lesions
Plummer–Vinson syndrome	Iron-deficiency syndrome with classic triad of esophageal web, spoon nail, and iron-deficiency anemia. Webs produce dysphagia, will regress with iron replacement
Polycystic kidney dz	Autosomal dominant bilateral dz; Si/Sx = onset in early or middle adult life with hematuria, nephrolithiasis, uremia, 33% of cases have cysts in liver, 10%–20% of pts have intracranial aneurysms, HTN is present in 70% of pts at Dx. Juvenile version is autosomal recessive, much rarer than adult type; almost all pts have cysts in liver and portal bile duct proliferation = "congenital hepatic fibrosis"

Dz	Description/Sx
Poncet's dz	Polyarthritis that occurs during active TB infxn but in which no organisms can be isolated from the affected joints; is thought to be autoimmune-mediated dz
Pott's dz	Tubercular infxn of vertebrae (vertebral osteomyelitis) leading to kyphoscoliosis 2° to pathologic fractures
Potter's syndrome	Bilateral renal agenesis; incompatible with fetal life, mother has oligohydramnios because fetus normally swallows large quantities of amniotic fluid and then urinates it out, but fetus cannot excrete swallowed fluid because it has no kidneys
Reed syndrome	Reed syndrome, also called multiple cutaneous and uterine leiomyomatosis (MCUL or MCUL1), is a genetic condition in which people develop benign (noncancerous) tumors containing smooth muscle tissue (leiomyomas) in the skin and, if female, also in the uterus. In some families, aggressive kidney cancer also occurs as part of the complex and is termed as hereditary leiomyomatosis and renal cell cancer (HLRRC). The complex is often referred to as MCUL/HLRRC (multiple cutaneous and uterine leiomyomatosis/hereditary leiomyomatosis and renal cell cancer) in the medical literature. The cause of both MCUL and HLRCC is a gene called fumarate hydratase (FH), an enzyme involved in the making of energy for the body. MCUL is inherited in an autosomal dominant pattern, which means that a person needs to inherit only one mutated copy of the FH gene to have symptoms of the condition. The symptoms vary from person to person, even within a family. Treatment is based on the person's specific symptoms.
Reflex sympathetic dystrophy (RSD) syndrome	Also known as complex regional pain syndrome (CRPS), a chronic neurologic syndrome characterized by severe burning pain, pathologic changes in bone and skin, excessive sweating, tissue swelling, extreme sensitivity to touch, usually 2° to an initiating noxious event or immobilization
Refsum's dz	Autosomal recessive defect in phytanic acid metabolism → peripheral neuropathy, cerebellar ataxia, retinitis pigmentosa, bone dz, ichthyosis (scaly skin)

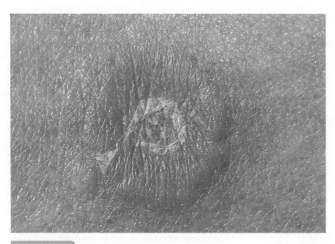

FIGURE A.4

Sweet's syndrome.

Rett's syndrome	Congenital retardation 2° to ↑ serum ammonia levels, more common in females. Sx = autism, dementia, ataxia, tremors
Schafer's dz	Defect in hexosaminidase B, in contrast to the A component of the enzyme that is defective in Tay–Sachs. Px is better for Schafer's
Schindler's dz	Defect in *N*-acetylgalactosaminidase
Schmidt's syndrome	Hashimoto's thyroiditis with diabetes and/or Addison's dz (autoimmune syndrome)
Sweet's syndrome	Recurrent painful reddish-purple plaques and papules (see Figure A.4) associated with fever, arthralgia, neutrophilia. Occurs more commonly in women, possibly due to hypersensitivity reaction associated with *Yersinia* infxn. Can also be seen in following upper respiratory infxn or with leukemia. Tx = prednisone, antibiotics if associated with *Yersinia* infxn
Syndrome X	Angina relieved by rest (typical) with a nml angiogram. Caused by vasospasm of small arterioles, unlike Prinzmetal's angina, which is vasospasm of large arteries

Dz	Description/Sx
Tarlov cysts	Tarlov cysts are fluid-filled sacs that most often affect nerve roots in the sacrum, the group of bones at the base of the spine. These cysts can compress nerve roots, causing lower back pain, sciatica (shock-like or burning pain in the lower back, buttocks, and down one leg to below the knee), urinary incontinence, headaches, sexual dysfunction, constipation, and some loss of feeling or control of movement in the leg and/or foot. Pressure on the nerves next to the cysts can also cause pain and deterioration of the surrounding bone. Tarlov cysts may become symptomatic following shock, trauma, or exertion that causes the buildup of cerebrospinal fluid. Women are at much higher risk of developing these cysts than are men.
Tay–Sachs dz	Autosomal recessive defect in hexosaminidase A, causing very early onset, progressive retardation, paralysis, dementia, blindness, cherry-red spot on macula, death by 3–4 yrs. Common in Ashkenazi Jews
Tropical spastic paraparesis	Insidious lower-extremity paresis caused by human T-cell leukemia virus (HTLV), which is endemic to Japan and the Caribbean, transmitted like HIV via placenta, body fluids, sex. Presents with mild sensory deficits, marked lower-extremity hyperreflexia, paralysis, urinary incontinence
Turcot's syndrome	Familial adenomatous polyposis with CNS medulloblastoma or glioma
Usher syndrome	Most common condition involving both hearing and vision impairment. Autosomal recessive dz → deafness and retinitis pigmentosa (form of night blindness)
Verner–Morrison syndrome	VIPoma = vasoactive intestinal polypeptide over-production. Leads to pancreatic cholera, increased watery diarrhea, dehydration, hypokalemia, hypo/achlorhydria
Von Recklinghausen's dz	Diffuse osteolytic lesions caused by hyperparathyroidism causing characteristic "brown tumor" of bone due to hemorrhage. Can mimic osteoporosis on X-rays
Wiskott–Aldrich syndrome	X-linked recessive defect in IgM response to capsular polysaccharides such as those of *Streptococcus pneumoniae,* but pts have ↑ IgA levels. Classic triad = recurrent pyogenic bacteria infxns, eczema, thrombocytopenia. Bloody diarrhea is often first Sx, then upper respiratory infxns; leukemia and lymphoma are common in children who survive to age 10

Wolman disease	Wolman disease is a type of lysosomal storage disorder. It is an inherited condition that causes a buildup of lipids (fats) in body organs and calcium deposits in the <u>adrenal glands</u>. Common symptoms in infants include enlarged liver and spleen, poor weight gain, low muscle tone, <u>jaundice</u>, vomiting, <u>diarrhea</u>, developmental delay, <u>anemia</u>, and poor absorption of nutrients from food. The condition is severe and life-threatening, however new therapies, such as <u>hematopoietic cell transplantation</u>, have shown promise in improving the outlook of children with this disease.
Xeroderma pigmentosa	Defect in repair of DNA damage caused by UV light (pyrimidine dimers). Pts highly likely to develop skin CA. Only Tx is avoidance of sunlight
Young syndrome	Young syndrome is a condition whose signs and symptoms may be similar to those seen in <u>cystic fibrosis</u>, including <u>bronchiectasis</u>, <u>sinusitis</u>, and obstructive azoospermia (a condition in which sperm are produced but do not mix with the rest of the ejaculatory fluid due to a physical obstruction, resulting in nonexistent levels of sperm in semen). The condition is usually diagnosed in middle-aged men who undergo evaluation for infertility. Although the exact cause has not been identified, it is believed to be a genetic condition. At this time, there is no known effective treatment or cure for Young syndrome.
Zellweger syndrome	Zellweger syndrome is the most severe form of a spectrum of conditions called <u>Zellweger spectrum disorders</u>. The signs and symptoms of Zellweger syndrome typically appear during the newborn period and may include poor muscle tone (hypotonia), poor feeding, seizures, hearing loss, vision loss, distinctive facial features, and skeletal abnormalities. Affected children also develop life-threatening problems in other organs and tissues, such as the liver, heart, and kidneys. Children with Zellweger syndrome usually do not survive beyond the first year of life. Zellweger syndrome is caused by <u>mutations</u> in any one of at least 12 <u>genes</u>; mutations in the <u>*PEX1*</u> gene are the most common cause. It is inherited in an <u>autosomal recessive</u> manner. There is no cure for Zellweger syndrome; treatment is generally symptomatic and supportive.

References

National Institute of Health Office of Rare Disease Research
http://rarediseases.info.nih.gov

QUESTIONS

1. A 32-yr-old G2P2 woman presents to the clinic and reports that she has not menstruated for 3 mos. She is a slender, athletically built, successful businesswoman. Which of the following is the most likely cause?

A. Turner's syndrome
B. Asherman's syndrome
C. Pregnancy
D. Tumor
E. Anxiety

2. A 65-yr-old African-American man has a Hx of benign prostatic hyperplasia and slow urinary stream. He develops increased frequency and dysuria. Urine microscopy shows 50–100 WBCs per high-power field. Gram stain reveals Gram-negative rods. You administer a 3-day course of trimethoprim/sulfamethoxazole (Bactrim) to treat a urinary tract infxn. However, 4 days later, the pt returns with fatigue. He notes a previous similar reaction to an antimalarial medication. Labs are as follows:

Hemoglobin: 8.5 g/dL

Hematocrit: 25.5%

Haptoglobin (serum): 20 mg/dL (nml: 50–220 mg/dL)

Which of the following diagnoses should be strongly considered?

A. Sickle cell anemia
B. Glucose-6-phosphate dehydrogenase (G6PD) deficiency
C. Hereditary spherocytosis
D. Paroxysmal nocturnal hemoglobinuria
E. Folic acid deficiency

3. A 64-yr-old man presents with painless jaundice and recent depressed mood. Abdominal CT is shown below. Which of the following is the most likely Dx?

A. Pancreatic adenocarcinoma
B. Pancreatic pseudocyst
C. Abdominal aortic aneurysm with compression of common bile duct
D. Splenic artery aneurysm with compression of common bile duct
E. Acute cholecystitis

4. A 4-yr-old with Down's syndrome who was previously active and able to run unassisted is brought to his primary care doctor by his parents because he has recently refused to walk. On PE, the pt is afebrile. There is no calor, rubor, or tumor on the legs. There is full range of motion passively and bilaterally, although the pt is irritable with the examination. No changes in the bones or soft tissues are seen on x-ray. White count is elevated to 50,000. What is the most likely Dx?

A. Leukemia
B. Septic arthritis
C. Toxic synovitis
D. Pauciarticular juvenile rheumatoid arthritis
E. A fussy child

5. A 20-yr-old man with no significant medical Hx presents to your office complaining of a HA. The HA is described as 9 out of 10 in intensity, usually occurs in the evening, lasts less than 30 minutes, and seems to be localized around the pt's right eye. The pt also notes that some tearing and redness of the right eye occur during these attacks. Drinking beforehand seems to worsen the Sx. The pt denies any visual changes and Hx of allergic rhinitis, polyuria, polydipsia, weight change, or recent respiratory illness. This pt most likely has which of the following?

A. Migraine
B. Subarachnoid hemorrhage
C. Simple partial seizure
D. Hypoglycemic episode secondary to new-onset diabetes
E. Cluster HA

6. A 25-yr-old woman undergoes surgery to repair a torn ACL. Her only medication is an oral contraceptive, which she continues to take during and after hospitalization. She has not been ambulatory since surgery. Her postoperative course is complicated by persistent fever of 38.1°C to 39.2°C that began 4 days after surgery. In addition, she has reported two episodes of transient shortness of breath. She denies urinary Sx. A chest radiograph and urinalysis are nml. What is the appropriate next course of action?

A. Lower extremity Utz to evaluate for deep venous thrombosis
B. Noncontrast chest CT to evaluate for atelectasis
C. Blood cultures to evaluate for bacteremia and initiation of broad-spectrum antibiotic Tx
D. D-dimer level to evaluate for deep venous thrombosis
E. Repeat urinalysis to evaluate for urinary tract infxn

7. A 20-yr-old man is giving his medical Hx to his new primary care physician. He is complaining of 1 wk of fever, accompanied by cough, arthralgias, and mild, nonbloody diarrhea. He is not taking any medication except for some acetaminophen for the fever. His review of systems is negative for hypertension, polyuria, polydipsia, fatigue, or weight changes. The pt does note, however, that when he was 8 yrs old, he had developed a 2-wk-long period of fever.

During the physical, the pt's new primary care physician notes that the pt has a grade 2/4 systolic ejection murmur heard best at the apex. The pt was not aware he had this condition. The physician also found that the pt has finger clubbing as well as swellings of the fingertips. These swellings are slightly tender to palpation. A funduscopic examination would most likely reveal which of the following?

A. Elevated, edematous disks with blurred margins and tortuous engorged veins

B. A nml-appearing disk with gray-folded elevations of the retina; over the elevations, the blood vessels appear tortuous, whereas elsewhere they appear nml

C. Small hemorrhagic spots, each with a central white area

D. The presence of extra, numerous, narrow, tortuous blood vessels superimposed over the nml vasculature

E. Grayish-white ovoid lesions with irregular, wool-like margins of varying sizes, some just slightly smaller than the size of the disk

8. A G3P0 woman at 12 wks of gestation presents to the clinic for her second prenatal visit. You had ordered labs on her first visit, and upon their review, you learn that the pt is rubella nonimmune. You recommend which of the following?

A. Voluntary interruption of the pregnancy

B. The vaccine should be withheld until the pt leaves the hospital.

C. Immediate vaccination

D. The vaccine should be withheld until after second trimester.

E. The vaccine should be withheld until after delivery.

9. An 82-yr-old woman presents to your primary care clinic with complaint of progressively worsening vision loss that is now preventing her from reading. You elicit a focused Hx of the course of her vision loss and you are concerned that she may have age-related macular degeneration (AMD). Which of the following is not a feature of AMD?

A. Vision loss
B. Presence of choroidal neovascular membranes
C. Hemorrhage
D. Pain

10. An 82-yr-old woman with a past medical Hx of hypertension presents with weight loss, HA, and generalized weakness. Head CT is obtained and reveals multiple enhancing masses. Of the following, which is the most likely Dx?

A. Glioblastoma multiforme
B. Primary CNS lymphoma
C. Cerebral metastases
D. Cerebrovascular accident
E. Meningioma

11. A 28-yr-old woman presents with soft, nonpainful, fleshy growths around her vulva and anus. You should initiate Tx with which of the following?

A. Topical podophyllin or trichloracetic acid
B. Benzathine penicillin G
C. A reminder to use condoms with every act of intercourse
D. Topical steroid
E. Surgery

12. A pt with COPD presents with some wheezing. His blood gas results are as follows:

pH: 7.37
pCO_2: 60 mm Hg
pO_2: 70 mm Hg
HCO_3: 37 mmol/L

What is this pt's acid-base disorder?

A. Acute respiratory acidosis
B. Chronic respiratory acidosis and metabolic alkalosis
C. Metabolic acidosis
D. Metabolic alkalosis
E. Chronic respiratory acidosis

13. A 48-yr-old female presents to the emergency department with a 2-wk Hx of sinus infxn that has worsened while on antibiotics. Her PE is concerning for medial orbit tenderness and edema. Which bone makes up the medial wall of the orbit?

A. Frontal
B. Ethmoid
C. Palatine
D. Zygomatic

14. A 25-yr-old female presents to the emergency room with a 1-wk Hx of left-sided unilateral frontal HA unresponsive to oxycodone. The pt is now developing left lid erythema, edema, and eye pressure. Pt denies any visual changes. CT scan is consistent with frontal sinusitis and preseptal cellulitis. What is the most appropriate Tx for this pt?

A. Continue oxycodone and discharge pt home on decongestants and nasal irrigations

B. Admit pt; give oral antibiotics, pain medications, and decongestants

C. Discharge pt home and follow-up in general ENT clinic

D. Admit pt; ENT consult; give IV antibiotics, pain medications, decongestants, and nasal irrigation; possible surgery if Sx continue to worsen

15. A 70-yr-old man who recently immigrated to the United States from a developing country presents with complaints of "electrical" radiating leg pain. He also reports sharp abd pains with nausea and vomiting, paroxysms of cough, and bladder and rectal spasms. On PE, a wide-based gait is observed. Labs include a positive VDRL. Pupillary examination would reveal which of the following?

A. Bilaterally nonreactive pupils

B. A left pupil that is larger than the right and reacts minimally to bright light but responds more to accommodation; administration of methacholine drops to both eyes results in prompt constriction of the left pupil but no response of the right

C. A left pupil that is smaller than the right pupil and is accompanied by left upper lid droop; administration of 4% cocaine in both eyes dilates the right pupil but not the left

D. Bilateral pinpoint pupils

E. Small pupils that are unreactive to a bright light but do accommodate to light

16. A 68-yr-old man presents to the emergency room with nausea, vomiting, and abdominal pain and distention. He has not passed gas or had a bowel movement for more than 24 hrs. He denies previous surgeries of any kind or serious medical illnesses. An abdominal plain film shows multiple dilated loops of small bowel. A nasogastric tube is placed, and IV fluids are administered. Which of the following is the most likely cause of small bowel obstruction in thispt?

A. Hernia

B. Peritoneal adhesions

C. Neoplasm

D. Crohn's dz

E. Gallstone ileus

17. An overweight 48-yr-old pt, who has had multiple incidences of vaginitis, presents with a global darkening of her skin color. The pt was previously on the Atkins diet but denies any abnormal eating habits now. Which of the following do you recommend?

A. Steroids
B. Hydroquinone cream
C. Insulin
D. Increased exposure to sunlight
E. Full disclosure of diet

18. A 34-yr-old man with diffuse alveolar infiltrates on CXR presents to the ER with severe hypoxia. Pulmonary function testing and arterial blood gas demonstrate the following: PCO_2 nml; large A–a difference; marked hypoxia, improving with oxygen administration; and decreased diffusing capacity of lung for carbon monoxide (DLCO). Which of the following is the cause of this pt's hypoxia?

A. Hypoventilation
B. Diffusion impairment
C. Decreased FiO_2
D. Ventilation–perfusion (V/Q) mismatch
E. Shunt

19. A thin, 82-yr-old woman presents to the emergency room complaining of uncontrollable back and chest pain. She reports coughing a lot recently as she was battling a cold and tried taking some oxycodone/acetaminophen, which did not relieve the pain. Her pain has been constant over the last week and does not seem to be associated with activity or eating. It starts between the shoulder blades and radiates around to the chest. She has a Hx of alcoholism and hip repair, when she fractured a hip falling off of a chair during one of her drinking binges. She had a stress test done 1 wk ago for the chest pain, which was reported as negative. Which of the following is most appropriate?

A. CT angiogram of the chest to rule out aortic dissection
B. Esophagram
C. Give aspirin and repeat stress test
D. Trial of NSAIDs
E. Thoracic spine x-ray

20. An 11-yr-old boy is in the clinic for a regular Hx and physical. He is concerned about how tall he will become and when puberty will start. Which of the following will be the first indication of puberty?

A. Pubic hair
B. Voice dropping

C. Testicular enlargement
D. Growth spurt
E. Increased penile length

21. An 88-yr-old woman with a Hx of osteoporosis and dementia is admitted for Tx of a community-acquired pneumonia. During the course of the evening, the pt becomes confused and frightened, begins to address people that are not present, and attempts to climb out of bed. Administration of which of the following is most likely to increase this pt's fall risk?

A. Haloperidol
B. Fluphenazine
C. Thiothixene
D. Chlorpromazine
E. Clozapine

22. An ambulance is called to an 82-yr-old woman's home for altered mental status. The pt is confused, her heart rate (HR) is 118, and her BP is 102/61. The pt is taken to the hospital and examined. Her examination reveals dry mucus membranes with decreased skin turgor. Lungs are clear to auscultation, and cardiac examination reveals a 2/6 systolic ejection murmur at the right upper sternal border. No edema or jugular venous distention is noted. Labs show the following:

Sodium: 117 mEq/L

Potassium: 3.6 mEq/L

Bicarbonate: 22 mEq/L

Glucose: 316 mg/dL

The pt's records are reviewed and show that she is on insulin, glyburide, and hydrochlorothiazide. Which of the following would be the best next step?

A. Administer DDAVP and check urine osmolality
B. Stop hydrochlorothiazide and give nml saline
C. Correct glucose with insulin and monitor sodium levels
D. Prescribe 40 mg IV Lasix
E. Replace sodium and potassium to nml levels over 2 hrs

23. A 32-yr-old G1P0 woman in the 8th week of her pregnancy presents to your office for an initial OBGYN appointment. She has a FHx of a mother who had cataracts as a child and is concerned about the possibility of her child having cataracts. Which of the following is not a cause of congenital cataracts?

A. Amblyopia
B. Rubella

C. Galactosemia
D. Toxoplasmosis

24. While turning in the kitchen to catch a can rolling off the counter, a 46-yr-old African-American man noted significant left hip pain and went to the emergency room for evaluation. A left hip x-ray was performed and shows a fracture of the femur.

Labs show:

Sodium: 138 mEq/L

Potassium: 4.2 mEq/L

Bicarbonate: 24 mEq/L

BUN: 34 mg/dL

Creatinine: 1.8 mg/dL

Calcium: 11.2 mEq/L

WBC: 10,600 /µL

Hemoglobin: 9.7 g/dL

Platelets: 297,000/µL

Which diagnostic study should be performed next to confirm the Dx?

A. Blood cultures
B. CXR
C. Colonoscopy
D. MRI of the left hip
E. SPEP/UPEP (serum protein electrophoresis/urine electrophoresis)

25. The family of a 91-yr-old woman is concerned about her change in mental status and brings her to the emergency room for evaluation. The pt was in the hospital for gout last week and was discharged with colchicine and short-acting morphine. She has been having difficulty sleeping the last two nights, shouting out that she cannot sleep because of pain. During the day, she can be calm and her "nml self," followed by periods of threatening behavior and kicking at her family. Prior to her hospital stay, she never exhibited these behaviors. She has also been seeing and talking to her husband, who passed away 5 yrs ago. Her examination is difficult because the pt will not cooperate, and she is only oriented to herself. Which of the following is most appropriate?

A. Give diphenhydramine for sleep at night.
B. Increase morphine to control pt's pain.
C. Prescribe haloperidol to give for agitation on an as-needed basis.
D. Order a CXR and urinalysis to rule out infxn and hold the morphine.
E. Reassure family that the pt is probably confused from her hospital stay and will likely return to baseline in a few days.

26. A 28-yr-old resident physician receives tuberculin skin testing as part of a routine health maintenance examination. He is generally healthy, is HIV negative, and has no known recent contacts with active tuberculosis (TB). When read at 48 hrs, the area of induration measures 6 mm. He has never received a BCG injection, and prior tuberculin skin tests have not resulted in induration. What is the Dx and course of action for this pt?

A. Negative tuberculin skin test; repeat in 1 to 2 yrs

B. Equivocal tuberculin skin test; obtain chest radiograph

C. Positive tuberculin skin test; obtain chest radiograph and treat with a 6-mo course of isoniazid

D. Positive tuberculin skin test; treat for active TB with isoniazid, ethambutol, pyrazinamide, and rifampin

E. Positive tuberculin skin test; treat only if Sx develop

27. A young mother brings in her 2-yr-old son for an appointment with you. During this visit, she tells you that her child snores very loudly at night, has no apnea or chronic nasal congestion, has a very nasally voice, and constantly has his mouth open because he cannot breathe through his nose. The child has no other Sx. On PE, he has nasal blockage despite no obvious findings on examination of the nose, clear rhinorrhea, mouth constantly opening while at rest, and nml tonsils. Lateral neck x-ray demonstrates a soft tissue mass completely obstructing the nasopharynx. Which of the following statements most applies to this case?

A. This pt must undergo endoscopic sinus surgery for removal of nasal polyps.

B. This pt suffers from allergies and must be started on allergy immunotherapy.

C. The pt is most likely suffering from adenoiditis and should be referred to an ENT.

D. This pt most likely has an osteoblastic tumor and will need immediate surgery.

28. The mother of a 6-wk-old brings the baby in to your clinic for a chief complaint of constipation. The baby is formula-fed. The mother brings the baby in now because the child has seemed weak and less active, including feeding less actively, but has been drooling more. The pt has maintained nml urine output throughout. You advise this parent to:

A. learn about nml developmental stages.

B. take the pt to hospital to be admitted.

C. give the pt half a child-size enema.

D. return to the clinic if her baby worsens.

E. send labs for urine organic acids

29. A 21-yr-old female presents to your office complaining of bloating and loose stools. Her Sx are worse after meals but persist throughout the day. She denies abdominal pain, fever, chills, nausea, or vomiting. She denies constipation and has four to five nonbloody, loose stools daily. Her vital signs are stable. Her examination is nml except for a papulovesicular rash on her shoulders, elbows, and knees. On lab evaluation, she is mildly anemic with an MCV of 75. Her electrolytes and liver function tests are nml. Which of the following tests would provide a definite Dx for her Sx?

A. Hydrogen breath test
B. Stool for Clostridium difficile
C. Small bowel biopsies
D. Trial of antidiarrheal agents
E. Colonoscopy

30. Your pt who has had multiple S. pyogenes infections in the past calls to tell you that she has had a sore throat for the past few days and now she is developing a rash. You ask her to come into the office and you are concerned that she may have scarlet fever based upon her description of the rash. Which of the following is not a physical finding of scarlet fever?

A. Follicular erythema
B. Strawberry tongue
C. Pastia's lines
D. "Sunburn with goose bumps"
E. Desquamation

31. A 52-yr-old woman with a long Hx of active rheumatoid arthritis undergoes emergency appendectomy while visiting relatives. She does not remember the names of her current medications. Following the surgery, she becomes persistently hypotensive and tachycardic, with BP of 80/55 mm Hg and HR of 120 bpm. Her hypotension does not respond to multiple fluid boluses of lactated Ringer's solution. She is severely fatigued and hyperkalemic (K = 5.3 mEq/L). Which of the following is the proper course of action in this pt?

a. Continue giving nml saline rapidly; obtain urgent nephrology consultation
b. Blood cultures, broad-spectrum antibiotics, and activated protein C to treat sepsis
c. Emergency echocardiogram to evaluate for congestive heart failure
d. Immediate abdominal CT to evaluate for abscess
e. Serum cortisol level and immediate administration of hydrocortisone 300 mg IV and nml saline

32. A 52-yr-old woman with a Hx of total abdominal hysterectomy is at her primary care physician's office for routine health maintenance. Which of the following is recommended for cancer screening for this pt?

A. Annual Pap smears
B. Annual transvaginal Utz
C. Breast examination and mammogram every 1–2 yrs
D. Annual transvaginal Utz with CA-125 testing
E. Colonoscopy every 3–5 yrs

33. A 4-yr-old boy, who was previously potty trained, is almost ready to enter pre-K. He is now drinking a lot and has wet himself several times. When asked by his mom if everything is all right, he says he is being teased about having "bug eyes" by the other children at his new school. Which of the following will most likely lead to the Dx of a histiocytosis X syndrome?

A. Splenomegaly
B. Hepatomegaly
C. Skull lesions
D. Hilar prominence
E. Sinus involvement

34. An otherwise healthy 55-yr-old man with hypercholesterolemia presents with an episode of right-sided hemiparesis. A continuous infusion of IV nml saline solution containing 5% dextrose is administered. The pt's Sx resolve in 12 hrs. Based on this description, the pt had, by definition, which of the following?

A. Transient ischemic attack (TIA)
B. Stroke
C. Simple partial seizure
D. Hypoglycemia
E. Migraine

35. A 23-yr-old man presents with a scaling rash on his elbows and knees. He also complains of dandruff that is not responsive to different Tx shampoos. Which of the following is (are) most likely involved as well?

A. Palms and soles
B. Fingernails
C. Face
D. Intertriginous areas
E. Pulmonary (lungs)

36. While working at home, a 67-yr-old man notices weakness and palpitations. He now presents to his primary care doctor for evaluation. His Hx is notable for a 20-pack-yr Hx of smoking and having a glass of wine daily. His last drink was 5 days ago. In the office, his HR is 132, and BP is 128/67. Cardiovascular examination reveals an irregularly irregular rhythm with no murmurs. The remainder of the examination is unremarkable. What is the next most appropriate step?

A. Admit the pt to the psychiatry ward for alcohol withdrawal.

B. Immediately shock the pt into nml sinus rhythm.

C. Reassure the pt that the heart rhythm is likely due to his old age and he needs no further evaluation.

D. Start a beta-blocker to slow the HR and follow up in 3 days.

E. Anticoagulate the pt and initiate a diagnostic workup for atrial fibrillation

37. A 24-yr-old woman develops an acute bout of bloody diarrhea accompanied by a low-grade fever. She takes ciprofloxacin for several days, and the diarrhea resolves. A few days after resolution, the pt begins to experience some weakness in her ankles, which makes it difficult to pick her feet up off the ground. Over the next several days, the weakness spreads up her legs so that she cannot flex her hips. Two days later, she develops the same weakness in her arms. She presents to the ER. The pt is profoundly weak in the lower extremities and somewhat less weak in the upper extremities. She is areflexic in the lower extremities and hyporeflexic in the upper extremities. You perform a lumbar puncture, and the CSF reveals CSF WBC 2/μL, red cells 10/μL, protein 150 mg/dL, and glucose nml. Which of the following is the correct Dx?

A. Aseptic meningitis

B. Bacterial meningitis

C. Neurosyphilis

D. Guillain-Barré syndrome

E. Amyotrophic lateral sclerosis

38. Your nurse fields a call from a parent of a 3-yr-old pt, whose older sibling has been home from school with chicken pox. The parent wants to know if the younger child needs to stay home from day-care. You ask the nurse to tell the parents that:

A. there is no reason to keep the child out of daycare.

B. the pt may return to daycare immediately but should be kept home while developing active lesions.

C. the pt may return to daycare after lesions start.

D. the pt may return to daycare after lesions crust over.

E. the pt may return to daycare after lesions clear.

39. A 45-yr-old woman with a Hx of Raynaud's syndrome and auto-immune thyroiditis presents to your clinic complaining of recent onset of itching and a slight yellow tinge to her skin. She denies having abdominal pain. PE reveals slight jaundice but is otherwise unremarkable. Preliminary labs are as follows:

AST (SGOT): 29 U/L

ALT (SGPT): 25 U/L

Alkaline phosphatase: 577 U/L

Bilirubin (total): 2.2 mg/dL

Bilirubin (direct): 1.7 mg/dL

CBC: Nml

Which of the following tests should be ordered to evaluate this pt?

A. Infectious hepatitis serologies

B. Antimitochondrial antibodies and liver Bx

C. Acetaminophen level

D. Direct Coombs' testing and serum haptoglobin

E. No further testing is indicated

40. You have been asked to evaluate a pt for possible alcohol abuse and dependence. You use the CAGE questionnaire to do a quick assessment. A more rigorous assessment is indicated when the pt replies "yes" when asked if he/she has ever:

A. consumed more than 8 drinks at one sitting.

B. felt Angered for no apparent reason.

C. felt Guilty about drinking.

D. felt more Energized after a drink.

E. felt more Eloquent after drinking.

41. An 85-yr-old man with known coronary artery dz is admitted to the hospital because of hematemesis and hypotension. After fluid resuscitation with nml saline, upper endoscopy reveals an oozing gastric ulcer that is treated endoscopically. However, following endoscopy, the pt complains of left-sided chest pain, diaphoresis, and dyspnea. An ECG is obtained and is unchanged from admission, showing occasional premature ventricular complexes but no new ST segment changes. The following additional lab values are obtained.

Hemoglobin: 7.2 g/dL

Hematocrit: 23.2%

Cardiac troponin T: 0.65 µg/L (nml: <0.1 µg/L)

Of the following interventions, which is indicated for this pt?

A. Emergent transfusion of four units of packed RBCs
B. Emergency administration of tissue plasminogen activator (tPA, a thrombolytic)
C. IV bolus of heparin followed by continuous heparin drip
D. Emergency coronary artery bypass grafting
E. Lidocaine drip to prevent ventricular fibrillation

42. A 33-yr-old man presents to the emergency room complaining of intense HA behind the left eye. He describes the pain as stabbing and denies any trauma. The pt relates that the pain began as he started to fall asleep and has been associated with tearing of the eye. On examination, the eyes are without any redness. Clear discharge is present involving the left eye with ptosis present. No other neurologic findings are present. What Tx would be best for abortive Tx?

A. Beta-blocker
B. Carbamazepine
C. NSAIDs
D. 100% oxygen
E. Verapamil

43. An 18-yr-old man presents to the emergency department with acute onset of testicular pain, nausea, and vomiting. He admits to multiple recent new sexual contacts. On examination, the testicle is extremely tender, swollen, and lying transverse in the scrotum. The cremasteric reflex is absent on the affected side. Doppler Utz to assess testicular blood flow is not immediately available. Which of the following is the proper course of action in this pt?

A. Discharge to home with a 7-day course of ciprofloxacin for epididymitis and ibuprofen for pain
B. Admit to the hospital with pt-controlled administration of IV narcotics and vigorous hydration
C. Order CBC, electrolytes, and urinalysis prior to determining disposition of the pt
D. Immediate urologic consultation for likely surgical decompression
E. Order pelvic CT with contrast to evaluate for anatomic abnormalities of the kidneys or ureters

44. JR, an 8-yr-old prepubescent boy, presents with a recent pruritic, erythematous rash on his face. He denies any Hx of insect bites or any systemic Sx. On detailed questioning, the boy's mother describes washing his clothes with a new generic detergent. Which of the following is the most appropriate initial Tx?

A. Hydrocortisone 2.5%
B. Hydrocortisone 1.0%

C. Triamcinolone 0.025%
D. Triamcinolone 0.1%
E. Betamethasone 0.1%

45. A 75-yr-old white woman presents to the emergency room after slipping on ice and falling onto her outstretched arms. She reports right wrist pain. Plain radiograph shows a distal radial (Colles') fracture. The pt weighs 105 lbs and is 5 feet tall. The only medications she is taking are atenolol and hydrochlorothiazide for hypertension, which she has taken for many yrs. She is 25 yrs postmenopausal and has not taken hormone replacement Tx. She smoked one pack of cigarettes per day for 30 yrs but quit smoking 20 yrs ago. Which of the following pt attributes decreases her risk for osteoporosis?

A. White race
B. Postmenopausal status
C. Thin build
D. Hydrochlorothiazide use
E. Hx of smoking

46. A 42-yr-old G5P5 woman presents at 36 wks of gestation with complaints of HA and leg swelling. On PE, you note a number of brown and purple nonblanching patches on her legs and arms. You also note sock marks on her shins. Which of the following do you recommend?

A. Referral to a shelter for abused women and their children
B. Admission to the hospital for monitoring, labs, and likely delivery
C. Bed rest
D. Avoidance of the sun
E. Stricter discipline to ensure that the older children pick up their toys so that your pt will not fall so often

47. Many different classes of antidepressants currently are available. If a pt is newly diagnosed with a major depressive episode and this pt has ongoing suicidal thoughts and a Hx of intentional drug overdose, which of the following antidepressants should absolutely be avoided as a first-line medication?

A. Imipramine
B. Fluoxetine
C. Sertraline
D. Bupropion
E. Paroxetine

48. A 68-yr-old man reports mild, increasing fatigue over the past several mos. PE is notable for cervical and axillary lymphadenopathy and splenomegaly. A CBC is ordered and reveals a WBC count of 234,000/μL. Other cell lines are within nml range. A peripheral blood smear shows multiple small, mature leukocytes with "soccer ball" nuclei. Which of the following statements is true for the Tx of this pt?

A. Early Tx with aggressive chemotherapy will likely be curative.

B. Immediate bone marrow transplantation is indicated.

C. Tx should focus on reducing Sx rather than on prolonging life.

D. The pt has a benign, infectious condition that will resolve spontaneously.

E. The pt will likely die within 3 mos.

49. A 27-yr-old woman presents to your office for a routine PE. She states that she is generally healthy and does not take any medications. She has no specific health concerns or new Sx. Her HR is 70 bpm. Her weight of 60 kg is unchanged from the previous year. However, her BP is found to be 160/95 mm Hg in each arm. One year ago, her BP was recorded as 120/75 mm Hg. PE reveals a high-pitched epigastric bruit. A pregnancy test is negative.

Serum electrolytes are as follows:

Na: 144.0 mEq/L

K: 2.8 mEq/L

HCO3: 34.0 mEq/L

BUN: 15.0 mg/dL

Creatinine: 1.0 mg/dL

Which of the following is the most likely Dx?

A. Primary (essential) hypertension

B. Renal artery stenosis

C. Aortic coarctation

D. Pheochromocytoma

E. Hyperthyroidism

50. A 9-mo-old previously happy baby is brought in by his maternal grandmother, in whose house he lives with his 15-yr-old mother and 13-yr-old maternal aunt. The grandmother is concerned because the child has started to cry when his paternal grandfather comes to visit. You suspect which of the following?

A. Inadequate exposure to men

B. Neglect

C. Nml development

D. Abuse

E. Colic

51. While working in the ophthalmology clinic you are asked about typical presentations of ophthalmological dz. Which disorder presents with leukocoria?

A. Viral conjunctivitis
B. Scleritis
C. Angle closure glaucoma
D. Retinoblastoma

52. A 75-yr-old man with a 100-pack-yr smoking Hx presents with 20-lb weight loss over the past 3 mos, generalized weakness, and fatigue. He also reports occasional hemoptysis. A chest radiograph is obtained and shows hyperinflation consistent with emphysema but no focal abnormalities. With regard to further studies indicated for this pt, which of the following statements is correct?

A. Absence of focal changes on chest radiograph essentially rules out the Dx of lung cancer.
B. High-resolution chest CT is indicated to further evaluate for malignancy.
C. Routine screening of pts who smoke with chest radiography is effective in the early detection of lung cancer.
D. Head CT and full-body CT are indicated to evaluate for malignancy.
E. Screening for antibodies associated with paraneoplastic syndromes is indicated at this time.

53. A 22-yr-old woman was arrested by police at a Broadway musical after suddenly screaming hysterically at the actors that there was a government plot to implant mind control devices into people's brains during the production and running onto the stage. The police investigation after the event revealed that the woman's friends and coworkers had noticed slight behavioral changes a few weeks prior. The pt's family knew of no Hx of psychiatric disorders, and the pt was not taking any psychiatric medications. A urine screen was negative for illicit drugs or alcohol. A preliminary medical examination was positive for the presence of resting and intention tremors, spasticity, and rigidity. The etiology of this woman's Sx was noted by which of the following physical findings of her eyes?

A. A ring of gold-brown pigment at the periphery of iris that is wider at the superior and inferior aspects than the medial and lateral aspects
B. Redness of the conjunctiva of one eye; pressing the lower lid against the globe produces a bulge above the point of compression

C. A raised, subconjunctival fatty structure growing in a horizontal band toward the pupil

D. Dots visible in the cornea without signs of inflammation

E. A gray band of corneal opacity 1.5 mm wide that is separated by a clear zone from the limbus

54. A 58-yr-old female presents with a sudden severe retro-orbital HA and extreme lethargy. She has been otherwise healthy and did not have any previous medical Hx. Her PE reveals a BP of 86/40, HR of 100, and respirations of 20, and she has a temperature of 99.1°F. Her examination is notable for decreased vision in her temporal fields upon confrontation. Noncontrast CT of her head shows a large mass with an area of hemorrhage in the sellar region. What should be done next?

A. Start IV pressor agents (norepinephrine)

B. Administer glucocorticoids

C. Take the pt emergently to surgery for decompression of the blood

D. Check prolactin, growth hormone, and TSH levels

E. Search for other causes of hypotension or sepsis with CXR and U/A

55. A 58-yr-old postmenopausal pt who recently suffered an L1 compression fracture would like to know what she should do for improved bone health. She is a smoker and has a Hx of a myocardial infarction. She had a DEXA scan with T-scores of –2.1 at her femoral neck and total hip, as well as a score of –2.3 in her lumbar spine. In addition to adequate vitamin D and calcium intake, you should prescribe which of the following medications?

A. Estrogen replacement Tx

B. Calcitonin

C. Running and jogging exercise

D. Bisphosphonate Tx

E. No Tx is necessary since her DEXA results show that she is in osteopenia range.

56. A 54-yr-old man presents to the dermatology clinic with brown scaly patches in his right axilla. Which of the following causes of intertriginous infxn fluoresces coral-red under Wood's lamp?

A. *Corynebacterium* spp.

B. *Candida albicans*

C. Tinea cruris

D. Tinea versicolor

E. *Malassezia furfur*

57. A male pt appears in your clinic inquiring whether or not he should receive a pneumonia vaccine. Which of the following profiles would indicate use of the vaccine?

A. A 50-yr-old pt who works in a daycare center

B. A 21-yr-old medical student with no medical problems

C. An otherwise healthy 35-yr-old pt with no spleen

D. A 60-yr-old with well-controlled hypertension

E. A 22-yr-old with no medical conditions who plans to go to Afghanistan on a photo assignment

58. A 28-yr-old woman presents to your clinic. You note weight gain since her last visit. She brushes this off with a sheepish grin and apologizes for less exercise and poorer eating habits since starting a new job. She does c/o hirsutism and reports missing several periods. She had hoped this was because she was pregnant, but a urine beta-human chorionic gonadotropin (hCG) is negative. You run some laboratories and find she has increased testosterone and luteinizing hormone (LH)/follicle-stimulating hormone (FSH) and nml dehydroepiandrosterone (DHEA). You call her back to the office to explain that she needs which of the following?

A. Hormonal contraceptives

B. Glucocorticoids

C. Mineralocorticoids

D. Exercise and food portion control

E. Exploratory surgery

59. A 17-yr-old boy presents to your office after being injured during a football game. He describes being hit on the lateral aspect of the knee while his foot was planted in the ground. He heard a pop and felt significant pain that required him to limp off the field and stop playing. Plain radiographs were negative for fracture. On PE, the knee is swollen, and the lower leg is easily pulled forward from the upper leg when the pt is supine. The pt is scheduled for an MRI of the knee.

Based on the H&P examination, which three structures are likely to have been damaged during this injury?

A. Anterior cruciate ligament, posterior cruciate ligament, and medial meniscus

B. Anterior cruciate ligament, medial collateral ligament, and medial meniscus

C. Anterior cruciate ligament, lateral collateral ligament, and lateral meniscus

D. Medial collateral ligament, lateral collateral ligament, and medial meniscus

E. Medial collateral ligament, lateral collateral ligament, and lateral meniscus

60. A 78-yr-old man is brought to the emergency room after 1 hr of abdominal pain, lightheadedness, nausea, and vomiting. He is unable to provide additional Hx because of his waxing and waning consciousness. BP is 90/50 mm Hg and HR is 130 bpm while the pt is supine. On PE, a large, pulsatile, mid-abdominal mass is detected. Which of the following is the correct immediate management of this pt?

A. Assess for orthostatic BP changes

B. Obtain STAT preliminary laboratory studies, including electrolytes, CBC, amylase, and lipase, and admit for observation

C. Obtain a STAT plain radiograph of the abdomen to rule out a bowel perforation or obstruction

D. Obtain a STAT abdominal CT with contrast to evaluate for ruptured abdominal aortic aneurysm

E. Immediately notify the surgical service and transfer the pt to the operating room for an emergency laparotomy

61. An 85-yr-old man with known coronary artery dz is admitted to the hospital because of hematemesis and hypotension. After fluid resuscitation with nml saline, upper endoscopy reveals an oozing gastric ulcer that is treated endoscopically. However, following endoscopy, the pt complains of left-sided chest pain, diaphoresis, and dyspnea. An ECG is obtained and is unchanged from admission, showing occasional premature ventricular complexes but no new ST segment changes. The following additional laboratory values are obtained.

Hemoglobin: 7.2 g/dL

Hematocrit: 23.2%

Cardiac troponin T: 0.65 µg/L (nml: <0.1 µg/L)

Of the following interventions, which is indicated for this pt?

A. Emergent transfusion of four units of packed RBCs

B. Emergency administration of tissue plasminogen activator (tPA, a thrombolytic)

C. IV bolus of heparin followed by continuous heparin drip

D. Emergency coronary artery bypass grafting

E. Lidocaine drip to prevent ventricular fibrillation

62. A 52-yr-old woman presents with a breast mass. Her first menarche occurred at age 12, and her first pregnancy was at 34 yrs of age. Menopause occurred at 48 yrs old. Her maternal grandmother had breast cancer at the age of 78 yrs. The pt drinks 2 to 3 cups of coffee daily and does not smoke. Which of the following places this pt at an increased risk for breast cancer?

A. Age of first menarche
B. Age of menopause
C. Age of first pregnancy
D. Caffeine intake
E. FHx

63. A 55-yr-old man with a prior Hx of alcoholism presents to the emergency department complaining of new-onset tremors. He claims that he has been alcohol abstinent for 10 yrs. A urine toxicology screen is negative for alcohol or illicit drugs. On PE, the pt is noted to have tremors and difficulty with finger-to-nose tasks and fine motor functions, such as writing. In addition, the pt has spider angiomata and noted asterixis. A mental status examination is notable for a defect in short-term memory. The pt is afebrile and denies bowel or bladder incontinence, and his WBC count is nml. Which of the following would be the next best test to order?

A. Serum ammonia level
B. Noncontrast head CT scan
C. EEG
D. Portable CXR
E. EMG

64. A pt presents to your office one autumn afternoon inquiring whether she should receive an influenza vaccine. Which of the following profiles would indicate giving the vaccine to your pt?

A. She is 25 yrs old, with no medical problems, and works in a publishing office.
B. She is a 45-yr-old federal judge with well-controlled hypertension.
C. She is a 25-yr-old medical student, with a documented allergy to chicken eggs
D. She is 17 yrs old, with mild, intermittent asthma, and is about to enter college.
E. She is a 66-yr-old retired teacher who has emphysema.

65. A 67-yr-old woman out shopping with her daughter complains of sudden-onset HA, lightheadedness, and right-sided weakness. Her daughter finds that her mother cannot move her right side.

You are on duty in the emergency department when the pt is brought in. A fingerstick glucose reads 125. The pt has no known seizure Hx and no known head trauma.

Which test should be ordered next?

A. Noncontrast head CT
B. PET scan

C. EEG
D. Head x-ray
E. Carotid Doppler Utz

66. A 24-yr-old graduate student in chemistry presents to the emergency department with severe burning pain in her right eye after an accident in the lab where she was splashed in the face with an unknown chemical. What is the most appropriate first step in the management of this pt with a suspected chemical burn involving the eye?

A. Check vision
B. Irrigation
C. Steroids
D. Call ophthalmologist

67. A 75-yr-old man with a Hx of hypertension and glaucoma presents to the clinic for a routine examination. During the Hx taking, the clinic physician finds that the pt's wife of 50 yrs passed away 1 yr ago. Since that time, he has had poor appetite, poor sleep, loss of weight, and feelings of despair and hopeless-ness, and he has become socially withdrawn. In addition, the pt has lost his meticulousness with his medications, including his eye drops. Gross challenge of the pt's visual field would likely reveal which of the following?

A. Loss of the central portion of the visual fields
B. Monocular blindness
C. Loss of the periphery of both eyes' visual fields
D. Bitemporal hemianopsia
E. Loss of the right upper quadrant of both visual fields

68. A 78-yr-old man has a past medical Hx significant only for gastro-esophageal reflux disease (GERD). He presents to the clinic complain-ing of mild abdominal pain, chronic fatigue, and increasing dyspnea on exertion. He denies hematemesis or black or bloody stools. PE reveals generalized and conjunctival pallor. Stool is guaiac negative.

Labs are as follows:

Hemoglobin: 8.4 g/dL

MCV: 77.8 μm3

Ferritin: 5.2 μg/L

Upper endoscopy reveals mild gastritis but is otherwise unremark-able. Which of the following is the most appropriate next course of action?

A. Colonoscopy
B. Ferrous sulfate 325 mg PO qd and reassurance

C. Ferrous sulfate 2 g IV × 1 and reassurance
D. Bone marrow Bx
E. Abdominal CT

69. The mother of a 3-yr-old boy calls because her child's temperature is 104°F. He has no rash or other Sx. The past medical Hx is significant only for recent adoption from Romania. The mother is concerned about preventing febrile seizures. Which of the following should you tell her?

A. Give acetaminophen right away.
B. Febrile seizures occur most often as the temperature is rising. Since his temperature is already high, he is less likely to have a febrile seizure.
C. Give ibuprofen right away.
D. Give aspirin right away.
E. As long as the child is not drowsy after a seizure, he will be fine.

70. A 25-yr-old pregnant woman undergoes a routine prenatal screening Utz. During the test, the technician incidentally notes the presence of multiple, small gallstones. The pt has never had any pain or other Sx related to gallstones, but seeks a surgical opinion on whether or not she should have her gallbladder removed. Which of the following would you advise?

A. Her lifetime risk of developing biliary colic is approximately 5%.
B. Her risk of developing biliary colic within the next year is approximately 20%.
C. Her lifetime risk of biliary colic is approximately 20%, and she should not undergo cholecystectomy unless Sx develop.
D. She should wait until after pregnancy before undergoing elective laparoscopic cholecystectomy.
E. She should undergo immediate laparoscopic cholecystectomy to prevent acute cholecystitis.

71. A 78-yr-old woman presents to the clinic with increasing shortness of breath on exertion. She has fainted on two occasions and often is lightheaded after standing up rapidly. PE reveals a midsystolic crescendo–decrescendo murmur at the right sternal border that radiates to the carotids. Peripheral pulses are weak and late when compared to heart sounds.

Which of the following is the proper course of action in this pt?

A. IV penicillin for Tx of presumed endocarditis with echocardiography to confirm the Dx
B. Atenolol 25 mg PO qd to relieve Sx of congestive heart failure and echocardiography to confirm the Dx in the near future

C. Lisinopril 10 mg PO qd to relieve Sx of congestive heart failure and echocardiography to confirm the Dx in the near future

D. Digitalis 1 mg PO ×1.0 and 0.1 mg PO qd to relieve Sx of aortic stenosis with echocardiography in the near future

E. Echocardiography to confirm aortic stenosis and referral to a cardiac surgeon

72. A 31-yr-old pt comes in with complaints of blistering on her skin. On PE, you realize that the pattern of distribution is consistent with areas of sun exposure. When you ask about sun exposure, the pt shows a picture of her at the beach with her family. You observe that all of the siblings are hirsute. Which of the following tests would most likely aid in the Dx?

A. Skin Bx

B. Skin Bx with immunofluorescence

C. Wood's lamp of urine

D. Serum chromosomes

E. Urine porphobilinogen

73. A 15-yr-old girl comes to see you for a routine physical required for school. At some point during the interview, she tells you that she is pregnant, has missed two periods, and tested positive on a home test kit. She asks that you not tell her parents. After the appointment, the girl's father, who is a long-time pt of yours, comes to your office to drive her home. He takes you aside and asks to speak to you in private. The father states that he is concerned that his daughter seems heavier than usual, has had some bouts of nausea with vomiting, and was wondering if she could be pregnant. Which of the following would you do?

A. You strike a balance between the need to maintain confidentiality with the daughter while upholding the trust between the father and yourself by stating that, "Even if she were, I couldn't tell you without her permission."

B. Because the pt is a minor, you are required to tell the father everything.

C. Because pt–doctor confidentiality can only be broken by order of a judge or in cases where someone's life is in immediate danger, you lie and tell him that his daughter could not possibly be pregnant.

D. Because not telling the father the truth would break the trust between physician and pt (here, the father), you tell the father that his daughter is pregnant but that he should not confront her with the knowledge.

E. You tell the father that you want to call in a family counselor.

74. A 38-yr-old female presents with mild hypercalcemia. She has been aSx without any Hx of bone fractures or kidney stones. There is no FHx of kidney stones or high calcium. Her examination is unremarkable. Her calcium level is 11.5 mg/dL. Her albumin, phosphorous, magnesium, and vitamin D levels are nml. What should be the next step in the evaluation or management of this pt?

A. Refer the pt for surgery of her parathyroid glands.
B. Observe and recheck calcium level in 3 mos.
C. Check a PTH level.
D. Start the pt on a loop diuretic in order to excrete more calcium.
E. Start the pt on a thiazide diuretic in order to decrease urinary calcium.

75. A 22-yr-old pregnant female at 10 wks' gestation has a Hx of Hashimoto's hypothyroidism and asks for advice about any changes in her thyroid medication. You should tell her which of the following?

A. She likely will not need to change the dose of her thyroid medication.
B. She will likely need to decrease the dose of her thyroid medication as her pregnancy progresses.
C. She likely will not need to take any thyroid medication during pregnancy.
D. She will likely have to increase the dose of her thyroid medication.
E. She will only need to increase the dose of her thyroid medication after she gives birth.

ANSWERS

1. **C.**

Pregnancy is actually the most likely cause of amenorrhea; it should always be the first consideration when a woman presents with a missing period. This is a case of amenorrhea. The pt's amenorrhea should persist for 6 mos since the last menstruation to be classified as secondary amenorrhea. Primary amenorrhea is diagnosed when the pt has not menstruated by age 16 yrs. Turner's syndrome would be a cause of primary amenorrhea. Asherman's syndrome, wherein the uterine cavity becomes scarred after a dilation and curettage, is the most common anatomic cause of secondary amenorrhea. Tumors, anxiety, and anorexia are all additional causes of amenorrhea but are all less common than pregnancy.

2. **B.**

This pt has hemolytic anemia that appears to coincide with administration of medications with oxidative properties. G6PD deficiency is an X-linked, recessive enzyme deficiency often observed in African-American men. It results in hemolytic anemia with administration of certain drugs, including antimalarials (e.g., primaquine, quinine), sulfonamides, and nitrofurantoin. In pts with G6PD deficiency, RBCs are unable to generate reduced glutathione, which protects hemoglobin from oxidative denaturation. Sickle cell anemia certainly would be a previously discovered disease in a 65-yr-old man and would not result in hemolysis only with medication administration. Hereditary spherocytosis results in a chronic hemolytic anemia not associated with medications. Paroxysmal nocturnal hemoglobinuria is an acquired stem cell disorder that predisposes RBCs to lysis by complement. It is not associated with medications. Folic acid deficiency results in macrocytic anemia rather than hemolysis.

3. **A.**

Painless jaundice and depressed mood in the elderly is suggestive of pancreatic cancer. CT shows a large, ill-defined mass in the body of the pancreas consistent with pancreatic adenocarcinoma. Jaundice is explained by blockage of biliary drainage. The mass is poorly defined and of high tissue density. Pancreatic pseudocyst results in a well-defined, low-density mass. Abd aortic aneurysm (AAA) with compression of common bile duct is incorrect because the mass is located in the pancreas and is not contiguous with the aorta. Splenic artery aneurysm with compression of common bile duct is incorrect because the mass is composed of tissue rather than blood vessels. Acute cholecystitis is incorrect because the gallbladder is visualized in this view and appears nml.

4. A.
Children with Down's syndrome are at an increased risk for leukemia. One would expect a neutrophil predominance and elevated ESR with septic arthritis, as well as unilateral findings and a fever. The x-ray should show joint space widening. Toxic synovitis would have a normal WBC count and ESR. Pauciarticular juvenile rheumatoid arthritis should not cause WBC count elevation. Fussiness would not elevate the WBC count and does not account for the refusal to walk.

5. E.
A unilateral, periorbital HA in a 20-yr-old man is a classic presentation for a cluster headache. Migraine typically involves the entire hemicranium and, in the classic form, involves visual field cuts (scotomas) accompanied by visual phenomenon such as scintillating lights. Subarachnoid hemorrhage presents as the "worst headache of my life." Causative mechanisms include head trauma, ruptured aneurysm, and arteriovenous malformation. Subarachnoid hemorrhage would not be expected to occur every evening. A simple partial seizure often presents with motor activity, aura, or visual disturbance—each of which would correlate to the region of the brain where the seizure occurs. Simple partial seizure do not commonly present with localized pain, tearing, and eye redness. Hypoglycemia can produce headache; however, the lack of Hx, polydipsia, or polyuria rule this out.

6. A.
Causes for postoperative fever include atelectasis, urinary tract infxn, wound infxn, deep venous thrombosis, and drug fever. In this pt who takes oral contraceptive pills and has not been ambulating, deep venous thrombosis with pulmonary embolism (PE) should be strongly considered. Lower extremity Utz is the test of choice to confirm the Dx and is the best answer available. V/Q scan or fine cut spiral CT with contrast then can be ordered if lower extremity Doppler results are suspicious or positive. In this setting of high clinical likelihood of DVT, some clinicians would choose to progress directly to a V/Q scan or fine cut spiral CT with contrast if available.

In the presence of a normal CXR, noncontrast chest CT likely will provide minimal additional information. Blood cultures may be obtained, but initiation of broad-spectrum antibiotics is not

indicated at this time because no source of infxn has been identified. D-dimer levels have very low specificity for deep venous
thrombosis, especially in postoperative pts. Repeating urinalysis
is unlikely to provide additional information in this pt without
urinary symptoms.

7. **C.**

The pt has bacterial endocarditis with a previous Hx of what
sounds like rheumatic fever. Funduscopic findings that are present
in a quarter of these pts are the classic Roth spots. Papilledema is
associated with increased ICP. There is no indication that this pt
has high ICP. Folded elevations describe a retinal detachment;
the elevations are the detached portions of the retina. The presence of extra, numerous, narrow, tortuous blood vessels superimposed over the normal vasculature describes the hyperproliferative
appearance of diabetic retinopathy. Given that the pt is not
taking diabetic medications and denies polydipsia, polyuria,
fatigue, or weight loss, this is unlikely. Grayish-white ovoid lesions
with irregular, wool-like margins of varying sizes, some just slightly smaller than the size of the disk, describe cotton-wool patches
(soft exudates) seen in HTN, which is not present in this pt.

8. **B.**

Rubella is one of the TORCH diseases. The measles mumps and
rubella (MMR) vaccine is a live vaccine, so it should not be given
while the mother is pregnant or could be around other pregnant
women. Although there is limited evidence of injury to children
of mothers who were inadvertently given this vaccine while pregnant, due to the theoretical risk of in utero infxn and damage
to the child, the use of live vaccines in pregnant pts is strongly
discouraged. While there have been reports of seroconversion in
infants that are breastfeeding when the mother is vaccinated with
MMR, infants do not become actively infected and the vaccine is
thought to be safe in mothers who are breastfeeding. Thus, it is
ideally given when the mother is leaving the hospital.

9. **D.**

Pain is not a feature of AMD. Severe vision loss can occur due to
the presence of choroidal neovascular membrane leaks and cause
subretinal hemorrhages.

10. **C.**

Cerebral metastases from unknown primaries are the most common cause of brain tumors in the elderly. In women, lung cancer
and breast cancer are common causes of cerebral metastases.

Glioblastoma multiforme would not result in multiple discrete lesions. Although primary CNS lymphoma may produce a similar appearance, with multiple enhancing lesions, it is far less common than metastatic disease. Cerebrovascular accidents do not have this appearance of multiple discrete masses. Meningiomas may be multiple, discrete masses but are located at the meninges rather than in the brain parenchyma.

11. A.

This is a case of human papillomavirus (HPV). Topical podophyllin or trichloroacetic acid is the initial Tx of choice. Refractory cases may require cryosurgery or excision. HPV-6 and HPV-11 are more commonly associated with anorectal and genital warts; HPV-16 and HPV-18 are more commonly associated with cervical cancer. Benzathine penicillin G is given for the Tx of syphilis, which can present with painless ulcers. Health professionals always recommend condoms as a form of barrier protection, but they may not cover enough of the anatomy to prevent the transmission of HPV. These growths may be mistaken for hemorrhoids, for which topical steroids can be prescribed. Only refractory cases may require cryosurgery or excision.

12. B.

This pt who suffers from COPD has chronic CO_2 retention (i.e., chronic respiratory acidosis), with a markedly elevated CO_2 level. Yet despite having a markedly elevated CO_2, the pt is not acidemic because his body is chronically retaining bicarbonate to compensate for the respiratory acidosis. Hence, there is a secondary, chronic metabolic alkalosis that has compensated for the chronic respiratory acidosis.

13. B.

The medial wall is composed of maxilla, lacrimal, ethmoid, and sphenoid bones; the zygomatic bone is part of the lateral wall and floor of orbit. The frontal bone is part of the orbital roof, and the palatine is a small bone in the posterior portion of the orbital floor. This information is important when considering potential extension of sinus disease.

14. D.

The possible spread of a frontal sinus infxn to the brain and to the orbit warrants an admission with antibiotics, decongestants, and nasal irrigation. Careful observation for changes in vision or mental status is absolutely indicated and therefore admission to the hospital is appropriate. The other choices would provide an inadequate response to this potentially life-threatening situation.

15. E.

This pt has tertiary syphilis, a rarity in the United States today but still found in the developing world. Part of the spectrum of symptoms seen in advanced syphilis are the classic Argyll Robertson pupils that do not react to light but do constrict when one asks the pt to track an object as it moves toward them. The pupils are usually, but not always, bilateral.

Bilaterally nonreactive pupils may be caused by bilateral optic nerve lesions (or brainstem death, although obviously not applicable here). A left pupil that is larger than the right and reacts minimally to bright light but responds more to accommodation describe the Holmes-Adie pupil, which results from degeneration of ciliary ganglion cells (etiology unknown). Unlike the Argyll Robertson pupil, this usually is unilateral.

A left pupil that is smaller than the right pupil and is accompanied by left upper lid droop is a description of Horner's syndrome pupil, hinted at by the drooping eyelid. Whether the Horner's is due to a lesion above or below the superior cervical ganglion, the response to 4% cocaine is the same in that the affected pupil will not dilate. Use of an adrenaline eye drop solution can distinguish lesions above the ganglion (pupil will dilate in response to adrenaline) versus lesions below the ganglion (no effect on the affected pupil). Bilateral pinpoint pupils are typical for opiate overdose. Narcan will reverse the effect.

16. A.

In adult pts, the three most common causes of small bowel obstruction are, in order, peritoneal adhesions (from past surgeries), incarcerated hernias, and neoplasms. In this pt without a Hx of abd surgery, incarcerated hernia becomes the most common cause. PE should include a careful examination for hernias. This pt has no Hx of surgeries that would result in adhesions. Incarcerated hernias are more common than malignancies as a cause of small bowel obstruction. This pt would likely have a prior Dx of Crohn's dz, if present. Gallstone ileus is an extremely rare cause of small bowel obstruction.

17. C.

This pt has bronze diabetes, or primary hemochromatosis, requiring early phlebotomy to improve pt survival. The classic triad indicating liver dz includes increased skin pigmentation, cirrhosis, and diabetes mellitus. Multiple bouts of vaginitis in a pt with acanthosis nigricans (skin darkening around the neck, flexor surfaces, and intertriginous areas) can be seen with diabetes. Steroids are used for pts with dermatomyositis and other dermatologic or rheumatologic conditions. Hydroquinone cream can be used generically to lighten hyperpigmentation. Sunlight can alleviate pityriasis rosea or psoriasis (for which one Tx is PUVA [psoralens and ultraviolet A light]). pts can get an orangey appearance with excessive consumption of foods rich in beta-carotene.

18. B.

This is a very unusual pt, with marked impairment of gas diffusion across his alveoli (in this case, likely from pulmonary alveolar pro-teinosis, a rare dz). Hypoventilation is ruled out by normal PCO_2. PCO_2 changes inversely and linearly with ventilation, so hypoven-tilation always causes CO_2 retention and vice versa. Pts inspiring low FiO_2 do not have increased A–a differences. V/Q mismatch and diffusion impairment can be distinguished only by pulmonary function testing, specifically measuring DLCO. In your career, you will see many, many more pts with V/Q mismatch than diffusion impairment. Hypoxia from shunts does not improve much with administration of exogenous oxygen.

19. E.

This pt has a previous Hx of fracture, which occurred with mild trauma. At this age, osteoporosis would be the most likely cause. The pt likely has a poor nutritional status and is thin, which would also support osteoporosis. Vertebral fractures are common among women with osteoporosis, and the pt likely suffered such a frac-ture during her coughing attacks. These fractures can be very painful. Her constant pain with a dermatomal distribution would support this condition. Aortic dissection would be unlikely given the time frame. Alcohol can predispose pts to peptic ulcer dz; however, the pt has other associated factors to suggest a more likely alternative Dx. This pt's recent negative stress test makes the Dx of cardiac dz less likely. NSAIDs would be possible as a Tx for low back pain but would not be diagnostic and in this clinical set-ting, it is important to identify the etiology of her pain. The pt in question is complaining of upper back pain and warrants further evaluation.

20. C.

You can advise your pt to first expect testicular enlargement (average age 11.5 yrs), followed by increased penile length, growth of pubic hair, and his growth spurt (approximately 2 yrs after testicular enlargement). When and how much a boy's voice will change varies from person to person.

21. D.

Chlorpromazine (Thorazine) is considered a "low-potency" neuroleptic (based on D2 affinity) that, on the positive side, reduces the likelihood of parkinsonian symptoms seen in the "high-potency" neuroleptics but also increases the alpha-blocking effects, which are responsible for lightheadedness and postural hypotension. Postural hypotension would increase the fall risk (and risk of hip fracture) in an elderly pt and therefore should be avoided in this pt population. Haloperidol (Haldol) and fluphenazine (Prolixin) are considered "high-potency" neuroleptics and would be appropriate for sedating this pt without increasing her risk of fall through postural hypotension. Thiothixene and clozapine are not as good of choices as haloperidol (Haldol) or fluphenazine because some orthostatic hypotension has been noted, but they still would be better in this pt than chlorpromazine.

22. B.

This pt has hyponatremia. After correcting for elevated glucose, the pt still has a low sodium, and this likely is the cause of her symptoms. The next step in evaluation is to monitor fluid status. The pt appears to be hypovolemic with hyperdynamic precordium and elevated heart rate to support the exam findings. Tx in this case would require stopping her diuretic, which may have contributed to the low sodium, and giving fluid resuscitation. DDAVP is a Tx for central diabetes insipidus, which causes hypernatremia, not hyponatremia. The pt's sodium is only mildly altered by the elevated glucose and will need more aggressive Tx than monitoring. The pt is hypovolemic and her condition would only worsen with diuretic Tx. Correction of the sodium has to be done slowly to avoid complications. The goal would be to correct half the deficit in the first 24 hours.

23. A.

Amblyopia can be caused by cataracts but is not a cause of congenital cataracts. Infections such as rubella, varicella, toxoplasmosis, and syphilis can cause congenital cataracts. Metabolic disorders such as galactosemia are also causes.

24. E.

This pt has fractured his left hip with minimal trauma and would suggest a pathologic fracture. As a result, further investigation is needed for cause of the fracture including possible bone dz. On lab evaluation, the pt has anemia, hypercalcemia, and renal failure. This combination would make multiple myeloma the leading Dx. To make the Dx, SPEP/UPEP would be the next study to order. Blood cultures would be appropriate if the pt were febrile, which he is not. A CXR may aid in evaluating other bones, but a skeletal survey would be more appropriate. To evaluate for lung cancer, which can metastasize to the bones, a CT scan of the chest would be more appropriate. Colon cancer usually does not metastasize to the bones first. Without any Hx of change in bowel habits, this test would not be high on the list. MRI may confirm a bone lesion, but in the setting of the lab abnormalities, this test would not be necessary.

25. D.

The pt is experiencing altered mental status with hallucinations and aggressive behavior after a recent hospital stay. The waxing and waning of symptoms is consistent with delirium. There are many causes of delirium, including infxn, electrolyte disturbances, and medications. Administration of sedatives, opiates, or other medications to elderly pts is particularly likely to induce delirium. Anticholinergics can exacerbate symptoms of delirium in the elderly and may cause more agitation; hence, diphenhydramine should not be given. Haloperidol is an appropriate Tx for this pt's aggressive behavior if she is a harm to herself or others, but infxn should first be ruled out and the morphine should be stopped.

26. A.

Criteria for a positive tuberculin skin testing are as follows: low-risk pts (not normally tested): >15 mm; high-risk pts (health care workers): >10 mm; and very high–risk pts (HIV, close contact): >5 mm. This pt/physician does not have HIV or a close contact with active TB, therefore an induration ≥10 mm is required for this tuberculin skin test to be considered positive. Chest radiography is required for pts with skin test conversion to evaluate for active dz. Isoniazid is only required for positive PPD. Multidrug Tx is only required for active tuberculosis. This pt's tuberculin skin test is not positive. In any case, new skin test conversions are treated with isoniazid prophylaxis, not just if symptoms develop.

27. C.

Sinus surgery for nasal polyps is not indicated because no polyps were seen on exam. The pt may have allergies, but because of difficulty breathing at night (loud snoring) and chronic mouth breathing, treating these allergies may not be enough, and an ENT should be consulted for removal of adenoids. Allergies and nasal polyps also do not explain the etiology of the neck mass. Lateral neck film was done to evaluate the size of the child's adenoid pad and how much of the nasopharyngeal airway it actually occupies. If greater than 50% of the airway is occupied by adenoid or the pt has very significant symptoms, then adenoidectomy is recommended. Osteoblastic tumor would not appear as a soft tissue mass on x-ray but instead as a bony mass.

28. B.

Children vary in activity level and food consumption as they go through stages, but the combination of this with constipation is concerning. This pt could well have infantile botulism. The parent probably followed folklore, giving the constipated child corn syrup or honey. These food additives have been linked to infantile botulism in pts younger than 1 yr. Infantile botulism can lead to acute, flaccid paralysis; because the pt may require intubation for respiratory support, the baby should be monitored in a hospital. Drooling is a developmental step, but there are more symptoms to note here that should cause a higher index of suspicion. Although constipation causes discomfort, there are more symptoms to note here that should cause a higher index of suspicion. The pt should return to the clinic if he were to develop these symptoms at home. He already is in your clinic, so admitting the pt to hospital is a better choice. Always be extra cautious in such a young infant, especially given the change in mental status. One would send for urine organic acids if one was concerned for a metabolic disorder; this is not the case in this pt.

29. C.

This pt likely has celiac sprue, which is an immune-mediated sensitivity to dietary gluten. It causes a chronic diarrhea with malabsorption due to small bowel villous atrophy. Pts may present with iron-deficiency anemia even before having malabsorptive symptoms. Pts may also have weight loss, failure to thrive, and growth retardation. A classic rash associated with celiac sprue is dermatitis herpetiformis, which is a pruritic, papulovesicular rash found commonly on the shoulders, elbows, and knees. Diagnostic tests include anti-tissue transglutaminase, antigliadin, and antiendomysial antibodies, but the definitive Dx is an endoscopy with small bowel biopsies revealing blunting of the small bowel villi. Tx is a gluten-free diet. Complications of celiac dz include intestinal lymphoma and ulcerative jejunoileitis. Hydrogen breath tests are used for the Dx of lactase deficiency and bacterial overgrowth. Although the pt could have Clostridium difficile–associated diarrhea, she does not provide a classic Hx of recent antibiotic use or hospitalization. Her symptoms and clinical features are more suggestive of celiac disease. Antidiarrheal agents usually should be avoided until a Dx is found. Additionally, they do not provide a Dx for her disease. Celiac disease is a disorder of the small bowel; therefore, the Dx will be missed with colonoscopy with biopsies.

30. A.
Follicular erythema refers to folliculitis. The other findings are seen in scarlet fever. The rash of scarlet fever usually begins on the head or neck with multiple 1–2 mm papules on top of diffuse, blanching erythema (often described as a sunburn with goose bumps). Strawberry tongue is an early finding. The rash then spreads to the trunk and then the extremities while sparing the palms and soles. Late in the course, desquamation is seen. The rash often has prominent lines of confluent petechiae found in the axilla and in the antecubital fossa, which are known as Pastia's lines.

31. E.
Adrenal crisis is the most likely Dx in this pt with a Hx of rheumatoid arthritis likely treated with corticosteroids. Hypotension and mental status changes that do not respond to fluid challenge are the hallmarks of this disease. Hyperkalemia may also be present. Immediate IV steroid administration is essential. Serum cortisol can confirm the Dx.

Fluids alone will not improve BP in pts with adrenal insufficiency. These must be administered in conjunction with corticosteroids. Whereas sepsis is a consideration, adrenal crisis is a more likely explanation for hypotension in this pt whose Hx probably included chronic corticosteroid use. Signs and symptoms that indicate congestive heart failure are not present. There is no reason to suspect abscess unless hypotension persists after adrenal insufficiency is treated.

32. C.
Cancer screening for healthy female adults includes Pap smears, mammograms, and colorectal cancer screening with colonoscopy, flex sigmoidoscopy, or stool guaiac cards. This pt has had a total abd hysterectomy and, therefore, no longer needs Pap smears (unless the pt had a Hx of abnormal cervical pathology warranting continued evaluation). Given her age, mammograms and breast exams should be performed every 1 to 2 yrs. Ovarian cancer screening is not performed due to the high false-positive rates. No combination of testing is currently recommended except in high-risk pts (e.g., FHx). Colonoscopy is warranted after the age of 50 yrs; however, the frequency is incorrect (once every 10 yrs would be correct).

33. C.

Hand–Schüller–Christian, the more chronic-progressive of the histiocytosis X syndromes, has the classic triad of exophthalmos, skull findings, and diabetes insipidus.

One can see splenomegaly with a variety of conditions, including sickle cell disease. One sees hepatomegaly with Letterer–Siwe disease (usually fatal in infants). One sees hilar prominence with a variety of diseases, including tuberculosis. Sinus involvement is not associated with histiocytosis.

34. A.

A TIA is a neurologic deficit resulting from a cerebral circulation defect. Unlike a stroke, however, in a TIA, the symptoms resolve within 24 hours. A simple partial seizure is certainly on the differential of stroke-like symptoms; the postictal state following a seizure may sometimes result in Todd's paralysis. In this case of an otherwise healthy 55-yr-old with hypercholesterolemia, a TIA is a more likely explanation of his presentation than new onset, unprovoked simple partial seizure resulting in Todd's paralysis. Hypoglycemia can produce stroke-like symptoms. However, if hypoglycemia had produced these symptoms, administration of a dextrose solution would have reversed the symptoms in less than the 12 hours described. Migraines can result in visual disturbances and dysarthria, but complete hemiparesis is uncommon.

35. B.

This pt has psoriasis, which commonly presents on extensor surfaces and with fingernail pitting. It can be associated with arthritis and is commonly identified clinically by the Auspitz Si (punctate bleeding when a psoriatic scale is scraped off) and the Koebner phenomenon (skin lesions along lines of trauma). Pts with psoriasis are treated with PUVA or immunosuppressants. Do not confuse psoriasis with sarcoidosis, which is primarily a pulmonary disease but can affect virtually any body system and can have a variety of rashes, including erythema nodosum. There are a number of causes for rashes present on palms and soles, including Rocky Mountain spotted fever, Kawasaki's disease, and other diseases. In infants, "cradle cap" (seborrheic dermatitis) can spread to the face. Intertriginous areas are affected by scabies, Candida, or tinea. Eczema is linked to asthma (the atopic pt).

36. E.

The pt is having symptoms likely related to his elevated heart rate and irregular rhythm. The irregularly irregular rhythm is indicative of atrial fibrillation. Although the exact cause is not identified, alcohol can contribute, as can hyperthyroidism or underlying valvular disease. Pts with chronic atrial fibrillation should be anticoagulated prior to attempting conversion to nml sinus rhythm, and if they cannot be converted, they need to receive long-term anticoagulation to prevent stroke. Elevated heart rate can be a Si of alcohol withdrawal; however, the pt does not have any other symptoms to support this Dx. In addition, the time frame would be unusual because symptoms usually begin in 2 to 3 days. Atrial fibrillation should not be converted without anticoagulation unless a transesophageal echocardiogram is performed to rule out the presence of an intra-atrial clot. Age is a risk factor for atrial fibrillation; however, many medical problems can lead to this arrhythmia, and the pt should be evaluated before Tx is begun. The elevated heart rate does need to be controlled; however, this does not obviate the need for anticoagulation.

37. D.

This is the classic presentation of Guillain–Barré syndrome. Typically an antecedent GI or upper respiratory illness is present, followed by steadily progressive ascending paralysis with loss of reflexes. The classic CSF finding is "cytoalbumin dissociation," which basically means high protein with few WBCs. Meningitis typically presents with headache, photophobia, neck pain, and neck stiffness. The ascending pattern of paresis and its rapid progression are not consistent with tabes dorsalis of neurosyphilis. Amyotrophic lateral sclerosis is a chronic degenerative disease and would not progress this quickly. It typically causes weakness with muscle fasciculations and often hyperreflexia.

38. D.

Pts with chickenpox (varicella zoster virus) are contagious until the lesions crust over. Parents may choose to expose their child to a contagious child, but the contagious child should not expose the other children in daycare unless asked. Ideally, this parent would not bring the child into the office because your entire practice would be exposed.

39. B.

This pt may have primary biliary cirrhosis, an autoimmune disease characterized by cholestasis resulting from destruction of the intrahepatic bile ducts. Primary biliary cirrhosis is associated with Raynaud's syndrome, scleroderma, Sjögren's syndrome, and autoimmune thyroiditis. It typically presents in middle-age women with elevated alkaline phosphatase in the early stages and elevated bilirubin and jaundice in later stages. It is diagnosed by antimitochondrial antibodies and confirmed by liver Bx. Liver transaminases (AST, ALT) are nml in this pt and would be markedly elevated in acute viral hepatitis. Significant hepatocellular damage from acetaminophen would result in elevated liver transaminases, which are not present in this pt. Hemolysis is not responsible for this hyperbilirubinemia, which is primarily direct (conjugated). Any pt with jaundice needs a complete workup to determine the etiology.

40. C.

The CAGE questions are: (1) Have you ever tried or felt the need to try to Cut down on your drinking? (2) Have you been Annoyed by people asking you about your drinking? (3) Have you ever felt Guilty about your drinking? (4) Have you ever taken an Eye opener in the morning? Answering "yes" to at least one of the four questions suggests possible alcohol dependence and/or abuse and should lead to further inquiries. Answering yes to two questions gives an 80% sensitivity to the pt having an alcohol problem. The other choices are not part of the CAGE questionnaire and therefore are incorrect.

41. A.

This pt is having a myocardial infarction, as indicated by typical signs and symptoms and positive cardiac enzymes. ECG changes are not necessary for the Dx of myocardial infarction. In this case, anemia is resulting in decreased oxygen supply to the myocardium and must be corrected immediately. While there is no consensus on a specific hemoglobin target in this setting, studies have demonstrated that pts with acute coronary syndrome are at a higher risk of myocardial damage and long-term morbidity with a hemoglobin below 11 g/dL. There is clear evidence that if the hemoglobin is <7 g/dL, pts will benefit from blood transfusion. Therefore, many clinicians would recommend that in the setting of symptomatic anemia and coronary artery disease, blood transfusions should be given with a goal of maintaining hemoglobin >10.0 g/dL although the specific target remains controversial. If BP permits, beta-blockade will decrease oxygen demand and so should also be initiated.

Thrombolytics are strictly contraindicated in this pt with recent GI bleeding. Heparin is not a good choice in a pt with recent bleeding. Coronary artery bypass grafting is not indicated acutely and cannot be performed until after coronary angiography. Lidocaine drips are not beneficial in reducing the incidence of ventricular fibrillation in pts with ectopy.

42. D.

One-hundred percent oxygen is used for acute Tx of cluster head-ache, from which this pt is suffering. Cluster headaches affect men more often than women, and the pain usually occurs around the onset of sleep. His description of pain is also consistent with this type of headache and has associated lacrimation in the eye to support the Dx. Beta-blockers are used for prophylaxis of migraine headaches. Carbamazepine is used for trigeminal neuralgia, which may cause similar pain but typically affects older adults. NSAIDs are used in migraine and tension headaches, which present with different pain symptoms. Verapamil is used for prophylaxis of cluster headaches, rather than acute Tx.

43. D.

Testicular torsion should be strongly considered in this pt and therefore is a surgical emergency. Doppler Utz will allow assess-ment of testicular artery flow, but surgical consultation and likely intervention should not be delayed. Delay of more than several hours in surgical decompression of testicular compression will result in infarction and will require removal of the testicle. CT will not provide additional information concerning testicular torsion.

Discharge to home with a 7-day course of ciprofloxacin for epididymitis and ibuprofen for pain describes the Tx of epididy-mitis, which may mimic testicular torsion. However, epididymitis cannot be presumed without first ruling out testicular torsion.

Admit to the hospital with pt-controlled administration of IV narcotics and vigorous hydration describes the early Tx of nephrolithiasis, which is not appropriate in this pt.

44. B.

This is likely a case of eczema or contact dermatitis. In either case, it is not appropriate to write a Rx for a steroid cream stronger than hydrocortisone 1% for use on the face because of the skin-thinning tendencies (and resultant telangiectasias) of stronger steroids. The weakest steroid that is effective should be used, particularly on the face. This question requires an understanding of the relative potencies of steroids. Steroids are categorized by class, which reflects their potency. The classes of steroids are: class I, super high potency; class II and III, high potency; class IV and V, medium potency; class VI and VII low potency. Hydrocortisone 2.5% is a group VII steroid but is too strong and would likely cause damage to the skin of the face. Triamcinolone 0.025% is a group VI steroid. Triamcinolone 0.1% is a group VI steroid but obviously too strong. Betamethasone 0.1% is a group V steroid.

45. D.

Thiazide-type diuretics decrease renal excretion of calcium. Whites and Asians are at increased risk for osteoporosis compared with African-Americans. Postmenopausal status is a major risk factor for osteoporosis. A thin build predisposes to osteoporosis, whereas obesity is protective against osteoporosis. Smoking is strongly associated with osteoporosis.

46. B.

Although it is possible that this mother has been tripping over toys, leading to bruises, or that the sock lines are indicative of regular leg swelling seen in pregnancy, one cannot afford to overlook a complication of severe pregnancy-induced HTN (PIH)—the HELLP syndrome (hemolysis, elevated liver enzymes, and low platelets). PIH progresses to this syndrome in 5% to 10% of pregnancies (more commonly in older, multiparous pts). The only cure is delivery, with supportive care as needed.

   Although abuse certainly is something one does not want to miss, having the pt admitted can afford precious time to further investigate the social setting if the medical workup is negative. Bed rest will not alleviate the problems presented by this pt. This condition has nothing to do with sunburn. Although it certainly would benefit this pt to have her children help pick up their toys, this will not address her medical situation.

47. A.

Imipramine is a tricyclic antidepressant (TCA). Agents in this class may cause fatal heart arrhythmias if taken in overdose. Fluoxetine, sertraline, and paroxetine are all selective serotonin reuptake inhibitors (SSRIs), which are excellent first-line agents for depression. Bupropion is a pure norepinephrine reuptake inhibitor. It can be used as a first-line agent except in pts with a seizure Hx.

48. C.

Chronic lymphocytic leukemia (CLL) is indolent and is not curable by chemotherapy. Most pts with this disease do not require immediate Tx; Tx should be deferred until pts develop significant symptoms. Bone marrow transplantation is not curative and is very risky in older pts. A benign, infectious condition that will resolve spontaneously describes infectious mononucleosis, a disease characterized by large, atypical lymphocytes on peripheral smear. CLL is not infectious and does not resolve spontaneously. The life expectancy in newly diagnosed CLL usually is 2 to 10 yrs, depending on stage at Dx.

49. B.

Renal artery stenosis should be strongly suspected when HTN develops at age younger than 30 yrs or older than 50 yrs. A characteristic bruit or refractory HTN makes the Dx more likely. In this female pt, the most likely cause of renal artery stenosis is fibromuscular dysplasia. Atherosclerosis is the most common cause of renal artery stenosis in older pts. Hypokalemia due to hyperaldosteronism is often observed in renal artery stenosis. Electrolyte abnormalities would not be expected in essential HTN.

Aortic coarctation is an exceedingly rare cause of secondary HTN in a person of this age.

Pheochromocytoma is a rare tumor that may cause secondary HTN but almost always is accompanied by other symptoms (tachycardia, diaphoresis, anxiety, etc.). Hyperthyroidism usually is accompanied by systemic symptoms such as weight loss, heat intolerance, and tachycardia.

50. C.

The baby is showing stranger anxiety, which is a nml stage in development that starts between 6 and 12 months. This is the point when the child realizes who his/her primary caretakers are and shies away from others who are "new" (even relatively). If neglect was suspected, in general, one would expect to see other manifestations of neglect, as well as less attachment to any figure or a general noncommittal response to any adult. The behavior does not indicate abuse. Colic, particularly in fussy babies, presents at approximately 3 wks and lasts until approximately 3 months of age.

51. D.

Viral conjunctivitis, scleritis, and angle closure glaucoma commonly present with a painful red eye. Viral conjunctivitis pts also have tearing, foreign body sensation, watery discharge, and preauricular adenopathy. Angle closure glaucoma pts have photophobia, blurry vision, and mid-dilated pupil. Pts with scleritis have severe pain with thinning of sclera (blue in appearance due to underlying choroid). Leukocoria (white pupil) is commonly seen in children with retinoblastoma and also in cataracts.

52. B.

The suspicion for malignancy should be very high in this pt with extensive weight loss and smoking Hx. Chest CT is reasonable when the suspicion of lung cancer is very high.

Routine screening by chest radiography of pts who smoke has not been shown to be effective in the early detection of lung cancer and does not improve outcomes or Px. Full-body CT is unnecessary in this pt until lung cancer is ruled out with chest CT. Antibody tests for antibodies associated with paraneoplastic syndromes are expensive and not indicated at this time.

53. A.

This woman has the psychiatric and neurologic manifestations of Wilson's disease. Her eye exam is notable for golden-brown rings known as Kayser–Fleischer rings. Redness of the conjunctiva of one eye and pressing of the lower lid against the globe produces a bulge above the point of compression describe chemosis, edema of the conjunctiva that is shown as a bulge when one uses the lower lid to press against it. A raised, subconjunctival fatty structure growing in a horizontal band toward the pupil describes a pterygium, an inflammatory structure forming secondary to chronic eye irritation, such as from wind and dust. Visible dots in the cornea are found in Fanconi syndrome, which results in cystine deposits in the cornea without an inflammatory component. A gray band of corneal opacity 1.5 mm wide that is separated by a clear zone from the limbus describes arcus senilis, a nml finding in the elderly.

54. B.

The pt in this case has pituitary apoplexy, a condition that occurs when there is sudden impairment in neurologic, endocrine, or neuro-ophthalmic function after a sudden hemorrhage into an existing pituitary adenoma. Often the pt will not have known that he or she had an adenoma prior to the apoplectic event. In this situation, her hypotension is likely due to acute adrenal insufficiency from ACTH deficiency secondary to the acute hemorrhage. As a result, before any further therapeutic or diagnostic measures are undertaken, IV glucocorticoids should be given in stress dose amounts (e.g., 100 mg IV hydrocortisone every 8 hours). IV pressor agents would not be the initial way to manage a pt with hypotension either with sepsis (IV fluids first) or in a case of apoplexy. Although the pt likely needs an urgent decompression of the hemorrhage in order to relieve the pressure on the optic chiasm, undergoing surgery in a pt who likely has acute adrenal insufficiency could be catastrophic. Checking the pituitary hormones is important in order to evaluate the functionality of the adenoma; however, this would not take precedence in the emergent situation of acute adrenal insufficiency. Given the CT findings of a pituitary mass and hemorrhage, sepsis is not the cause of her hypotension.

55. D.

A pt with a lumbar compression fracture has a Dx of osteoporosis regardless of her bone mineral density results. The best Tx for this pt that has been proven to reduce future fracture rates in lumbar and hip areas is bisphosphonates. Estrogen Tx would not be a prudent choice even though it does prevent further fractures. Estrogen Tx has been shown to increase the risk of cardiovascular disease, and in this pt who smokes and has a Hx of cardiovascular disease, it should not be given. Calcitonin is sometimes used for bone pain in the acute event; however, the effects of this may wear off with chronic use, and calcitonin is considered second-line Tx. Running and jogging should not be prescribed immediately after a lumbar fracture because this may predispose this pt to further fractures. While exercising against gravity is a good way to improve bone health, this should be done in a way that minimizes high-impact stressors to the pt. As mentioned earlier, although the BMD results are not consistent with osteoporosis, this pt has osteoporosis given her L1 compression fracture and should be started on Tx.

56. A.

Erythrasma is an intertriginous infxn caused by a Corynebacterium, which fluoresces coral-red under Wood's lamp. It is otherwise difficult to distinguish this infxn from tinea cruris or Candida. Tinea versicolor does not cause intertriginous infections. Malassezia furfur is a species name of the organism that causes tinea versicolor.

57. C.

Asplenic pts are less effectively able to control infections from encapsulated organisms such as Streptococcus pneumoniae. Therefore, this pt would be an appropriate recipient of the vaccine, even given his young age. The 50-yr-old pt is not at high risk. The age cutoff is age 65+. The medical student is not at high risk, even though he works with pts. Being below the age cutoff and having well-controlled HTN are not risk indications for the vaccine. Travel to Afghanistan does not warrant administration of the vaccine.

58. D.

This pt is suffering from polycystic ovarian syndrome, the most common cause of androgen excess and hirsutism. For a pt who hopes to become pregnant, weight loss is the first step in improving the androgen excess and its associated effects. One expects the LH/FSH ratio to be approximately 3:1. In pts who do not desire to become pregnant, hormonal contraceptives can help interrupt the feedback cycle, leading to decreased LH production.

Glucocorticoids are used for congenital adrenal hyperplasia, in which case the DHEA would have been elevated. Mineralocorticoids have no role in this pt. Surgery would be indicated if a tumor, such as a Sertoli-Leydig cell tumor (causing testosterone secretion but decreased LH/FSH), was present.

 B.

These structures are known as the "unhappy triad" and often are injured during football games. High-impact force to the lateral knee stretches the structures that provide stability to the medial knee: the anterior cruciate ligament (ACL), medial collateral liga-ment (MCL), and medial meniscus. The anterior drawer Si indicates likely ACL injury and is present in this pt.

Posterior cruciate ligament is more often injured during bent-knee trauma such as motor vehicle accidents. The posterior drawer Si is present rather than the anterior drawer Si. The lateral collateral ligament and lateral meniscus are unlikely to be dam-aged by trauma to the lateral knee. They are injured less often than the medial structures. Damage to both collateral ligaments is rare during a single injury. The lateral collateral ligament is the least-injured knee ligament because it is under less tension than the MCL.

 E.

This pt has signs and symptoms that are highly suggestive of ruptured AAA. In hemodynamically unstable pts with symptoms suggestive of ruptured AAA, immediate surgical intervention is essential and should not be delayed for radiologic evaluation. In hemodynamically stable pts, immediate CT occasionally is obtained in consultation with the surgical service in order to plan emergent AAA repair. However, this pt is clearly hemodynamically unstable, and surgery should not be delayed. It would not be appropriate to delay the surgical management of this condition for orthostatics or lab work-up as this pt is hemodynamically unstable.

 A.

This pt is having a myocardial infarction, as indicated by typical signs and symptoms and positive cardiac enzymes. ECG changes are not necessary for the Dx of myocardial infarction. In this case, anemia is resulting in decreased oxygen supply to the myo-cardium and must be corrected immediately. While there is no consensus on a specific hemoglobin target in this setting, studies have demonstrated that pts with acute coronary syndrome are at a higher risk of myocardial damage and long-term morbidity with a hemoglobin below 11 g/dL. There is clear evidence that if the hemoglobin is <7 g/dL, pts will benefit from blood transfusion. Therefore, many clinicians would recommend that in the setting of symptomatic anemia and coronary artery disease, blood transfusions should be given with a goal of maintaining hemoglobin >10.0 g/dL although the specific target remains controversial. If BP permits, beta-blockade will decrease oxygen demand and so should also be initiated.

Thrombolytics are strictly contraindicated in this pt with recent GI bleeding. Heparin is not a good choice in a pt with recent bleeding. Coronary artery bypass grafting is not indicated acutely and cannot be performed until after coronary angiography. Lidocaine drips are not beneficial in reducing the incidence of ventricular fibrillation in pts with ectopy.

62. C.

The two most important risks of breast cancer are age and gender. Risk is also related to hormone exposure and having a first pregnancy at greater than 30 yrs old. Her risk would be increased because of this factor. An early age for onset of menarche (<11 yrs old) is considered an increased risk factor. Late menopause (>50 yrs old) is an increased risk factor. Caffeine intake dose not impact breast cancer risk. The pt's FHx is not significant enough to increase her risk. There is no suggestion of an autosomal dominant pattern, and no Hx of a first-degree relative with breast cancer is given.

63. A.

This man likely has hepatic encephalopathy as indicated by the H&P. The presence of asterixis helps to distinguish a metabolic disturbance from a neurologic disturbance. The main use for an ammonia level here is to follow its downward course with Tx rather than for diagnostic purposes. CT scan would be best for diagnosing a hemorrhagic stroke. EEGs are better used for diagnosing seizures. Portable CXR might be able to diagnose pulmonary disease with secondary sequelae of mental status changes but would not explain the tremors or asterixis. EMG would be indicated if the pt had noted muscular weakness.

64. E.

Criteria for receiving influenza vaccine include age >50 yrs, presence of heart disease/lung disease, and those who work in high-risk environments, such as health care workers. This pt fulfills both the age cutoff and the pulmonary disease criteria. Controlled HTN would not place her at risk and is not a criterion for the vaccine. The 25-yr-old medical student would qualify if not for her allergy; the vaccine is made in eggs and is contraindicated in those with a chicken egg allergy. Well-controlled minor asthma is not a criterion for the vaccine.

65. A.

A stroke must be ruled out. To evaluate for a potential intracranial bleed, a head CT without contrast should be performed after a quick fingerstick to rule out hypoglycemia and a seizure Hx. PET scans are used to evaluate brain activity centers and would not be appropriate in this emergent situation. EEG would be used better for nonemergent evaluation of brain activity, especially in the case of seizures. Head x-rays are no longer routinely performed because of the poor sensitivity and specificity of such a scan. Carotid Doppler Utz scans are best used for evaluating anterior blood flow going into the brain, not for intracranial flow itself.

66. B.

Always irrigate first to remove the offending material. Visual Px is directly related to duration of chemical exposure to offending material. Remove any debris, and irrigate multiple times if needed. An ophthalmologist must then be called to evaluate pt, assist with visual exam, and consult on potential treatments such as steroids.

67. C.

Visual field loss in glaucoma is insidious because pts often do not notice loss of the peripheral visual field until late in the course of the disease. Loss of the central portion of the visual fields describes a central scotoma. This may occur if there is an occipital lesion corresponding to the central portion of the visual field or if there is compression of the nerve bundles to both eyes, as the nerves corresponding to central vision are most vulnerable to extrinsic compression. Optic neuritis will also classically cause a central scotoma.

Monocular blindness explains a lesion of one optic nerve. Bitemporal hemianopsia is the classic presentation of a lesion of the optic chiasma, such as from a pituitary tumor. Loss of the right upper quadrant of both visual fields is the result of a lesion of the left temporal lobe, where the optic radiations corresponding to the right upper quadrant visual field travel.

68. A.

Iron-deficiency anemia in adults must be assumed to result from occult GI bleeding until proved otherwise. Colorectal cancer is an important cause of iron-deficiency anemia that should be ruled out by colonoscopy in this pt. Even if upper endoscopy reveals a possible source of bleeding, colonoscopy should also be performed to evaluate for iron-deficiency anemia. Because bleeding is likely to be intermittent, stool guaiac testing is insufficient to rule out colorectal cancer. Iron replacement alone does not evaluate the cause of bleeding. Bone marrow Bx is unnecessary for the Dx of iron-deficiency anemia. Abd CT is insensitive for the detection of colorectal cancer unless it has metastasized to the liver or outside the bowel lumen.

69. B.

It is accurate to state that febrile seizures occur most often as the temperature is rising and can be a presenting Sx of an illness. Since his temperature is already high, he is less likely to have a febrile seizure. It is important to remember that although febrile seizures most often occur at the beginning of an illness (in the first day) as the child's temperature rises, febrile seizures can happen also as the temperature declines. Acetaminophen and ibuprofen are fine adjuvants and may make the child more comfortable, but placebo control trials have not shown evidence that antipyretics can prevent febrile seizures. Aspirin should only be given under doctor's orders (as in the case of Kawasaki's syndrome). Many children are drowsy after a seizure; this has no known prognostic value.

70. C.

aSx gallstones are common, and the vast majority of pts with them will not develop pain or other symptoms. However, there is a 2% to 3% yearly risk and 20% lifetime risk of developing biliary colic. Surgical intervention is not necessary unless symptoms arise.

71. E.

This pt has symptoms and examination findings that are classic for aortic stenosis (AS). Digitalis may be effective for mild AS, but surgery is required for anything more than mild disease. Pts with severe AS require surgical valve replacement or, if unable to tolerate surgery, percutaneous balloon valvuloplasty. Echocardiography is useful to confirm the Dx of AS prior to referral to a cardiac surgeon.

This pt does not have evidence of endocarditis. In any case, blood cultures rather than echocardiography are the gold standard for Dx of endocarditis. Beta-blockade is contraindicated in symptomatic AS because it will likely increase symptoms by decreasing cardiac output. Afterload reduction with an ACE inhibitor will also exacerbate symptoms in AS, because vasoconstriction is required to preserve adequate BP. This pt is too severely symptomatic for digitalis to result in any significant improvement.

72. C.

This pt has porphyria cutanea tarda, which is characterized by blistering, increased hair on temples and cheeks, and no abd pain. The disease is transmitted via an autosomal dominant pattern, thus the similarity in her siblings. The urine of these pts fluoresces an orange-pink color under the Wood's lamp as a result of increased uroporphyrins. A skin Bx, which is often the gold standard for Dx in dermatology, would not be helpful in this case. Pemphigus vulgaris has immunofluorescence surrounding epidermal cells, showing a "tombstone" pattern; immunofluorescence in bullous pemphigoid shows a linear band around the basement membrane, with increased eosinophils in the dermis. Therefore, a skin Bx with immunofluorescence would not be helpful in this case. Although some dermatologic conditions have known chromosomal abnormalities, Dx usually is obtained clinically or through Bx and only confirmed by chromosomal analysis. Urine porphobilinogen is the test for acute intermittent porphyria, which is associated with abd pain.

73. A.

Factors to balance here are (a) confidentiality to the daughter and (b) maintaining therapeutic trust between doctor and father. This choice provides the best balance between these two conflicting needs. A doctor is not required by law to tell the parents everything (although some states require parental consent for a minor who wishes an abortion). Although patient–doctor confidentiality can only be broken by order of a judge or in cases where someone's life is in immediate danger, lying to the father does not maintain the trust between the doctor and the father. Telling the father that the pt is pregnant response violates the confidentiality of the pt. Calling in a family counselor does not uphold trust with the father and serves no purpose except to pressure the daughter to reveal her pregnancy.

74. C.

The first step in the evaluation of hypercalcemia is to determine whether it is a PTH-dependent or -independent hypercalcemia. The most likely cause in this young female without a FHx of hypercalcemia or kidney stones is primary hyperparathyroidism due to a parathyroid adenoma. A high or inappropriately nml PTH level would be typical of a pt with primary hyperparathyroidism. A urinary calcium would help distinguish a parathyroid adenoma from another PTH-dependent disease (e.g., familial hypocalcuric hypercalcemia [FHH]). If the pt did have an evaluation that led to the Dx of parathyroid adenoma, then surgery would be indicated. While observation is a possibility in a pt with very mild hypercalcemia due to parathyroid adenoma or FHH, a Dx should still be made because the differential and Tx differ drastically if this is a PTH-independent disease, in which case diseases like sarcoidosis, hypercalcemia of malignancy, and vitamin D toxicity would be on the differential. Treating hypercalcemia with a loop diuretic may be an option for severe hypercalcemia during a hospitalization; however, in this case, there is no Dx, and it is certainly not severe hypercalcemia. A thiazide diuretic would decrease urinary calcium at the expense of increasing her serum calcium. In any event, this would not be the next choice for the pt described here without a clear Dx.

75. D.

During a typical pregnancy, the dose of thyroid medication often requires a 33% increase in total dose. Her TSH should be checked within 6 wks of conception and rechecked during regular intervals to keep the TSH within the nml range and, if possible, in the low-nml range. Maternal complications are rare but are seen with severe hypothyroidism, including placental abruption, pre-eclampsia, increased rate of caesarian section, and postpartum hemorrhage. Additionally, high TSH levels are associated with lower intelligent quotients in the future for the child. In Graves' disease, antithyroid medication can be lowered and sometimes tapered completely off. Her thyroid medication requirements will likely be increased during the end of the first trimester into her second trimester, not after she delivers.

INDEX

Page numbers followed by *f* refer to figures; page numbers followed by *t* refer to tables.

A

AAA. *See* Abdominal aorta aneurysms
Abandonment, 486t
ABCDE diagnosis, 148–152, 151f, 414t
Abdomen surgery, 158–159, 158f–160f
Abdominal aorta aneurysms (AAA), 208, 211f
   rupture of, 209
Abdominal infection, 125t
ABG. *See* Arterial blood gas
ABI. *See* Ankle–brachial index
α-blockers, 3t
Abortion, 241–242
   chromosomal abnormalities causing, 241
   completed, 242t
   definition of, 241
   incomplete, 242t
   inevitable, 242t
   missed, 242t
   recurrent, 242t
   risk factors of, 241
   threatened, 242t
   types of, 242t
   vaginal bleeding with, 241
Abscess, 378, 397
   amebic, 67
   bacterial, 67
   Bezold's, 275
   dermatology, 397
   hepatic, 67
   peritonsillar, 313
   retropharyngeal, 314–316
   subperiosteal, 275
Absence, 382, 383t
Abuse. *See also* Child abuse
   sexual, 301
   substance, 303
Acantholysis, 389
Acanthosis nigricans, 408–410, 413f
Accountable Care Organizations (ACO), 493
ACE. *See* Angiotensin-converting enzyme
Acetaminophen, 471t
Achalasia, 165
Achilles tendonitis, 343
Achondroplasia, 495
Acid-base disorder, 128
ACL. *See* Anterior cruciate ligament tear
Acne, 396
ACO. *See* Accountable Care Organizations
ACOG. *See* American College of Obstetricians
   and Gynecologist
Acoustic neuroma, 310t
Acquired immunodeficiency syndrome (AIDS),
   324–328
   epidemiology of, 324
Acromegaly, 79
ACS. *See* Acute coronary syndrome
ACTH. *See* Adrenocorticotropic hormone

Acting out, 358
Acute adrenal crisis, 85
Acute coronary syndrome (ACS), 4
   occurrence of, 4
   risk stratification for, 8t
Acute dystonia, 355t
Acute endocarditis, 35
   causes of, 35
Acute lymphoblastic leukaemia (ALL), 121–122
Acute myelogenous leukemia (AML), 122
Acute pancreatitis, 172–173
   causes of, 172
   classic physical findings, 172
   complications of, 173
Acute renal failure (ARF), 70
   causes of, 70
   characteristics of, 71t
   definition of, 553
   postrenal, 70
   prerenal failure, 70
Acute respiratory distress syndrome (ARDS), 40,
   42–45, 45f, 154
Acute stress disorder, 357. *See also*
   Posttraumatic stress disorder (PTSD)
Acute tubular necrosis (ATN), 70, 71
   causes of, 71
Addison's disease, 84
   causes of, 84
Adenocarcinoma, 47t
Adenoiditis, 280, 282f
Adenoma sebaceum, 295
Adenomyosis, 255
Adenosine diphosphate (ADP), 142
ADH. *See* Antidiuretic hormone
ADHD. *See* Attention-deficit hyperactivity disorder
Adjustment disorder, 369
Adie syndrome, 495
Adolescence
   anorexia nervosa, 304
   confidentiality, 304
   eating disorders, 304
   epidemiology, 303–304
   HEADSSS assessment, 304
   injuries, 303
   morbidity in, 303
   screening, 304
   sex, 303
   substance abuse, 303
   suicide, 303
ADP. *See* Adenosine diphosphate
Adrenal cortical hyperfunction, 86
Adrenal disorders, 84–86
   adrenal cortical hyperfunction, 86
   adrenal insufficiency, 84–86
   adrenal medulla, 86
   Cushing's syndrome, 84, 85f
Adrenal hyperplasia, 258t

Adrenal insufficiency, 84–86
Adrenal medulla, 86
    pheochromocytoma, 86
Adrenergics, 450t
Adrenocorticotropic hormone (ACTH), 84
Adrenoleukodystrophy, 495
Adult respiratory distress syndrome (ARDS),
    42, 44, 45f, 457t
Advance directives, 488
Advanced maternal age (AMA), 233
Advanced Trauma Life Support (ATLS), 151
A-fib. See Atrial fibrillation
AFP. See Alpha-fetoprotein
Age-related macular degeneration, 442
α–glucosidase inhibitors, 83t
Agoraphobia, 355–356. See also Anxiety
    disorders
AIDS. See Acquired immunodeficiency syndrome
AIN. See Allergic interstitial nephritis
Akathisia, 355t
Alanine aminotransferase (ALT), 61, 170
Albers-Schönberg disease, 495
Albinism, 405–406
Albumin-cytologic dissociation, 380
Alcohol, 367t
Alkali agents, 471t
Alkaptonuria, 495
Allergic conjunctivitis, 437t
Allergic interstitial nephritis (AIN), 70
Alpha-fetoprotein (AFP), 221
Alport syndrome, 433, 495
ALS. See Amyotrophic lateral sclerosis
ALT. See Alanine aminotransferase
Altruism, 358
Alzheimer's disease, 385–386
AMA. See Advanced maternal age
Amantadine, 387
Amaurosis fugax, 373t
Amblyopia, 431
Amenorrhea, 255–256, 366
    causes of, 256
    definition of, 256
    pregnancy causing, 256
    treatment of, 256
American College of Obstetricians and
    Gynecologist (ACOG), 233
α-methyldopa, 3t
Aminoglycoside, 323
Amitryptiline, 557
AML. See Acute myelogenous leukemia
Amnesia, 369
Amoxicillin, 271
Amphetamines, 351
Amylin analog, 83t
Amyloidosis, 458t
Amyotrophic lateral sclerosis (ALS), 388, 534
ANA. See Anti-nuclear antibody
Anal cancer, 186
    risk factors of, 186
Anal fissure, 185–186
Anemia, 111–117, 112f–113f
    hemolytic, 60, 118t, 119f
    hypoproliferative, 118t
    iron deficiency, 111–112

    megaloblastic, 116–117
    microcytic, 111–116
    normocytic, 117
    sickle cell, 115–116
    sideroblastic, 112–114
    thalassemias, 114–115
Anesthetics, 449t
Aneurysm occlusion, 204f
Aneurysms, 208–209, 210f, 211f
Angina
    pectoris, stable, 2–4
    Prinzmetal's, 10
    treatment of, 5t
    unstable, 4–5
Angiotensin-converting enzyme (ACE), 10
Angiotensin receptor blocker (ARB), 3t, 30
Angle-closure glaucoma, 438t, 445
Anhedonia, 349
Ankle–brachial index (ABI), 213
Ankle injuries, 343. See also Sports medicine
    complaints
    achilles tendonitis, 343
    ankle sprains, 343
Ankle sprains, 343
Ankylosing spondylitis, 102
Anorexia and bulimia nervosa, 366
Anorexia nervosa, 304
    child and adolescent psychiatry, 366
Anovulation, 260
Anterior cruciate ligament tear (ACL), 341t
Anterior uveitis, signs of, 441f. See also Keratitis
Antibacterials, 450t
Antibiotics, 450t
Anticholinergic, 450t, 471t
Antidiuretic hormone (ADH), 71
Anti-nuclear antibody (ANA), 98, 481
Antipsychotic-associated movement disorders, 355t
Antisocial personality disorders, 359t
Antistreptolysin O (ASO), 37
Antiviral, 450t
Anxiety disorders, 354–357. See also Psychiatry
    agoraphobia, 355–356
    generalized, 357
    obsessive–compulsive disorder, 356
    panic disorder, 354–355
    posttraumatic stress disorder, 356–357
Aorta, coarctation of, 297–299. See also
    Congenital heart disease
Aortic dissection, 209–212
Aortic regurgitation (AR), 32–34, 33t
    Corrigan's pulse, 32
    de Musset's sign, 33
    Duroziez's sign, 33
    Müller's sign, 33
    murmurs in, 32
    occurrence of, 32
    Quincke's sign, 32
    signs of, 32–33
    Traube's sign, 32
    water hammer pulse, 32
Aortic sclerosis, 33t
Aortic stenosis (AS), 33t, 35
    occurrence of, 35
Aphasia, 373t
Aplastic anemia, 118t

Appendicitis, 162t
Apple core lesion, 166, 460t
Apraxia, 373t
APUDoma, 59
AR. See Aortic regurgitation
ARB. See Angiotensin receptor blocker
ARDS. See Acute respiratory distress syndrome
5-α-Reductase deficiency, 87t
ARF. See Acute renal failure
Argyll Robertson Pupil, 433
Argyria, 495, 496f
Aripiprazole, 354t
Arnold–Chiari malformation, 293
Arrest disorders, 237
Arsenic, 471t
Arterial blood gas (ABG), 154
Arteriovenous malformations (AVM), 502
Arthritis, reactive, 102–103
Arthropathies and connective tissue disorders,
        97–108
    Behçet's syndrome, 100
    gout, 106–108, 107f, 109f
    mixed connective tissue disease, 106
    polymyalgia rheumatica, 108
    rheumatoid arthritis, 97–98
    sarcoidosis, 104–106
    scleroderma, 103–104
    septic arthritis, 108, 127t
    seronegative spondyloarthropathy, 100–103
    Sjögren's syndrome, 100
    systemic lupus erythematosus, 98–100, 99f
Artificial tears, 437t
AS. See Aortic stenosis
ASD. See Atrial septal defect
Aseptic avascular necrosis, 284t
Asherman's syndrome, 256
ASO. See Antistreptolysin O
Aspartate aminotransferase (AST), 61, 170
Asperger syndrome, 363–364. See also Child
        and adolescent psychiatry
Aspiration pneumonia, 125t
Aspirin, 471t
Assault, 486t
AST. See Aspartate aminotransferase
Asterixis, 381
Asthma, 41t
Ataxia-telangiectasia, 496
Ataxic cerebral palsy, 388
Atelectasis, 148
Athetoid cerebral palsy, 388
ATLS. See Advanced Trauma Life Support
ATN. See Acute tubular necrosis
Atopic dermatitis, 402
Atrial ectopy, 26
Atrial fibrillation (A-fib), 26
    characteristics of, 27
    complications of, 28
    etiology of, 27
Atrial flutter, 28–29
Atrial septal defect (ASD), 296
Atrioventricular (AV), 25
Atrophic gastritis, 56–57
Attention-deficit hyperactivity disorder (ADHD),
        365

Audiogram, 312
Auricular hematoma, 477t
Auspitz sign, 400
Autism, 363–364. See also Child and
        adolescent psychiatry
Autoimmune hemolysis, 118t
Avastin, 184
AVM. See Arteriovenous malformations
A-V nicking, 444
Avoidant personality disorders, 360t
Azathioprine, 59
Azidothymidine (AZT), 172
Azithromycin, 271
Azotemia, 70, 73
AZT. See Azidothymidine

B
B_1 (Thiamine), 345t
B_2 (Riboflavin), 345t
B_3 (Niacin), 345t
B_5 (pantothenate), 345t
B_6 (Pyridoxine), 346t
B_{12} (Cyanocobalamin), 346t
Bacillary angiomatosis, 423–424
Bacterial abscesses, 455t
Bacterial conjunctivitis, 437t
Bacterial meningitis, 377t
Bacterial prostatitis, 324
Bacterial tracheitis, 277t
Baker's cyst, 339. See also Sports medicine
        complaints
Bamboo spine, 102, 102f
Banti's syndrome, 496
Barbiturates, 368t
Bariatric surgery, 186–189, 187f
Barium enema, 181
Barlow's syndrome, 32
Barrett esophagus, 165, 166
Barrett's esophagus, 319–320, 319f
Bartonella henselae, 423
Bartonella quintana, 423
Bartter's syndrome, 496
Basal cell carcinoma, 414t
Basilar skull fractures, 204–205, 205f
Bat's wing shadow, 457t
Battery, 486t
Battle's sign, 204, 205
β-blockers, 471t
B_{12} deficiency, 381
Becker's dystrophy, 110
Beckwith–Wiedemann syndrome, 496
Bee/wasp sting, 475t
Behçet's syndrome, 100
Bell's palsy, 127t
Bence-Jones proteinuria, 95
Benign cysts, 265t
Benign gynecology, 247–256
    contraception, 249–250
    endometriosis, 253–255
    HPV vaccine, 252–253
    menstrual cycle, 247–249, 248f,
        249t
    Pap smear, 250–252
    vaginitis, 253

Benign positional vertigo, 310t
Benign prostatic hyperplasia (BPH), 70, 328–329
Benign tumors, 169
Benzodiazepine, 66, 354, 357, 371, 471t
Bereavement, 350. See also Mood disorders
Berger's disease, 76t
Bernard–Soulier syndrome, 496
Bevacizumab, 184
Bezold's abscess, 275
Bifid uvula, 291
Biguanide, 83t
Bilateral hilar adenopathy, 105
Bilaterally elevated diaphragm, 459t
1° biliary cirrhosis, 61–63. See also Liver disorders
Biliary colic, 161t, 170
Bilirubin-induced neurologic dysfunction (BIND), 553
BIND. See Bilirubin-induced neurologic dysfunction
Binswanger's disease, 497
Biofeedback, 357
Biostatistics, 479–480, 479t–480t
    case-control study, 480
    clinical trial, 479
    cohort study, 480
    definition, 479t–480t
    study types, 479–480
Biotin, 346t
Bipolar disorder, 351
Birth defects, drug influencing, 219t
Bishop score, 237, 237t
Bisphosphonate, 93
Bitemporal hemianopsia, 431, 432f
Bites and stings, 125t, 475t–476t
    bee/wasp, 475t
    black widow spider, 475t
    brown recluse spider, 475t
    cats, 475t
    dogs, 476t
    human, 476t
    snake, 475t
Bitot's spots, 437t
Black widow spider bite, 475t
Blastomyces dermatiditis, 55t
Bleeding, 472
    abnormal uterine, 262
    anal, 186
    disorder, preoperative evaluation of, 142–143
    dysfunctional uterine, 257
    intracranial, 374
    lower GI, 182f
    rectal, 186
    site, 202t
    third-trimester, 243
    vaginal, 221
Blepharitis, 435t
Blistering disorders, 420–423
    bullous pemphigoid, 421
    erythema multiforme, 421
    pemphigus vulgaris, 420–421
    porphyria cutanea tarda, 421

Blizzard's syndrome, 256
Blood product replacement, surgery, 142–144
    bleeding disorder, preoperative evaluation of, 142–143
    normal hemostasis, 142
    transfusion, 143–144, 144t
Blood urea nitrogen (BUN), 70, 145
Blowout fracture, 448t
Blue bloater. See Chronic bronchitis
Blue sclera, 440
Blumer's shelf, 167
Blunting of costophrenic angles, 457t, 463f, 464f
Blunt laryngeal trauma, 477t
BMI. See Body mass index
BMT. See Bone marrow transplantation
BNP. See Brain natriuretic peptide
Body dysmorphic disorder, 362. See also Somatoform disorder
Body mass index (BMI), 186, 344
Body surface area (BSA), 154, 155f
    in burns, 155t
Bone marrow transplantation (BMT), 97
Bone tumors, 94–97, 95t
    multiple myeloma, 94–97, 96f
Bone within bone sign, 456t
Borderline personality disorders, 359t
Borrelia burgdorferi, 424
Botulism, infant, 268
Bow-leggedness. See Genu varum
BPH. See Benign prostatic hyperplasia
Bradycardia, 231
Bradykinesia, 387
Brain abscess, 125t, 378
Brain natriuretic peptide (BNP), 540
Branchial cleft cyst, 156t
Braxton Hicks contractions, 233
BRBPR. See Bright-red blood per rectum
Breast-feeding, 240
Breast surgery, 189–198
    cancer risks, 190
    gynecomastia, 190
    mammography, 198
    mastalgia, 189–190
    tumors, 191–198, 192f
Breech presentation, 238, 238f
Bright-red blood per rectum (BRBPR), 181
Broca's aphasia, 374
Bronchial carcinoid tumors, 47t
Bronchiectasis, 42t
Bronchiolitis, 275
Bronchitis, 125t
    chronic, 41t
Bronchoalveolar carcinoma, 47t
Bronze diabetes, 410–413
Brown recluse spider bite, 475t
Brudzinski's sign, 376
Brugada syndrome, 497
Brushfield spots, 293
Bruton's agammaglobulinemia, 497
Bruton's lines, 114
BSA. See Body surface area
Budd–Chiari syndrome, 68–69

Buffalo hump, 84, 85f
Bulimia nervosa, child and adolescent psychiatry, 366
Bulla, 389, 394f
Bullous myringitis, 275
Bullous pemphigoid, 421, 422f
BUN. See Blood urea nitrogen
Burkitt's lymphoma, 124
Burns, surgery, 154–155
Bursitis, 339–340. See also Sports medicine complaints
    pes anserine, 340
    prepatellar, 339

C
CABG. See Coronary artery bypass graft
CAD. See Ischemic heart disease
CADASIL (Cerebral Autosomal Dominant Arteriopathy with Sub-cortical Infarcts and Leukoencephalopathy), 497
Café-au-lait spots, 418f, 500
CAH. See Congenital adrenal hyperplasia
Caisson's disease, 497
Calcinosis, 104, 104f
Calcium pyrophosphate dihydrate (CPPD), 107
CAN. See Contrast associated nephropathy
Cancer
    anal, 186
    basal cell carcinoma, 414t
    breast, 347t
    cervical, 264–265, 326t
    cervix, 347t
    colon, 183–184, 347t
    cutaneous T-cell lymphoma, 415t
    Kaposi's sarcoma, 415t
    malignant melanoma, 414t
    parenchymal lung, 47t
    prostate, 200–201, 201f, 329
    skin, 414t–415t, 415f–417f
    squamous cell carcinoma, 414t
    vaginal, 266
    vulvar, 266
Candida, 429t
CAP. See Community-acquired pneumonia
Capillary hemangioma, 446
Carbamazepine, 383, 384t
    bipolar disorder treated with, 351
    birth defects due to, 219t
    seizure therapy with, 383t
Carbon monoxide, 471t
    poisoning, 380–381
Carbonic anhydrase inhibitors, 451t
Carbuncle, 397, 397f
Carcinoembryonic antigen (CEA), 47t, 184
Carcinoid syndrome, 35, 59
    occurrence of, 59
Cardiology, 1–38
    acute coronary syndrome, stratification for, 8t
    angina treatment, 5t
    cardiomyopathy, 31
    congestive heart failure, 30–31
    EKG findings and arrhythmias, 10–30

hypercholesterolemia, therapy for, 6t
hypertension, 1–2, 1t–4t
ischemic heart disease, 2–10
    myocardial infarction, evolution of, 9f
    pericardial disease, 37–38
    P-QrS-T complex, 10, 11f–24f
    unstable angina, 7t
    valvular disease, 31–37
Cardiomyopathy, 31, 31t
Cardiopulmonary Resuscitation (CPR), 489
Caroli's disease, 497
Carotid atheroma, 373
Carotid body tumor, 156t
Carotid Doppler ultrasound, 453t
Carotid vascular disease, 215–216
Carpal tunnel syndrome, 337–338
Case control study, 480
Cat bite, 475t
Cataract, 440
Catheterization, 8t
Cat-scratch disease, 423
Cauda equina syndrome, 332t, 333
Causation, 486t
Cavernous hemangioma, 445
Cavity, 458t, 467f
CBD. See Common bile duct
CBT. See Cognitive behavioral therapy
CCP. See Cyclic citrullinated peptides
CEA. See Carcinoembryonic antigen
Cellulitis, 126t, 397
Central alveolar hypoventilation. See Pickwickian syndrome
Central pontine myelinolysis, 380. See also Demyelinating diseases
Central venous pressure (CVP), 148
Cephalosporin, 53, 323
Cerebral infarction, 375f
Cerebral palsy, 388
    ataxic, 388
    athetoid, 388
    dyskinetic, 388
    spastic, 388
Cerebrospinal fluid (CSF), 52, 152, 289, 376
Cerebro vascular accidents (CVA), 216
Cervical cancer, 264–265
    risk factors of, 264
    signs and symptoms of, 265
Cervical intraepithelial neoplasia (CIN), 250
Cervical lymphadenitis, 157t
CFU. See Colony-forming units
CGD. See Chronic granulomatous disease
Chadwick's sign, 218
Chagas disease, 165
Chalazion, 435t
Chancroid, 327t
Charcot–Marie–Tooth disease, 498
Charcot's triad, 171
Chédiask-Higashi syndrome, 498
Cheilosis, 346t
Chemical burns, 447t
Cherry-red spot on macula, 444
Cheyne–Stokes respirations, 205, 498
CHF. See Congestive heart failure

Child abuse, 299–303. See also Trauma
  burns, 301
  classic findings of, 301
  epidemiology of, 299
  injury, 299
  sexual abuse, 301
  signs and symptoms of, 299
  skeletal survey in, 300f
  treatment of, 301
Child and adolescent psychiatry, 363–366
  anorexia nervosa, 366
  Asperger syndrome, 363–364
  attention-deficit hyperactivity disorder, 365
  autism, 363–364
  bulimia nervosa, 366
  conduct disorder, 364–365
  depression, 364
  oppositional defiant disorder, 364–365
  psychological testing, 363
  separation anxiety, 364
  Tourette's disorder, 365–366
Child Protective Services (CPS), 299
Chip fracture, 301
Chlamydia, 200, 219
Chlamydia psittaci, 54t
Chlamydophila pneumoniae, 54t
Chlamydia trachomatis, 260, 275, 553
Chloasma. See Melasma
Chlorpromazine, 354t
Chocolate cysts, 255
Cholangitis, 126t, 161t
  ascending, 171
Cholecystitis, 161t, 170–171
Choledocholithiasis, 60, 161t, 171
Cholelithiasis, 169–170
Cholinesterase inhibitors, 386
Chromium, 346
Chronic bronchitis, 41t
Chronic gastritis (Atrophic gastritis), 56–57
Chronic granulomatous disease (CGD), 498
Chronic lymphocytic leukaemia (CLL),
      122–124
  signs and symptoms of, 122
Chronic myelogenous leukemia (CML), 122
Chronic obstructive pulmonary disease (COPD),
      29, 40–42, 41t–42t, 145, 551
  asthma, 41t
  bronchiectasis, 42t
  chronic bronchitis, 41t
  emphysema, 41t
Chronic renal failure, 73
Ciguatera, 473
Cilostazol, 213
Ciprofloxacin, 450t
CIN. See Cervical intraepithelial neoplasia
Circinate balanitis, 103
Cirrhosis, 63–66
  ascites differential diagnosis, 63t
  causes of, 63
  encephalopathy, 65
Classic Beck's triad, 37
Clavicle fracture, 335. See also Sports medicine
      complaints
Cleft lip, 291, 292f
Cleft palate, forms of, 292f

Clinical studies, 479–494
  biostatistics, 479–480
  study types, 479
Clinical trial, 479
Clomiphene, 260
Clonorchis sinensis, 172
Clostridium botulinum, 268
Clonazepam, 308t
Clozapine, 354t
Cluster headache, 307t
CML. See Chronic myelogenous leukemia
CMV. See Cytomegalovirus
CNS malignancy, 206t
Coagulation disorders, 117–120
  hypercoagulable disease, 120t
  inherited disorders, 120
  thrombocytopenia, 117, 119t, 120t
Coarctation of aorta, 293
Cobblestone mucosa, 58
Cocaine, 351
Coccidioides, 378
Coccidioides immitis, 408
Codman's triangle, 95t
Coffee bean sigmoid volvulus, 459t, 469f
Cognitive behavioral therapy (CBT), 349
Cog-wheel rigidity, 386
Cohort study, 480
Cold-agglutinin disease, 118t
Collagen vascular disease, 285–287
Collateral ligament tear, 341t
Colles. See Distal radius fracture
Colon cancer, 183–184
  epidemiology of, 183–184
  screening of, 184
Colonic polyps, 177–178
  familial adenomatous polyposis, 178
  hyperplastic polyps, 178
  Juvenile polyposis syndromes, 178
  neoplastic polyps, 177–178
  Peutz–Jeghers syndrome, 178, 179f
Colon, surgery, 177–184
  colon cancer, 183–184
  colonic polyps, 177–178
  diverticular disease, 180–181
  GI hemorrhage, 181–182, 182f
  large intestine obstruction, 182–183
  volvulus, 183
Colonic polyps, 177–178
Colony-forming units (CFU), 324
Colposcopy, 250–252
Comedonecrosis, 195
Common bile duct (CBD), 170
Common good, 486t
Community-acquired pneumonia (CAP), 53–56,
      54t–55t, 126t
  anaerobes, 55t
  atypical, 54t
  fungal pneumonia, 54t–55t
  typical bacterial, 54t
  viral, 55t
Comparative negligence, 486t
Complex regional pain syndrome (CRPS), 508
Conduct disorder, 364–365. See also Child and
      adolescent psychiatry
Condylomata lata, 413

Confidentiality, 304
Congenital adrenal hyperplasia (CAH), 88t, 258t
Congenital heart disease, 296–299
    aorta, coarctation of, 297–299
    atrial septal defect, 296
    great arteries, transposition of, 297
    patent ductus arteriosus, 299
    tetralogy of fallot, 297–299
    ventricular septal defect, 296–297
Congenital hyperbilirubinemia, 60t
Congenital hypothyroidism, 287–288. See also
        Metabolic disorder
Congenital pyloric stenosis, 295–296
Congestive heart failure (CHF), 1, 296–297, 535
    causes of, 30
    definition of, 30
    etiology of, 30
    signs and symptoms of, 30
    treatment of, 30–31
Conjugated hyperbilirubinemia, 288, 289t
Conjunctivitis, 103
Conn's syndrome, 2t, 73, 86
Consent, 486t
Contact dermatitis, 402–403
Continuous positive airway pressure (CPAP), 40,
        371, 525
Contraception, 249–250
Contractions, 221
Contrast associated nephropathy (CAN), 146
Conversion disorder, 362. See also Somatoform
        disorder
COPD. See Chronic obstructive pulmonary
        disease
Copper, 346
Copper wiring, 444
Corneal abrasion, 438t
Coronary artery bypass graft (CABG), 5t, 8
Coronary artery disease (CAD), 2
    risk factors for, 2
Corrigan's pulse, 32
Corticotropin releasing hormone (CRH), 84
Courvoisier's law, 172
Coxsackie A virus, 272t
CPAP. See Continuous positive airway pressure
CPK. See Creatine phosphate kinase
CPPD. See Calcium pyrophosphate dihydrate
CPR. See Cardiopulmonary Resuscitation
CPS. See Child Protective Services
Crabs. See Pediculosis pubis
Craniofacial abnormalities, 291–292
Craniotabes, 93
CRASH mnemonic, 286
Creatine phosphate kinase (CPK), 110
Creeping eruption. See Cutaneous larva migrans
Crescentic glomerulonephritis, 76t
CREST syndrome, 104
CRH. See Corticotropin releasing hormone
Crigler–Najjar syndrome, 60t, 553
Crohn's disease, 58–59, 58t, 176
Cronkhite–Canada syndrome, 178
Croup (Laryngotracheobronchitis), 276t, 278f
CRPS. See Complex regional pain syndrome
Cryptococcus neoformans, 55t
CSF. See Cerebrospinal fluid
CTCL. See Cutaneous T-cell lymphoma

Cullen's sign, 164, 172
Cultural medicine, 492
Culture-negative endocarditis, 36
    causes of, 36
Cupping, 491–492
Curling's ulcer, 155
Cushing's syndrome, 2t, 84, 85f
Cushing's triad, 205
Cutaneous larva migrans, 427f, 428
Cutaneous T-cell lymphoma (CTCL), 124, 415t
CVA. See Cerebro vascular accidents
CVP. See Central venous pressure
Cyanide, 472t
Cyclic citrullinated peptides (CCP), 98
Cyst, 389
    benign, 265t
    branchial cleft, 156t
    dermoid, 156t
    hydatid, 460t
    thyroglossal duct, 156t
Cystic fibrosis, 456t
Cystic hygroma, 156t
Cysticercosis, 379t, 455t
Cystinuria, 498
Cytomegalovirus (CMV), 56

D

Dacrocystorhinstomy (DCR), 440
Dacryocystitis, 435–440, 442f
Damages, 486t
Danazol, 255
Danon disease, 498
DCIS. See Ductal cancer in situ
DCR. See Dacrocystorhinstomy
Death, 488
Decongestants, 450t
Deep tendon reflex (DTR), 380, 498
Deep venous thrombosis (DVT), 45, 225, 297
Degenerative diseases, 385–388
    Alzheimer's disease, 385–386
    amyotrophic lateral sclerosis, 388
    cerebral palsy, 388
    dementia vs. delirium differential, 386t
    Huntington's chorea, 387
    multiinfarct dementia, 386–387
    Parkinson's disease, 387
    Picks's disease, 387
Delirium tremens (DT), 65
Delivery, 233–239
    abnormal labor, 236–238
        arrest disorders, 237
        indications for induction, 237
        management of, 237
        passage, 236
        passenger, 236
        power, 236
    Bishop score, 237t
    Braxton Hicks contractions, 233
    breech presentations, 238, 238f
    disseminated intravascular coagulation, 239
    initial presentation, 233–234
    postpartum hemorrhage, 238
    retained placenta, 239
    stages of labor, 234–236
    uterine atony, 239

Delusional disorder, 353t
Delusions, 352
Dementia vs. delirium differential, 386t
de Musset's sign, 33
Demyelinating diseases, 378–380
    central pontine myelinolysis, 380
    Guillain–Barré syndrome, 380
    multiple sclerosis, 378–380
Denial, 358
Dental infections, 126t, 317. See also
        Outpatient medicine
Dependent personality disorders, 360t
Depo-Provera contraception, 251t
Deposition, 486t
Depression, 356, 364. See also Child and
        adolescent psychiatry
    pharmacologic therapy for, 350t
De Quervain's tenosynovitis, 499
De Quervain's thyroiditis, 89–90
Dermatology, 389–430
    blistering disorders, 420–423
    common disorders, 399–413
    fungal cutaneous disorders, 429t, 430f
    infections, 396–399
    neurocutaneous syndromes, 418t
    parasitic infections, 424–428
    skin cancer, 414t–415t, 415f–417f
    terminology, 389, 390f–395f
    topical steroids, 396t
    vector–borne diseases, 423–424
Dermatomyositis, 110, 408
Dermographism, 403
Dermoid cyst, 156t, 446
DES. See Diethylstilbestrol
DEXA. See Dual energy X-ray absortiometry
DI. See Diabetes insipidus
Diabetes, 79–84
    type I, 79–81
    type II, 81–84, 83t
Diabetes insipidus (DI), 71
Diabetic foot, 126t
Diabetic ketoacidosis (DKA), 80
Diabetic retinopathy, 442, 443f
Diamond–Blackfan syndrome, 499
Diaphoresis, 86
Diarrhea, 320, 321t–323t
    infectious causes of, 323t
Diazepam, 385t
DIC. See Disseminated intravascular
        coagulation
Diethylstilbestrol (DES), 250
Diflorasone, 396t
DiGeorge's syndrome, 499
Digital rectal exam (DRE), 181
Digoxin, 31, 472t
Dilated small bowel, 459t, 468f, 469f
DIP. See Distal interphalangeal
Diphtheria, tetanus, pertussis (DTaP), 538
Diphyllobothrium latum, 117
Displacement, 358
Disproportionate means, 486t
Disseminated intravascular coagulation (DIC),
        45, 119t, 143, 239
Disseminated tuberculosis. See Miliary tuberculosis

Dissociative amnesia, 369
Dissociative disorder, 369
Dissociative fugue, 369
Distal interphalangeal (DIP), 554
Distal radius fracture, 336, 337f
Diverticular disease, 180–181
    characteristics of, 180
    diverticulitis, 180–181
    diverticulosis, 180
Diverticulitis, 180–181
Diverticulosis, 180
Dizygotic twins, 246
DKA. See Diabetic ketoacidosis
DNI. See Do not Intubate
DNR. See Do Not Resuscitate
Doctoring, 489–492
    cultural medicine, 492
    HEADSSS interviewing mnemonic, 489–491
    identifying abuse, 491–492
    interpreter, 492
    interview technique, 489–491, 490t
    trust in patient doctor relationship, 489
Dog bite, 476t
Donepezil, 557
Do not Intubate (DNI), 489
Do Not Resuscitate (DNR), 489
Dorsiflexion, 331
Double-wall sign on abdominal plain film, 459t
Down's syndrome, 221, 233, 292–293
    child with, 294t
Doxycycline, 53
DRE. See Digital rectal exam
Dressler's syndrome, 499
Drop attack, 373t
Drospirenone and ethinyl estradiol
        contraception, 251t
Drug abuse, 367–368. See also Psychiatry
    drug intoxications and withdrawal,
        367t–368t
Drug-induced mania, 351–352. See also Mood
        disorders
Dry eye, 451t
DT. See Delirium tremens (DT)
DTaP. See Diphtheria, tetanus, pertussis
DTR. See Deep tendon reflex
Dual energy X-ray absortiometry (DEXA), 93
Dubin–Johnson syndrome, 60t
Duchenne muscular dystrophy, 110
Ductal cancer in situ (DCIS), 195, 196f
Due care, 486t
Duke criteria, 36
Dumping syndrome, 187
Duodenal ulcer, 57–58
    H. pylori in, 57
    smoking and, 57
Durable power of attorney, 488
Duroziez's sign, 33
Duty, 486t
DVT. See Deep venous thrombosis
Dyschezia, 9
Dysfibrinogenemia, 120t
Dysfunctional uterine bleeding, 256
Dyshidrotic eczema, 404
Dyskinetic cerebral palsy, 388

Dysmenorrhea, 255
Dyspareunia, 255
Dyspepsia, 56, 318
Dysphonia, 317
Dyssomnias, 370–371
Dysthymic disorder, 350
Dystocia, 236

E
Eagle syndrome, 499
Early repolarization, 22f
Ears, nose, and throat (ENT), 306–317
    dental infection, 317
    epistaxis, 312–313
    hearing loss, 311–312
    hoarseness, 317
    inner ear disease, 310, 310t
    Lemierre's syndrome, 314
    otitis externa, 306–310, 309f
    peritonsillar abscess, 313
    pharyngitis, 313, 316t
    retropharyngeal abscess, 314–316
    sinusitis, 313, 314t
EBV. See Epstein–Barr virus
ECC. See Endocervical curettage
Echocardiography, 297
Eclampsia, 226t
ECT. See Electroconvulsive treatment
Ectopic pregnancy, 162t, 243
    differential diagnosis of, 243
    signs and symptoms of, 243
    treatment of, 243
Eczema, 402–403
Eczematous Dermatitis. See Eczema
EDC. See Estimated date of confinement
EDTA. See Ethylene diaminetetraacetic
        acid
Edward's Syndrome, 292
EGD. See Esophagogastroduodenoscopy
Ego defenses, 358–360
    acting out, 358
    altruism, 358
    denial, 358
    displacement, 358
    humor, 358
    identification, 358
    intellectualization, 358
    introjection, 358
    projection, 358
    rationalization, 360
    reaction formation, 360
    regression, 360
    sublimation, 360
    suppression, 360
Ehlers–Danlos syndrome, 499, 519, 548
Ehlers–Danlos syndrome vascular type, 499,
        500f
EKG findings, 12f–24f, 45
    arrhythmias, 10, 25–27
Eisenmenger's complex, 296
Elbow injuries, 335–336. See also Sports
        medicine complaints
    dislocation, 336
    epicondylitis, 335

olecranon bursitis, 336
    olecranon fracture, 335–336
Electroconvulsive treatment (ECT), 349
Electrolyte disorders and management, 135–138
Ellis–van Creveld, 499
Emergency medicine, 471–478
    bites and stings, 475t–476t
    ENT trauma, 476t–478t
    fish and shellfish toxins, 473t–474t
    toxicology, 471t–473t
Emphysema, 41t
Encephalitis, 127t, 378, 379t
Encephalopathy, 65
    acute, 289
Endocarditis, 35–37, 126t
    acute, 35
Endocarditis diagnosis, duke criteria for, 36t
Endocervical curettage (ECC), 252
Endocrine pancreatic neoplasm, 175
Endocrinology, 79–92
    adrenal disorders, 84–86
    diabetes, 79–84
    gonadal disorders, 86
    hypothalamic pituitary axis, 79
    multiple endocrine neoplasia syndromes, 92
    thyroid, 87–91
    thyroid malignancy, 91–92
Endometrial carcinoma, 262–264
Endometrioma, 255
Endometriosis, 253–255, 260
Endoscopic retrograde cholangiopancreatography
        (ERCP), 61, 453t, 537
Endotracheal (ET) tube, 148
ENT. See Ears, nose, and throat
Entaemoeba histolytica, 67
ENT trauma, 476t–478t
    auricular hematoma, 477t
    blunt laryngeal trauma, 477t
    facial fracture, 478t
    foreign body, 476t
    mandible fx, 478t
    nasal fx, 477t
    TM perforation, 476t
Eosinophilic esophagitis, 57
Eosinophilic granuloma, 287
Ephelis. See Freckle
Epicanthal folds, 293
Epicondylitis, 335
    lateral, 335
    medical, 335
Epididymitis, 126t, 198, 200
Epiglottitis, 277t, 279f, 280
Epistaxis, 312–313
Epithelial cell tumor, 265t
EPO. See Erythropoietin
Epstein–Barr virus (EBV), 124
Erb's paralysis, 499
ERCP. See Endoscopic retrograde
        cholangiopancreatography
Erysipelas, 397–398
Erythema infectiosum (fifth disease), 272t
Erythema multiforme, 421, 423f
Erythema nodosum, 408, 411f
Erythematous maculopapular rash, 408

Erythrasma, 399, 400f
Erythrocyte sedimentation rate (ESR), 37
Erythromycin, 437t
Erythropoietin (EPO), 49
Escherichia coli, 320, 377t
Esophageal diverticula, 165
Esophageal dysmotility, 104
Esophageal sphincter tone, 222
Esophageal tumors, 165–166
Esophagogastroduodenoscopy (EGD), 533
Esophagus surgery, 159–166
    achalasia, 165
    esophageal diverticula, 165
    esophageal tumors, 165–166
    hiatal hernia, 159–165
ESR. See Erythrocyte sedimentation rate
Essential hypertension, 1
Essential thrombocythemia, 121t
Estimated date of confinement (EDC), 219
Estrogen, 249
Ethics and law, 479–494
    abandonment, 486t
    assault, 486t
    battery, 486t
    biostatistics, 479–480, 479t–480t
    calculation of statistical values,
        480–485, 481t
    causation, 486t
    common good, 486t
    comparative negligence, 486t
    consent, 486t
    damages, 486t
    deposition, 486t
    disproportionate means, 486t
    doctoring, 489–492, 490t
    due care, 486t
    duty, 486t
    fiduciary, 487t
    futility, 487t
    good Samaritan law, 487t
    health care delivery, 492–494
    human dignity, 487t
    informed consent, 487t
    law and ethics, 485–489, 486t–487t
    privilege, 487t
    settlement, 487t
    wrongful death, 487t
Ethosuximide, 384t
Ethylene diaminetetraacetic acid (EDTA),
        114
Ethylene glycol, 472t
Evan's syndrome, 499
Ewing's sarcoma, 95t
Exanthems, 272t
Exocrine pancreas, 172–175
    acute pancreatitis, 172–173
    endocrine pancreatic neoplasm, 175
    pancreatic cancer, 175
    pancreatic pseudocyst, 173–174
Exposure desensitization, 356
Extended care facilities, 493. See also Health
        care delivery
Extracerebral hematoma, 203f
Extrapulmonary disease, 43t

Eye colors, 440
    blue sclera, 440
    blue vision, 440
    opaque eye, 440
    yellow eye, 440
    yellow vision, 440
Eyelid laceration, 447t
Ezetimibe, 6t

F
FA. See Fibroadenoma
Fabry's disease, 500
Facial fracture, 478t
Factitious disorder, 360–361
    definition of, 361
Failure to thrive (FTT), 290–291
Familial adenomatous polyposis (FAP), 178
Familial polyposis syndromes, 178
Family history (FH), 489
Family medicine. See Outpatient medicine
Fanconi's anemia, 500
Fanconi syndrome, 500
FAP. See Familial adenomatous polyposis
Farber's disease, 500
Fasciitis, necrotizing, 398–399. See also
        Infection
FAST. See Focused Assessment with
        Sonography for Trauma
FDA. See Food and Drug Administration
Febrile seizures, 289–290
Felbamate, 385t
Felty's syndrome, 501
Femoral hernia, 168, 168f
Femoral neck fracture, 339, 340f
Fenofibrate, 6t
Fetal alcohol syndrome, 296
Fetal assessment/intrapartum surveillance,
        227–233
    fetal growth, 227–228
    fetal maturity, tests of, 228–229
    fetal well-being, 228
    genetic testing, 233
    intrapartum fetal assessment, 229–232
    isoimmunization, 232–233
FHR, 228, 231, 231f
Fetal maturity, tests of, 228–229
FEV. See Forced expiratory volume
Fever
    intraoperative, 147
    postoperative, 148
FFP. See Fresh-frozen plasma
FH. See Family history
FHR. See Fetal heart rate
Fibroadenoma (FA), 190
Fibrocystic disease, 192–195, 193f–194f
Fibrolamellar CA, 501
Fibrous dysplasia, 94, 446. See also
        Nonneoplastic bone disease
    types of, 94
Fibrous histiocytoma, 446
Fibrous pseudo-lump, 195
Fiduciary, 487t
Filling defects in stomach on upper GI series, 459t
Fine-needle aspiration (FNA), 195, 537

Fingernail pitting, 400, 401f
Fish and shellfish toxins, 473t–474t
  ciguatera, 473t
  neurotoxic shellfish, 474t
  paralytic shellfish, 474t
  scombroid, 473t–474t
  tetrodotoxin, 474t
Fistula-in-ano, 185
Fitz-Hugh-Curtis syndrome, 161t, 501
Flaccid epidermal bullae, 420
Flaccid paralysis, 268
Flame hemorrhages, 444
Fluid and electrolytes, surgery with,
        138–141
  common disorders, 139–141,
        140t–141t
  fluid management, 138
  hydration of patients, 139
  physiology, 138, 139f
Fluocinonide (Lidex), 396t
Fluoroquinolone, 323
FNA. See Fine-needle aspiration
Focal segmental glomerulosclerosis, 74t
Focused Assessment with Sonography for
        Trauma (FAST), 151
Foley catheter, 176
Folic acid, 118t
Follicle-stimulating hormone (FSH), 247
Folliculitis, 396–397
Food and Drug Administration (FDA), 259
Forced expiratory volume (FEV), 40, 551
Forced vital capacity (FVC), 40, 551
Foreign body, 476t
Foreign-body aspiration, 277t
Foreign body orbital trauma, 447t
Fournier's gangrene, 200
Fraction of inspired O_2 (FIO$_2$), 40
Fracture, 332t
Fragile X Syndrome, 293
Freckle, 406
Fresh-frozen plasma (FFP), 144
FSH. See Follicle-stimulating hormone
FTT. See Failure to thrive
Fugue, 369
Fungal cutaneous disorders, 429t, 430f
  Candida, 429t
  onychomycosis, 429t
  tinea, 429t
  tinea versicolor, 429t
Furuncle, 398, 398f
Fusobacterium necrophorum, 314
Futility, 487t
FVC. See Forced vital capacity

G

Gabapentin, 384t
Galactosemia, 501
Gallbladder surgery, 169–172
  ascending cholangitis, 171
  biliary colic, 170
  cancer, 171–172
  cholecystitis, 170–171
  choledocholithiasis, 171
  cholelithiasis, 169–170

Gangrene
  dry, 212
  Fournier's, 200
Gardnerella, 253, 254f
Gardner's syndrome, 178, 501
GAS. See Group A Streptococcus
Gas in portal vein, 460t
Gasless abdomen on abdominal plain film,
        459t, 468f
Gastric tumor surgery, 166–167
Gastric ulcer (GU), 57
  H. pylori in, 57
Gastrinoma, 175
Gastritis, chronic, 56–57
Gastroenteritis, 126t, 164t, 380
Gastroenterology and hepatology, 56–70
  gastroesophageal disease, 56–57
  large intestine, 59
  liver, 59–70
  small intestine, 57–59
Gastroesophageal disease
  chronic gastritis, 56–57
  dyspepsia, 56
  eosinophilic esophagitis, 57
  gastric ulcer, 57
Gastroesophageal reflux disease (GERD), 159,
        318–320
  causes of, 318
  signs and symptoms of, 318
Gastrointestinal complaints, outpatient, 318–320
  diarrhea, 320
  dyspepsia, 318
  GERD, 318–320
Gastrointestinal hemorrhage, 181–182, 182f
Gaucher's disease, 501
GBS. See Group B Streptococcus
GDM. See Gestational diabetes mellitus
Gemfibrozil, 6t
Generalized anxiety disorder, 357
Genetic and congenital disorder, pediatrics,
        290–299
  aorta, coarctation of, 297–299
  Arnold–Chiari malformation, 293
  atrial septal defect, 296
  brushfield spots, 293
  congenital heart disease, 296–299
  congenital pyloric stenosis, 295–296
  craniofacial abnormalities, 291–293
  Down's syndrome, 292, 294f
  Edward's syndrome, 292
  failure to thrive, 291
  fetal alcohol syndrome, 293
  Fragile X Syndrome, 293
  great arteries, transposition of, 297
  neural tube defects, 293
  Patau's syndrome, 293
  patent ductus arteriosus, 297
  tetralogy of fallot, 297–299
  tuberous sclerosis, 295
  Turner syndrome, 293, 295f
  unilateral cleft lip, 291
  ventricular septal defect, 297
Genu valgum, 283, 283f
Genu varum, 281

GERD. See Gastroesophageal reflux disease
Germ cell tumor, 265t
Gestational diabetes mellitus (GDM), 223–224
    causes of, 224
    risk factors of, 223
Gestational trophoblastic neoplasia (GTN), 267
GFR. See Glomerular filtration rate
Ghon complex, 49
Giant cell tumor, 95t
GI hemorrhage, 181–182, 182f
    causes of, 181
Gilbert syndrome, 60t
Glanzmann's thrombasthenia, 501
Glasgow Coma scale, 148, 152t
Glaucoma, 444–445, 451t
    angle-closure, 445
    open-angle, 444–445
Glomerular disease, 73–75
    nephritic syndrome, 75
    nephrotic syndrome, 73–74
    urinalysis in, 75, 77t
Glomerular filtration rate (GFR), 75, 220
Glucagonoma, 175
Glucola screening test, 224
Glucose-6-phosphate dehydrogenase (G6PD), 288
Glycogenoses, 501
GNR. See Gram-negative rods
GnRH. See Gonadotropin-releasing hormone
Goiter, 157t
Goldman cardiac risk index, 145, 146t
Golfer's elbow, 335
Gonadal disorders, 86
    hypogonadism of either sex, 86, 88t
    male gonadal axis, 86, 87t
Gonadotropin-releasing hormone (GnRH), 247
Good Samaritan law, 487t
Gottron's papules, 110
Gout, 106–108, 107f, 109f
G6PD. See Glucose-6-phosphate dehydrogenase
Gradenigo syndrome, 310
Graham Steell murmur, 35
Gram-negative rods (GNR), 56
Grand mal seizure, 541
Granuloma inguinale (Donovaniasis), 327t
Grasp reflex, 373t
Grave's disease, 89f
Gravidity, 218
Great arteries, transposition of, 297–299. See also Congenital heart disease
Grey Turner's sign, 164, 172
Ground glass opacities on lung CT, 456t
Group A Streptococcus (GAS), 398
Group B Streptococcus (GBS), 221, 227
GTN. See Gestational trophoblastic neoplasia
GU. See Gastric ulcer
Guillain–Barré syndrome, 380
Guttate psoriasis, 400
Gynecology, 247–267
    benign, 247–255
    contraception, 249–250
    hirsutism, 257, 258t
    infertility, 255–260
    menstrual cycle, 247–249, 248f, 249t
        oncology, 262–267
        Pap smear, 250–252
        reproductive endocrinology, 255–260
        urogynecology, 260–262
        virilization, 257, 258t
Gynecomastia, 190

H
HAART. See Highly active antiretroviral treatment
Haemophilus influenzae, 376, 377t, 435
Hairy cell leukemia, 122, 123f
Hallucinations, 352
Haloperidol, 352, 354t
Hampton's hump, 45
Hand, foot, and mouth disease, 272t
Hand–Schüller–Christian disease, 287
HAP. See Hospital-Acquired Pneumonia
Harris–Benedict equation, 344
Harrison's groove, 93
Hartnup's disease, 501
Hashimoto's disease, 91
Hb. See Hemoglobin
HbA₁c. See Hemoglobin A₁c
HBV. See Hepatitis B virus
HCAP. See Health Care-Associated Pneumonia
hCG. See Human chorionic gonadotropin
HCV. See Hepatitis C virus
Head injury, 202–204, 261f
Headache, 306, 307t
    treatment of, 308t
Head Louse. See Pediculosis capitis
HEADSSS interviewing mnemonic, 489–491
Health Care-Associated Pneumonia (HCAP), 56
    causes of, 56
Health care delivery, 492–494
    ACO, 493
    extended care facilities, 493
    HMO, 492–493
    hospice, 493
    hospital personnel, 494
    hospitals, 492
    hospital safety, 494
    medicare/medicaid, 493
Health Maintenance Organizations (HMO), 492–493
Hearing loss, 311–312
    Alport's syndrome, 311
    conductive, 311
    diagnostic hearing tests, 311–312
    sensorineural, 311
Hegar's sign, 218
Helicobacter pylori, 318
HELLP syndrome, 226
Hemangioma, 169, 407–408, 407f
    capillary, 407
    cherry, 408
    strawberry, 408
Hemangiosarcoma, 169
Hematology, 111–125, 112f
    anemia, 111–117
    coagulation disorders, 117–120
    leukemias, 121–124
    lymphoma, 124–125
    myeloproliferative disease, 121, 121t

Hematuria, 328. See also Urogenital complaints
Hemiplegia, 373t
Hemochromatosis, 66
    causes of, 66
Hemoglobin A$_{1c}$ (HbA$_{1c}$), 82
Hemoglobin (Hb), 111
Hemolytic anemia, 60, 118t, 288
Hemolytic-uremic syndrome (HUS), 119t
Hemopericardium, 37
Hemophilia, 120
Hemophilus influenzae, 271
Hemorrhoids, 184–185
Henoch–Schönlein purpura (HSP), 76t, 287
Heparin, 472t
Hepatic abscess, 67
    causes of, 67
Hepatic adenoma, 169
Hepatic encephalopathy, 381
Hepatic tumor surgery, 169
    benign tumors, 169
    malignant tumors, 169
Hepatitis, 61, 161t
    diagnosis and treatment of, 62t–63t
Hepatitis B virus (HBV), 63, 64f
Hepatitis C virus (HCV), 63, 143
Hepatobiliary iminodiacetic acid (HIDA), 170
Hepatocellular cancer, 169
Hepatolenticular degeneration. See Wilson's
    disease
Hepatoma, 169
Hepatopulmonary syndrome, 502
Hepatorenal syndrome, 501
*Hereditary nonpolyposis colorectal cancer
    (HNPCC), 184*
Hernia sugery, 167–168, 167t
Heroin (Opioids), 368t
Herpangina, 316t
Herpes simplex virus (HSV), 325t, 379t
Herpes zoster, 127t, 306, 438t, 439f
Hesselbach's triangle, 167
HFE gene, 66
HHNK. See Hyperosmolar hyperglycemic
    nonketotic coma
HHV-8. See Human herpes virus-8
Hiatal hernia, 159–165
    types of, 159–165
HiB. See H. influenzae type B (HiB)
HIDA. See Hepatobiliary iminodiacetic acid
Hidradenitis Suppurativa, 399
High-density lipoprotein (HDL), 10
*High-grade squamous intraepithelial lesion
    (HSIL), 519*
*Highly active antiretroviral treatment (HAART),
    328*
Hilar adenopathy, 458t
H. influenzae type B (HiB), 280
Hip osteoarthritis, 339. See also Sports
    medicine complaints
Hip problems, 338–339. See also Sports
    medicine complaints
    dislocations, 339
    femoral neck fracture, 339, 340f
    hip osteoarthritis, 339
    trochanteric bursitis, 338

Hirsutism, 257, 258t
Histiocytosis X, 287
Histoplasma capsulatum, 55t
History of present illness (HPI), 489
Histrionic personality disorders, 360t
HIV. See Human immunodeficiency virus
HLA. See Human leukocyte antigen
HMO. See Health Maintenance Organizations
HNPCC. See Hereditary nonpolyposis colorectal
    cancer
Hoarseness, 317
Hodgkin lymphoma, 125
Hollenhorst plaque, 444
Holt–Oram syndrome, 502
Homocystinemia, 120t
Homocystinuria, 502
Homonymous hemianopia, 373t
Homosexuality, 369
Honeycomb lung, 456t
Hordeolum, 435t, 436f
Hormone replacement treatment (HRT), 258
Horner's syndrome, 46, 48f
Hospice, 493
Hospital, 492
    community, 492
    intermediate, 492
    safety, 494
    tertiary medical center, 492
Hospital-Acquired Pneumonia (HAP), 56
    causes of, 56
Hospital personnel, 494
Hot and Cold Theory, 492
HPA. See Hypothalamic-pituitary-adrenal
HPI. See History of present illness
HPL. See Human placental lactogen
HPRT. See Hypoxanthine-Guanine
    Phosphoribosyl Transferase
HPV. See Human papilloma virus
HRT. See Hormone replacement treatment
HSIL. See High-grade squamous intraepithelial
    lesion
HSP. See Henoch–Schönlein purpura
HSV. See Herpes simplex virus
HTLV. See Human T-cell leukemia virus
Human bite, 476t
Human chorionic gonadotropin (hCG), 218
Human dignity, 487t
Human herpes virus-8 (HHV-8), 327
Human immunodeficiency virus (HIV), 324
    retinitis in, 127t
Human leukocyte antigen (HLA), 144
*Human papilloma virus (HPV), 252–253, 317,
    326t, 413*
Human placental lactogen (HPL), 224
Human T-cell leukemia virus (HTLV), 124, 510
Humor, 358
Hunter's disease, 502
Huntington's chorea, 387
Hurler's disease, 502
HUS. See Hemolytic-uremic syndrome
Hydatid cyst, 460t
Hydatidiform mole, 267
Hydrocephalus, 206–208, 207f
Hydrocortisone, 147

Hydrops fetalis, 232
Hyperbilirubinemia
    conjugated, 288, 289t
    unconjugated, 288
Hypercalcemia, 94
Hypercholesterolemia, therapy for, 6t
Hypercoagulable disease, 120t
Hypercoagulable states, 45
Hyperdense tissue, 452
Hyperemesis gravidarum, 227
Hyperkalemia, 84, 136t, 135f
    evaluation of, 138
Hyperkeratosis, 389
Hypernatremia, evaluation of, 133
Hyperosmolar hyperglycemic nonketotic coma
        (HHNK), 82
Hyperparathyroidism, 188
Hyperpigmentation, 84, 223, 406–413
    acanthosis nigricans, 408–410
    bronze diabetes, 410–413
    dermatomyositis, 408
    erythema nodosum, 408
    freckle (ephelis), 406
    hemangioma, 407–408
    lentigo, 406
    melasma (chloasma), 407
    mongolian spot, 406
    nevocellular nevus, 406
    pityriasis rosea, 408
    seborrheic keratosis, 408
    xanthoma, 408
Hyperplastic polyps, 178
Hypersomnia, 371
Hypertension (HTN)
    causes of, 1
    causes of secondary, 2t
    definitions of, 1t
    essential, 1
    malignant, 1–2
    medical treatment of, 3t–4t
    treatment, 2
    treatment indications of, 1t
Hypertensive emergency, 1–2
Hypertensive urgency, 1
Hyperthyroidism, 87–90, 90
    signs and symptoms of, 87
Hypertrophic cardiomyopathy (HCM), 35
Hypertrophic obstructive cardiomyopathy, 35
Hypertrophic subaortic stenosis, 35
Hypertrophy, 27
Hyperviscosity syndrome, 95
Hyphema, 437t, 439f, 448t
Hypocalcemia, 73
Hypochondriasis, 362. See also Somatoform
        disorder
Hypodense tissue, 452
Hypogonadism, genetic, 88t
Hypokalemia, 135t
    evaluation of, 134
Hyponatremia, 84, 380
    evaluation of, 132
Hypopigmentation, 404–406
    albinism, 405–406
    pityriasis alba, 406
    vitiligo, 404–405

Hypopnea, causes of, 39
Hypoproliferative anemia, 118t
Hypothalamic deficiency, 256
Hypothalamic-pituitary-adrenal (HPA), 86
Hypothalamic pituitary axis, 79
    acromegaly, 79
    prolactinoma, 79
Hypothyroidism, 90–91
    causes of, 90
    signs and symptoms of, 90
Hypotonia, 288
Hypoxanthine-Guanine Phosphoribosyl
        Transferase (HPRT), 504
Hypoxemia
    causes of, 38–40
    DDx, 38
    mechanisms of, 38t
    presentation of, 40
    Tx, 40
Hysterectomy, 264
Hysterosalpingogram, 260

I

IBW. See Ideal body weight
Ice-cream scoop falling off cone, 285t
ICF. See Intermediate care facilities
ICP. See Intracranial pressure
IDC. See Invasive ductal cancer
Ideal body weight (IBW), 344
Identification, 358
Idiopathic hypertrophic subaortic stenosis, 35
Idiopathic myelofibrosis, 121t
Idiopathic thrombocytopenic purpura (ITP), 119t
IFN-γ. See Interferon-γ
IgG. See Immunoglobulin G
IGT. See Impaired glucose tolerance
IMA. See Inferior mesenteric artery
I-MIBG. See Iodine
        131-metaiodobenzylguanidine
        (I-MIBG)
Immunoglobulin G (IgG), 232
Immunization, 273f–274f
Impaired glucose tolerance (IGT), 82
Impetigo, 396
    crusted bullous, 397f
Impotence, 330–331. See also Urogenital
        complaints
    causes of, 330
    occurrence of, 330
    treatment of, 330–331
Impulse-control disorders, 369–370
    intermittent explosive disorder, 369–370
    kleptomania, 370
    pyromania, 370
    trichotillomania, 370
Inactivated poliovirus (IPV), 538
Incontinentia pigmenti, 502
Independent Practice Association (IPA), 492,
        493
Indomethacin, 299
Infant botulism, 268. See also Pediatrics
Infection, 332t, 396–399
    acne, 396
    empiric antibiotic treatment for, 125t–127t
    erythrasma, 399

folliculitis, 396–397
  hidradenitis suppurativa, 399
  impetigo, 396
  scarlet fever, 399
  SubQ infection, 397–399
Inferior mesenteric artery (IMA), 209
Inferior surface rib notching, 456t
Inferior vena cava (IVC), 46
Infertility, 259–262
  anatomic disorder, 260
  anovulation, 260
  causes of, 259
  definition of, 259
Infiltrative ophthalmopathy, 88, 89f
Inflammation, 52, 58t, 89, 438t, 456t
  infection and, 376–378
  palpebral, 435t
  tear duct, 435, 440
Inflammatory bowel disease, 58–59
  comparison of, 58t
Informed consent, 487t
Inguinal hernia, 167–168, 168f
Inherited disorders, 120
Inner ear disease, 310, 310t
Insomnia, 370–371
Insulinoma, 175
Interferon-γ (IFN-γ), 52
Intermediate care facilities (ICF), 493
Intermittent explosive disorder, 369–370
Internal medicine
  cardiology, 1–38
  endocrinology, 79–92
  gastroenterology and hepatology, 56–70
  hematology, 111–126, 112f
  musculoskeletal disorders, 93–111
  nephrology, 70–79
  pulmonary, 38–56
Internuclear ophthalmoplegia, 431
Interpreter, 492
Interstitial fibrosis, 43t
Interview technique, 489–491, 490t
Intestinal lymphangiectasia, 323t
Intracranial bleeding, 374
Intracranial hemorrhage, 202t, 203f–204f
Intracranial pressure (ICP), 151, 306, 378
Intraductal Hyperplasia, 195
Intraductal Papilloma, 195
Intrahepatic cholestasis, 60
  causes of, 60
Intraocular pressure (IOP), 444
Intrapartum fetal assessment, 229–232
Intrapartum surveillance, 227–233
  fetal growth, 227–228
  fetal maturity, tests of, 228–229
  fetal well-being, 228
  genetic testing, 233
  intrapartum fetal assessment, 229–232
  isoimmunization, 232–233
Intrauterine device contraception, 251t
Intrauterine growth retardation (IUGR), 229
Intrauterine pressure catheter (IUPC), 235
Intravenous pyelogram (IVP), 453t
Introjection, 358
Intussusception, 162t
Invasive ductal cancer (IDC), 195, 196, 197f

Invasive lobular cancer, 196, 199f
Inverse psoriasis, 400
Iodine, 157t
Iodine 131-metaiodobenzylguanidine (I-MIBG),
    86
IOP. See Intraocular pressure
IPA. See Independent Practice Association
IPV. See Inactivated poliovirus
IRAK-4 deficiency, 503
Iron, 472t
Ischemia, 20f, 27
Ischemic heart disease (CAD)
  acute coronary syndrome, 4
  NSTEMI, 5–7
  Prinzmetal's angina, 10
  risk factors for, 2
  stable angina pectoris, 2–4
  ST Elevation MI, 7–10
  unstable angina, 4–5
Isoimmunization, 232–233
Isoniazid, 472t
Isosorbide dinitrate, 31
Isovalinic acidemia, 503
ITP. See Idiopathic thrombocytopenic purpura
IUGR. See Intrauterine growth retardation
IUPC. See Intrauterine pressure catheter
IVC. See Inferior vena cava
Ivermectin, 428
Ivory vertebral body, 456t
IVP. See Intravenous pyelogram; IV pyelogram
IV pyelogram (IVP), 323

J
Janeway lesions, 36
Jaundice, 59–61
  congenital hyperbilirubinemia, 60t
  extrahepatic, 60–61
  hemolytic anemia, 60
  intrahepatic cholestasis, 60
  occurrence of, 59
JCAHO. See Joint Commission on Accreditation
    of Healthcare Organizations
Jervell and Lange-Nielsen syndrome, 503
Job's syndrome, 503
Joint Commission on Accreditation of Healthcare
    Organizations (JCAHO), 494
Jugular venous pressure (JVP), 30
Juvenile polyposis syndromes, 178
Juvenile rheumatoid arthritis, 285–286
  types of, 286t
JVP. See Jugular venous pressure

K
Kallmann's syndrome, 88t
Kaposi's sarcoma, 327, 415t
Kasabach–Merritt, 503
Kawasaki's disease, 285–287
Kayser–Fleischer ring, 381, 382f, 433, 559
Keflex, 440
Keloid, 389, 395f
Keratitis, 438t, 439f–441f
Keratoconjunctivitis (Sjögren's disease), 437t
Keratoderma blennorrhagicum, 103
Kerley B lines, 457t, 465f
Kernig's sign, 376

Keshan's disease, 503
Kidney, ureter, bladder x-ray (KUB), 453t
Klatskin's tumor, 172
Klebsiella pneumoniae, 54t
Kleptomania, 370
Klinefelter's syndrome, 87t, 190
Klippel–Trénaunay–Weber syndrome, 503
Klumpke's paralysis, 503
Knee injuries, 341t
Knee problems, 339–341, 341t. See also Sports
    medicine complaints
    Baker's cyst, 339
    bursitis, 339–340
    ligament injuries, 340–341
Knock-knees. See Genu valgum
Köbner's phenomenon, 400
Krukenberg tumor, 166
KUB. See Kidney, ureter, bladder x-ray
Kussmaul hyperpnea, 80

L
Labor/delivery, 233–239
    abnormal, 236–238
    Braxton Hicks contractions, 233
    breech presentations, 238, 238f
    initial presentation, 233–234
    postpartum hemorrhage, 238–239
    stages, 234–236, 234f
    stages of, 234–236
Labyrinthitis, viral, 310t
Lactase deficiency, 322t
Lactation, 240
Lacunar infarct, 373
LAE. See Left atrial enlargement
LAFB. See Left anterior fascicular block
Lambert–Eaton syndrome, 48, 111
Lamotrigine, 384t
Laplace's law, 209
Large cell carcinoma, 47t
Large intestine, 59
    obstruction, 182–183
        causes of, 182
        signs and symptoms of, 182
Larva currens, 428
Laryngomalacia, 280, 281f
Larynx, 317
Last menstrual period (LMP), 219
Lateral collateral ligament (LCL), 340
Lateral decubitus chest plain film, 453t
Laurence–Moon–Biedl syndrome, 88t, 444
Law and ethics, 485–489, 486t–487t
    advance directives, 488
    beneficence, 488
    confidentiality, 488
    death, 488
    DNR orders, 489
    informed consent, 485–487
    malpractice, 485
    nonmaleficence, 488
LBBB. See Left bundle branch block
LCA. See Leber's congenital amaurosis
LCIS. See Lobular carcinoma in situ
LCL. See Lateral collateral ligament
LDL. See Low density lipoprotein

Lead, 472t
Lead pipe sign on barium enema, 460t, 470f
Leber's congenital amaurosis (LCA), 503
Lecithin, 229
Left anterior fascicular block (LAFB), 26
Left atrial enlargement (LAE), 27
Left atrium (LA), 32
Left bundle branch block (LBBB), 26
Left lower quadrant (LLQ), 158, 163t
Left posterior fascicular block (LPFB), 26
Left upper quadrant (LUQ), 158, 163t
Left ventricular hypertrophy (LVH), 27
Legal issues
    abandonment, 486t
    assault, 486t
    battery, 486t
    causation, 486t
    common good, 486t
    comparative negligence, 486t
    consent, 486t
    damages, 486t
    deposition, 486t
    disproportionate means, 486t
    due care, 486t
    duty, 486t
    fiduciary, 487t
    futility, 487t
    good Samaritan law, 487t
    human dignity, 487t
    informed consent, 487t
    privilege, 487t
    settlement, 487t
    wrongful death, 487t
Legg–Calvé–perthes disease, 284f
Legionella pneumoniae, 54t
Leigh's disease, 503
Leiomyoma, 177
Leiomyosarcoma, 264
Lemierre's syndrome, 314
Lens dislocation, 433
Lentigo, 406
Leopold maneuvers, 234
Leriche syndrome, 212
LES. See Lower esophageal sphincter
Lesch–Nyhan syndrome, 504
Letterer–Siwe disease, 287
Leukemia, 121–124, 446
    acute lymphoblastic leukemia, 121–122
    acute myelogenous leukemia, 122
    chronic lymphocytic leukemia, 122–124
    chronic myelogenous leukemia, 122
    lymphocytic, 446
    myelogenous, 446
Leukocoria, 444
Leukocyte adhesion deficiency, 504
LFT. See Liver function test
LH. See Luteinizing hormone
Lhermitte sign, 504
Libman-Sacks endocarditis, 36, 98
Licensed practical nurse (LPN), 494
Licensed vocational nurse (LVN), 494
Lichenification, 389, 395f
Liddle's disease, 504
Li–Fraumeni's syndrome, 504

Ligament injuries, 340–341, 341t. See also
        Sports medicine complaints
    anterior cruciate injury, 340
    MCL and LCL, 340
    meniscal tears, 341–342
Likelihood ratio (LR), 482–485
    calculation of, 482
    usage of, 483–484
Limp, pediatric, 284, 284t–285t
Linitis plastica, 166
Listeria monocytogenes, 278, 377t
Lithium
    bipolar disorder treated with, 351
    birth defects due to, 219t
Liver abscess, 126t
Liver calcifications, 460t
Liver disorders, 59–70
    1° biliary cirrhosis, 61–63
    Budd–Chiari syndrome, 68–69
    cirrhosis, 63–66
    hemochromatosis, 66
    hepatic abscess, 67
    hepatitis, 61, 62t–63t
    jaundice, 59–61
    nonalcoholic steatohepatitis, 66
    portal HTN, 67–68, 69f
    veno-occlusive disease, 70
    Wilson's disease, 66–67
Liver function test (LFT), 145
Living will, 488
LLQ. See Left lower quadrant
LMP. See Last menstrual period
Lobular carcinoma in situ (LCIS), 196
LOC. See Loss of consciousness
Loop diuretics, 31
Lorazepam, 385t
Loss of consciousness (LOC), 382
Loteprednol, 449t
Lou Gehrig's disease, 388
Low back pain, 331–333. See also Sports
        medicine complaints
    red flags, 332t
    signs and symptoms of, 331
Low density lipoprotein (LDL), 9
Lower esophageal sphincter (LES),
        165
LPN. See Licensed practical nurse
LR. See Likelihood ratio
Lucent lesion, 452
Ludwig's Angina, 317
Lumbar puncture, 380
Lung abscess, 126t
Lung nodules, 458t, 466f
Lung tissue, 43t
LUQ. See Left upper quadrant
Luteinizing hormone (LH), 247
LVH. See Left ventricular hypertrophy
LVN. See Licensed vocational nurse
Lyme disease, 424
Lymphangio-leiomyomatosis, 47t
Lymphangioma, 446
Lymphangitis carcinomatosa, 457t
Lymphogranuloma venereum, 327t
Lymphoid tumors, 446

Lymphoma, 124–125, 166
    angiocentric T-cell, 124
    Hodgkin lymphoma, 125
    non-Hodgkin lymphoma, 124
Lynch syndromes I and II, 184
Lysergic acid diethylamide, 353t

M
MAC. See Mycobacterium aviumintracellulare
        complex
Macroglossia, 293
Macula, cherry-red spot on, 382, 444
Macular degeneration, age-related, 442
Macule, 389, 390f
Magnetic resonance CP (MRCP), 61
Magnetic resonance imaging (MRI)
    bone tumors, 462f
    CT v., 453t
    knee injuries, 341t
Major depressive disorder (MDD), 349
Major histocompatibility complex (MHC), 144
Malassezia genus, 403
Malignant hypertension, 1–2
    hypertensive emergency, 1–2
    hypertensive urgency, 1
Malabsorption diarrhea, 320
Malignant melanoma, 414t, 444
Malignant tumors, 169
Malpractice, 485
Mammography, 198
Mandible fx, 478t
Manic depression. See Bipolar disorder
Maple syrup urine disease, 504
Marantic endocarditis, 36
Marchiafava–Bignami syndrome, 504
Marcus Gunn Pupil, 431
Marfan's disease, 504
Marfan's syndrome, 32, 208, 433
Marijuana, 304
Marjolin's ulcer, 155
Mask-like facies, 386
Mastalgia, 189–190
McCune–Albright's syndrome, 94
MCD. See Minimal change disease
MCL. See Medial collateral ligament
McMurray test, 341
MCP. See Metacarpophalangeal
MCTD. See Mixed connective tissue disease
MCV. See Mean corpuscular volume
MDD. See Major depressive disorder
Mean corpuscular volume (MCV), 541
Measles, mumps, rubella (MMR), 538
Measles (Rubeola), 272t
Mechanical destruction, 118t
Meckel's diverticulum, 162t, 176
Medial collateral ligament (MCL), 340
Medial epicondylitis (Golfer's elbow), 335
Medial meniscus, tear of, 342f
Mediastinal tumors, 49f, 49t
Medicare/medicaid, 493
Medullary cancer, 92
Megaloblastic anemia, 116–117, 116f
    causes of, 116–117
    folic acid deficiency, 117

Melanocytes, 404
Melanoma, malignant, 414t, 455t
Meglitinides, 83t
Melanosis coli, 504
Melasma, 407
MELAS syndrome. See Mitochondrial
    encephalopathy and lactic acidosis
    syndrome
Memantine, 386, 557
Membranoproliferative glomerulonephritis, 74t
Membranous glomerulonephritis, 74t
Mendelson's syndrome, 505
Ménière's disease, 310t
Meningismus, 376
Meningitis, 126t, 376–378
    bacterial, 377t
    cerebrospinal fluid findings in, 376t
    community acquired, 377t
Meniscal tears, 341–342. See also Ligament
    injuries
Meniscus tear, 341t, 549
Menopause, 257–259
    definition of, 257
    signs and symptoms of, 257–258
Menorrhagia, 257
Menstrual cycle, 247–249, 248f
    phases of, 249t
Mental retardation, 295
Meralgia paresthetica, 505
Mercaptopurine, 59
Mercury, 472t
MERRF. See Myoclonic Epilepsy associated with
    Ragged Red Fibers
Mesenchymal tumor, 446
Mesenteric ischemia, 217
    acute intestinal ischemia, 217
    chronic intestinal ischemia, 217
Metabolic acidosis, 129
Metabolic alkalosis, 130
Metabolic and nutritional disorders, 380–382
    B_{12} deficiency, 381
    carbon monoxide poisoning, 380–381
    hepatic encephalopathy, 381
    Tay–Sachs disease, 382
    thiamine deficiency, 381
    Wilson's disease, 381
Metabolic bone disease, 93–94
    osteoporosis, 93
    Paget's bone disease, 93–94
    rickets/osteomalacia, 93
    scurvy, 93
Metabolic disorder, 287–290. See also Pediatrics
    congenital hypothyroidism, 287–288
    febrile seizures, 289–290
    newborn jaundice, 288–289
    Reye syndrome, 289
Metacarpophalangeal (MCP), 98, 524
Methanol, 472t
Methicillin-resistant Staphylococcus aureus
    (MRSA), 36, 398
Methicillin-susceptible Staphylococcus aureus
    (MSSA), 36
Methylmalonic acid (MMA), 541
Metritis, 241

Metronidazole, 67
MG. See Myasthenia gravis
MHC. See Major histocompatibility complex
MI. See Myocardial infarction
Microcytic anemia, 111–116
    iron deficiency anemia, 111–112
    lead poisoning, 114
    sickle cell anemia, 115–116, 115f
    sideroblastic anemia, 112–114
    thalassemia, 114–115, 114t–115t
Midline differential diagnosis, 164t
Migraine headache, 307t
Miliary tuberculosis, 51, 51f
Minamata disease, 505
Minimal change disease (MCD), 74t
Mitochondrial encephalopathy and lactic acidosis
    syndrome (MELAS syndrome), 505
Mitral regurgitation, 33t
Mitral stenosis (MS), 32, 33t
Mitral valve prolapse (MVP), 31–32, 33t
    occurrence of, 31
Mitral valve regurgitation (MVR), 32
Mixed connective tissue disease (MCTD), 106
MMA. See Methylmalonic acid
MMR. See Measles, mumps, rubella
Mobitz block, 25
Molar pregnancy, 267
Mönckeberg's arteriosclerosis, 505
Mondor's disease, 190
Mongolian spot, 406
Monoamine oxidase inhibitors (MAOI), 350t
Monoarticular arthritis, 106, 108
Mononucleosis (Ebstein-Barr virus), 316t
Monozygotic twins, 246
Mood disorders, 349–352, 350t, 353t. See also
    Psychiatry
    bereavement, 350
    bipolar disorder, 351
    drug-induced mania, 351–352
    dysthymic disorder, 350
    major depressive disorder, 349
Moon facies, 84, 85f
Moraxella catarrhalis, 271
Motor Neuron disease, 388
MRCP. See Magnetic resonance CP
MRSA. See Methicillin-resistant Staphylococcus
    aureus
MS. See Multiple sclerosis
M-spike, 95
MSSA. See Methicillin-susceptible
    Staphylococcus aureus
Mucocele, 446
Mucocutaneous lymph node syndrome,
    285–287
Müller's sign, 33
Multifocal atrial tachycardia (MFAT), 26, 29
Multiinfarct dementia, 386–387
Multiple contrast-enhancing lesions, 455t, 461f
Multiple endocrine neoplasia syndromes, 92, 92t
Multiple gestations, 246–247
    congenital anomalies with, 246
    dizygotic twins, 246
    fetal complications, 246
    incidence of, 246

maternal complications, 246
monozygotic twins, 246
spontaneous abortions with, 246
twin-twin transfusion syndrome with, 247
Multiple lung small soft tissue, 457t
Multiple myeloma, 77t, 94–97, 96f
Multiple personality disorder. See Dissociative
disorder
Multiple sclerosis (MS), 378–380
Münchhausen's syndrome, 505
Murmurs, 33t
differential diagnosis for, 34t
Murphy's sign, 170
Muscle disease, 108–111
Duchenne muscular dystrophy, 110
myasthenia gravis, 110–111
myopathic disease, 110
neurogenic disease, 108
polymyositis and dermatomyositis, 110
types of, 108
Musculoskeletal disorders, 93–111
arthropathies and connective tissue disorders,
97–108
bone tumors, 94–97
metabolic bone disease, 93–94
muscle disease, 108–111
nonneoplastic bone disease, 94
MVP. See Mitral valve prolapse
MVR. See Mitral valve regurgitation
Myasthenia gravis (MG), 48, 110–111
causes of, 48
Mycobacterium aviumintracellulare complex
(MAC), 327
Mycobacterium leprae, 408
Mycoplasma pneumoniae, 118t, 127t
Myeloproliferative disease, 121, 121t
causes of, 120
Myocardial infarction (MI), 5, 163t, 209, 354
evolution of, 9f
Myoclonic Epilepsy associated with Ragged Red
Fibers (MERRF), 505
Myxedema, 90, 91f
Myxedema coma, 91

N

N-acetylcysteine, 146
Nägele's rule, 219
Naphazoline hydrochloride, 450t
Narcissistic personality disorders, 360t
Narcolepsy, 371
Nasal cannula (NC), 40
Nasal fx, 477t
NASH. See Nonalcoholic steatohepatitis
Nasogastric (NG) tube, 158
National Institutes of Health (NIH), 186
Neck mass differential diagnosis, 156t–157t
Necrotizing fasciitis, 126t, 200, 398–399
Negative Predictive Value (NPV), 482
Neisseria gonorrhoeae, 200, 219, 260
Neisseria meningitidis, 376, 377t
Neonatal jaundice, diagnosis of, 289t
Neoplastic polyps, 177–178
classification of, 177
occurrence of, 177

Nephritic glomerulonephropathies, 75, 76t–77t
Nephritic syndrome, 75
Nephrolithiasis, 78
ammonium magnesium phosphate stones, 78
calcium pyrophosphate stones, 78
uric acid stones, 78
Nephrology, 70–79
glomerular disease, 73–75
renal artery stenosis, 75–77
renal tubular and interstitial disorders, 70–73
tumors of kidney, 78–79
urinary tract obstruction, 77–78
Nephrotic glomerulopathies, 74t
Nephrotic syndrome, 73–74
systemic glomerulonephropathies, 75t
Neural tube defects, 293. See also Genetic and
congenital disorder, pediatrics
Neuroblastoma, 446
Neurocutaneous syndromes, 418t
Neurofibromatosis (NF), 418t, 419f
Neuroleptic malignant syndrome, 355t
Neurology, 373–388
degenerative diseases, 385–388
demyelinating diseases, 378–380
infection and inflammation, 376–378
metabolic and nutritional disorders, 380–382
seizures, 382, 383t
stroke, 373–374
Neurosurgery, 202–208
basilar skull fractures, 204–205
head injury, 202–204
hydrocephalus, 206–208
temporal bone fractures, 204
tumors, 205–206
Neurotoxic shellfish, 474t
Neutropenic fever, 126t
Nevocellular nevus, 406
blue nevus, 406
dysplastic nevus, 406
spitz nevus, 406
Nevoid basal cell carcinoma syndrome, 506,
506f
Newborn jaundice, 288–289. See also
Metabolic disorder
NF. See Neurofibromatosis
NHL. See Non-Hodgkin lymphoma
Niacin, 6t
Niemann–Pick's disease, 506
Night terror, 371. See also Parasomnias
Nightmares, 372
Nigro protocol, 186
Nikolsky's sign, 420, 420f
NIH. See National Institutes of Health
Nitroglycerin, 2
Nitroprusside, 2
Nocturnal penile tumescence, 330
Nonalcoholic steatohepatitis (NASH), 66
occurrence of, 66
Non-bizarre delusions, 353t
Non-Hodgkin lymphoma (NHL), 124, 328
Nonmaleficence, 488
Nonneoplastic bone disease, 94
fibrous dysplasia, 94
osteomyelitis, 94

Non–rapid eye movement (NREM), 370
Nonsclerotic skull lucency, 455t
Non-ST-elevation myocardial infarction (NSTEMI), 4–7
Nonsteroidal anti-inflammatory drugs (NSAID), 37, 142, 285
Nonstress test (NST), 228
Noonan's syndrome, 506
Normocytic anemia, 117, 118t
Norplant contraception, 251t
Norwalk virus, 321t, 323t
Nosocomial pneumonia, 127t
NPV. See Negative Predictive Value
NREM. See Non–rapid eye movement
NSAID. See Nonsteroidal anti-inflammatory drugs
NST. See Nonstress test
NT. See Nuchal translucency
Nuchal translucency (NT), 221
Nursemaid's elbow, 336
Nutrition, 343–347. See also Outpatient medicine
    assessment, 343–345
    vitamins and nutrition, 345–347

O

Obsessive–compulsive disorder (OCD), 356
Obsessive–compulsive personality disorders, 360t
Obstetrical complications, 241–247
    abortion, 241–242
    ectopic pregnancy, 243
    multiple gestations, 246–247
    preterm labor, 244–245
    PROM, 245–246
    third-trimester bleeding, 243, 244t
Obstetrics, 218–247
    fetal assessment and intrapartum surveillance, 227–233
    gestational week, height of uterus with, 220t
    labor and delivery in, 233–239
    obstetrical complications, 241–247
    postpartum care, 240–241
    pregnancy, medical conditions in, 223–227
    pregnancy, physiologic changes in, 222–223
    prenatal care, 218–221
    terminology, 218
    umbilical cord compression in, 229
    vaginal bleeding with, 221
Obstructive sleep apnea (OSA), 554
OCD. See Obsessive–compulsive disorder
OCP. See Oral contraceptive pills
Octreotide scanning, 558
Ocular melanoma, 449t
Ogilvie's Syndrome, 183, 556
Olanzapine, 354t
Olecranon bursitis, 336
Olecranon fracture, 335–336
OM. See Otitis media
Onychomycosis, 429t
Opaque eye, 440
Open-angle glaucoma, 444–445
Ophthalmic medications, 449t–451t
    adrenergics, 450t
    anesthetics, 449t
    antibacterials, 450t

anticholinergics, 450t
antiviral, 450t
decongestants, 450t
dry eye, 451t
glaucoma, 451t
NSAID, 450t
steroids (topical), 449t
Ophthalmology, 431–451
    classic syndromes/symptoms, 431–435, 432f
    dacryocystitis, 435–440, 442f
    eye colors, 440
    glaucoma, 444–445
    ophthalmic medications, 449t–451t
    orbital trauma, 447t–449t
    orbital tumors, 445–446
    palpebral inflammation, 435t
    red eye, 435, 437t–438t
    retina, 442–444
Opioids, 472t
Oppositional defiant disorder, 364–365. See also Child and adolescent psychiatry
Optic Neuritis, 434
Oral contraceptive pills (OCP), 219
Oral contraceptives
    alternatives to, 251t–252t
    risks and benefits of, 250t
Oral hypoglycemic agents, 83t
Oral hypoglycemics, 224
Oral thrush, 127t
Orbital cellulitis, 435t, 436f
Orbital trauma, 447t–449t
    blowout fracture, 448t
    chemical burns, 447t
    eyelid laceration, 447t
    foreign body, 447t
    hyphema, 448t
    ocular melanoma, 449t
    retinal detachment, 448t
    retrobulbar hemorrhage, 449t
    ruptured globe (open globe injury), 448t
    traumatic optic neuropathy, 448t
Orbital tumors, 445–446
    capillary hemangioma, 446
    cavernous hemangioma, 445
    dermoid cyst, 446
    fibrous dysplasia, 446
    fibrous histiocytoma, 446
    leukemia, 446
    lymphangioma, 446
    lymphoid tumors, 446
    metastases, 445
    mucocele, 446
    neuroblastoma, 446
    rhabdomyosarcoma, 446
    schwannoma, 446
Organophosphate, 472t
Orthopedic surgery, 283
Ortner's syndrome, 507
OSA. See Obstructive sleep apnea
Osler's nodes, 36
Osteitis deformans. See Paget's bone disease
Osteoarthritis, 100–102, 101f
    noninflammatory arthritis, 100
Osteochondroma, 95t
Osteogenesis imperfecta, 507

Osteomalacia. *See* Rickets
Osteomyelitis, 94, 127t, 285t. *See also*
    Nonneoplastic bone disease
  causes of, 94
  signs and symptoms of, 94
Osteopetrosis, 495
Osteoporosis, 93
  causes of, 93
  signs and symptoms of, 93
Osteosarcoma, 95t
Otitis externa, 306–310, 309f
Otitis media (OM), 268–275
  definition of, 268
Ottawa Rules, 549
Outpatient medicine, 306–347
  ears, nose, and throat, 306–317
  headache, 306, 307t, 308t
  nutrition, 343–347
  outpatient gastrointestinal complaints,
    318–320
  sports medicine complaints, 331–343
  urogenital complaints, 320–331
Ovarian dysfunction, 256
Ovarian neoplasms, 264, 265t–266t
Ovarian torsion, 162t

P
Packed Red Blood Cells (pRBCs), 143
Paget breast disease, 198
Paget's bone disease, 93–94
  complications in, 94
  signs and symptoms of, 94
Paget's disease, 456t
Palpebral inflammation, 435t
  blepharitis, 435t
  chalazion, 435t
  hordeolum, 435t, 436f
  orbital cellulitis, 435t, 436f
Palpitations, 86
Pancoast tumor, 46–49, 48f
Pancreatic cancer, 175
  epidemiology of, 175
  occurrence of, 175
Pancreaticojejunostomy, 173
Pancreatic pseudocyst, 173–174, 174f
Pancreatitis, 100, 164t, 173, 453t
Panic disorder, 354–355. *See also* Anxiety
    disorders
  occurrence of, 354
  signs and symptoms of, 354
Pap. *See* Papanicolaou
Papanicolaou (Pap), 219
Papilledema, 444
Pap smear, 250–252
Papillary cancer, 92
Papilledema, 444
Papule, 389, 391f
Paraganglioma, 156t
Parakeratosis, 389
Paralytic shellfish, 474t
Paramyxovirus, 272t
Paranoid personality disorders, 359t
Parasitic infections, 424–428
  cutaneous larva migrans, 428
  larva currens, 428

pediculosis capitis, 425
pediculosis pubis, 428
scabies, 424, 425f
Parasomnias, 371–372
  nightmares, 372
  night terror, 371
  restless leg syndrome, 372
  sleepwalking, 372
Parasympathomimetics, 451t
Parenchymal disease, 43t
Parenchymal lung cancer, 46, 47t
Parinaud's syndrome, 431
Parity, 218
Parkinsonism, 355t, 387
Parkinson's disease, 387
Paronychia, 398
Parvovirus B19, 272t
Paroxetine, 557
Partial thromboplastin time (PTT), 63, 142,
    225, 301
Pastia's lines, 399
Past medical history (PMH), 489
Past surgical history (PSH), 489
Patau's Syndrome, 291
Patch contraception, 251t
Patent ductus arteriosus (PDA), 297
Pathognomonic palpable purpura, 287
Patient Protection and Affordable Care Act, 493
Patient Safety and Quality improvement Act of
    2005, 494
PCC. *See* Prothrombin complex concentrate
PCL. *See* Posterior cruciate ligament tear
PCP. *See* *Pneumocystis* pneumonia
PCR. *See* Polymerase chain reaction
PDA. *See* Patent ductus arteriosus
PDE5. *See* Phosphodiesterase 5
PDGF. *See* Platelet-derived growth factor
PE. *See* Pulmonary embolism
Pediatric painful limp, 284t–285t
  aseptic avascular necrosis, 284t
  osteomyelitis, 285t
  septic arthritis, 127t, 284t
  slipped capital femoral epiphysis, 285t
  toxic synovitis, 284t
Pediatrics, 268–305. *See also* Adolescence
  bullous myringitis, 275
  child abuse, 299–303
  congenital disorder, 290–299
  developmental milestones, 269t
  genetic disorder, 290–299
  immunization schedules, 273f–274f
  infant botulism, 268
  infections, 268
  metabolic disorder, 288–290
  musculoskeletal, 281–287
  painful limp, 284t–285t
  puberty, 269t
  respiratory disorders, 268–280
  subperiosteal abscess, 275
  tanner stages, 269t
  ToRCHS, 270t–271t
  toxicology, 302t
  trauma and intoxication, 299–303
  upper respiratory disorders, 276t–277t
  viral exanthems, 272t

Pediculosis capitis, 425
Pediculosis pubis, 428
PEEP. See Positive end-expiratory pressure
Pel–Ebstein fevers, 126
Peliosis hepatis. See Bacillary angiomatosis
Pelvic inflammatory disease (PID), 127t, 243,
    325t
Pelvic relaxation, 260
Pemphigus vulgaris (PG), 420–423, 420f
Penicillamine, 67
Peptic ulcer, 57–58, 163t
Peptic ulceration, operations for, 159f
Peptide analogues, 83t
Percutaneous balloon angioplasty (PTA), 213
Percutaneous transluminal coronary angioplasty
    (PTCA), 5t, 8
Pericardial disease, 37
    pericardial fluid, 37
    pericarditis, 38
Pericardial effusion, 37
Pericardial fluid, 37
Pericarditis, 27, 38
    causes of, 38
Peripartum cardiomyopathy, 227
    occurrence in, 227
    risk factors of, 227
    treatment of, 227
Peripheral aneurysms, 209
Peripheral vascular disease (PVD), 212–214
Peritonsillar abscess, 313
Permethrin, 424, 425
Pernicious anemia, 57, 346t
Persistent Vegetative State (PVS), 488
Personality disorders, 357–360
    altruism, 358
    antisocial, 359t
    avoidant, 360t
    borderline, 359t
    characteristics of, 357–358
    clusters, 358
    dependent, 360t
    ego defenses, 358–360
    histrionic, 360t
    narcissistic, 360t
    obsessive–compulsive, 360t
    paranoid, 359t
    schizoid, 359t
    schizotypal, 359t
Pertussis, 276t
Pervasive developmental disorder, 363
Petechiae, 389
Peutz–Jeghers syndrome, 178, 179f
PG. See Pemphigus vulgaris
Phalen's test, 338
Pharyngitis, 127t, 313, 316t
Phenobarbital, 384t, 472t
Phenylephrine hydrochloride, 450t
Phenytoin, 383, 384t
Pheochromocytoma, 86
Phlegmasia alba dolens, 214
Phlegmasia cerulea dolens, 215
Phosphatidylglycerol, 229
Phosphodiesterase 5 (PDE5), 330
Phrenic nerve palsy, 458t

Picks's disease, 387
Pickwickian syndrome, 371, 515
PID. See Pelvic inflammatory disease
Pigeon breast, 93
PIGN. See Postinfectious glomerulonephritis
PIH. See Pregnancy-induced hypertension
Pinching, 491–492
Pinguecula, 434, 434f
Pink puffer. See Emphysema
PIP. See Proximal interphalangeal
Pituitary dysfunction, 256
Pityriasis alba, 406
Pityriasis rosea, 408, 410f
Placenta previa and placental abruption,
    comparison of, 244t
Placenta separation, signs of, 235–236
Plantar fasciitis, 331
Plaque, 389, 392f
Platelet-derived growth factor (PDGF), 142
Platelet destruction
    causes of, 119t
    labs in, 120t
Pleural effusion, 42, 43t
    lab analysis of, 44t
Plummer's disease, 89
Plummer–Vinson syndrome, 346t, 507
PMH. See Past medical history
PMN. See Polymorphonuclear leukocytes
Pneumocystis jiruveci, 54t
Pneumocystis pneumonia (PCP), 324
Pneumonia, 161t, 275–279
    community-acquired pneumonia, 53–56,
        54t–55t
    HCAP and HAP, 56
Pneumoperitoneum, 459t
Poisonings, pediatric, 302–303
Polycystic kidney disease, 507
Polycystic ovarian disease, 258t
Polycythemia vera, 121t
Polymerase chain reaction (PCR), 424
Polymorphonuclear leukocytes (PMN), 59
Polymyalgia rheumatica, 108
Polymyositis, 110
Poncet's disease, 508
Porphyria cutanea tarda, 421
Portal hypertension, 67–68, 69f
    causes of, 68t
    definition of, 67
Port-wine hemangioma of face, 418t
Positive end-expiratory pressure (PEEP), 44
    purpose of, 44
Positive Predictive Value (PPV), 482
Postcoital contraception, 252t
Posterior cruciate ligament tear (PCL), 341t
Postinfectious glomerulonephritis (PIGN),
    76t
Postpartum care, 240–241
    breast-feeding, 240
    contraception, 240
    depression, 240
    immunizations, 240
    lactation, 240
    uterine infection, 240–241
Postpartum depression, 240

Postpartum hemorrhage, 238–239
  causes of, 238
  definition of, 238
  disseminated intravascular coagulation, 239
  retained placenta, 239
  uterine atony, 239
Poststreptococcal glomerulonephritis (PSGN), 76t
Posttraumatic stress disorder (PTSD), 356–357,
    530
Potter's syndrome, 508
Pott's disease, 51, 508
Power of attorney, 488
PPD. See Purified protein derivative
PPO. See Preferred Provider Organization
PPV. See Positive Predictive Value
P-QrS-T Complex, 10, 11f–24f
Prader–Willi syndrome, 88t
pRBCs. See Packed Red Blood Cells
Prednisone, 287
Preeclampsia, 546
Preferred Provider Organization (PPO), 492, 493
Pregnancy
  anemia of, 222
  diastolic murmurs in, 222
  disease, 218
  ectopic, 243
  medical conditions in, 223–227
  PE in, 225
  physiologic changes in, 222–223
  test, 218
Pregnancy-induced hypertension (PIH), 221
  epidemiology of, 225
  signs and symptoms of, 225
  treatment of, 225–226
  types of, 226t
Premature delivery, 218
Premature rupture of membranes (PROM),
    244–246
Premature ventricular contraction (PVC), 29
Prenatal care, 218–221
  contraceptive history in, 219
  estimated date of confinement in, 219
  first-trimester visits, 220–221, 220t
  first visit, 218–220
  medical history in, 219
  obstetrical history in, 218–219
  pregnancy disease in, 218
  second-trimester visits, 221
  third-trimester visits, 221
Preoperative care, 145
Preterm labor (PTL), 221, 244–245
  cause of, 244
  definition of, 244
  risk factors of, 244
  signs and symptoms of, 244
Pretibial myxedema, 88–90
Primum non nocer, 488
Primidone, 384t
PR interval, 10
Prinzmetal's angina, 10
Privilege, 487t
Progesterone, 249
Progestin, 249
Progestin-only pills contraception, 251t

Progressive multifocal leukoencephalopathy
    (PML), 379t
Progressive optic neuropathy, 444
Progressive Systemic Sclerosis (PSS), 103–104
Projection, 358
Prolactinoma, 79
PROM. See Premature rupture of membranes
Proparacaine hydrochloride, 449t
Propionibacterium acnes, 396
Propylthiouracil (PTU), 90
Prostate, 328–329. See also Urogenital
    complaints
  benign prostatic hyperplasia, 328–329
  prostate cancer, 329
  prostatitis, 329
Prostate cancer, 200–201, 201f, 329
Prostate-specific antigen (PSA), 200, 329, 515
Prostatitis, 126t, 329. See also Urogenital
    complaints
Prosthetic valve endocarditis, 36
Proteinuria, 2t
Prothrombin complex concentrate (PCC), 144
Prothrombin time (PT), 63, 142, 301
Proton pump inhibitor, 57
Proximal interphalangeal (PIP), 98, 524
PSA. See Prostate-specific antigen
Pseudomonas aeruginosa, 397
Pseudotumor cerebri, 208
PSGN. See Poststreptococcal
    glomerulonephritis
PSH. See Past surgical history
Psoriasis, 399–402
  Auspitz sign, 400
  guttate, 400
  inverse, 400
  Köbner's phenomenon, 400
  pustular, 400, 402f
  signs and symptoms of, 399–400, 401f
  treatment of, 402
  variants, 400
Psoriatic arthritis, 103
PSS. See Progressive Systemic Sclerosis
Psychiatry, 348–372
  adjustment disorder, 369
  anxiety disorders, 354–357
  child and adolescent, 363–366
  dissociative disorder, 369
  drug abuse, 367–368, 367t–368t
  DSM-IV classifications, 348, 348t
  impulse-control disorders, 369–370
  mood disorders, 349–352
  personality disorders, 357–360
  principles for USMLE of, 348
  prognosis of disorders of, 349t
  psychosis, 352–354
  sexuality and gender identity disorders,
      368–369
  sleep, 370–372
  somatoform and factitious disorders,
      360–362
Psychological testing, child/adolescent, 363t
Psychosis, 352–354, 353t–355t
  delusions, 352
  hallucinations, 352

PT. See Prothrombin time
PTA. See Percutaneous balloon angioplasty
Pterygium, 433–434, 433f
PTL. See Preterm labor
PTSD. See Posttraumatic stress disorder
PTT. See Partial thromboplastin time
PTU. See Propylthiouracil
Pulmonary, 38–56
    COPD, 40, 41t–42t
    hypoxemia, 38–40
    mediastinal tumors, 49
    pneumonia, 53–56
    pulmonary vascular disease, 42–46
    respiratory tract cancer, 46–49
    restrictive lung disease and pleural effusion, 42
    tuberculosis, 49–53
Pulmonary capillary wedge pressure, 44
Pulmonary edema, 42–45, 45f, 457t
Pulmonary embolism (PE), 30, 45–46, 225
    lung infarctions and, 45
    prevention of, 46
    risk factors of, 45
Pulmonary hypertension, 46
    definition of, 46
Pulmonary hypoplasia scoliosis, 458t
Pulmonary regurgitation, 35
Pulmonary stenosis, 35, 270t
Pulmonary valve disease, 35
Pulmonary vascular disease
    PE, 45–46
    pulmonary edema and ARDS, 42–45
    pulmonary hypertension, 46
Pulsatile hematomas, 208
Purified protein derivative (PPD), 52, 535
    interpretation of, 52
Purpura, 389
Pustular psoriasis, 400, 402f
PVC. See Premature ventricular contraction
PVD. See Peripheral vascular disease
PVS. See Persistent Vegetative State
Pyelonephritis, 127t, 320
Pyromania, 370

Q
Quetiapine, 354t
Quincke's sign, 32
Quinidine, 473t
Q wave, 10

R
Rachitic rosary, 93
Radiculopathy, 332t, 333
Radioiodine, 90
Radiology, 452–470, 461f–470f
    chest x-ray, approach to, 453, 454f
    common findings, 455t–460t
    common radiologic studies, 453t
    radiopaque vs. radiolucent, 452
    terms and concepts, 452
RAE. See Right atrial enlargement
Raloxifene, 259
Ranson's criteria, 173t
Rapid eye movement (REM), 370

Rationalization, 360
Raynaud's phenomenon, 104
RBBB. See Right bundle branch block
RDS. See Respiratory distress syndrome
Reaction formation, 360
Reactive arthritis, 102–103
Rectal cancer, 186
Rectum and anus surgery, 182f, 184–186
    anal cancer, 186
    anal fissure, 185–186
    fistula-in-ano, 185
    hemorrhoids, 184–185
    rectal cancer, 186
Recurrent laryngeal nerve (RLN), 317
Red eye, 435, 437t–438t
    allergic conjunctivitis, 437t
    angle closure glaucoma, 438t
    bacterial conjunctivitis, 437t
    corneal abrasion, 438t
    hyphema, 437t, 439f
    keratitis, 438t, 439f–441f
    subconjunctival hemorrhage, 438t, 440f
    uveitis, 438t, 441f
    viral conjunctivitis, 437t
    xerophthalmia, 437t
Reed–Sternberg (RS) cells, 126
Reflex sympathetic dystrophy (RSD) syndrome, 508
Refsum's disease, 508
Regression, 360
REM. See Rapid eye movement
Renal amyloidosis, 75t
Renal artery stenosis, 2, 75–77, 217
    classic dyad, 75–77
Renal cell cancer, 78
Renal tubular acidosis (RTA), 71, 72t
Renal tubular and interstitial disorders, 70–73
    acute renal failure, 70, 71t
    acute tubular necrosis, 71
    chronic renal failure, 73
    drug-induced AIN, 71
    renal tubule functional disorders, 71–73
Renal tubule functional disorders, 71–73
    DI, 71–72
    RTA, 71
    SIADH, 72–73
Renovascular hypertension, 216–217
Reproductive endocrinology, 255–260
    amenorrhea, 255–256
    dysfunctional uterine bleeding, 257
    hirsutism, 257, 258t
    infertility, 259–262
    menopause, 257–259
    virilization, 257, 258t
Respiratory acid-base differential, 131
Respiratory disorders, 268–280, 278f
    adenoiditis, 280
    bronchiolitis, 275
    bullous myringitis, 275
    epiglottitis, 280
    immunization schedules, 273f–274f
    otitis media, 268–275
    pediatric upper, 276t–277t
    pneumonia, 275–279

stridor, 280–282
subperiosteal abscess, 275
upper respiratory disease, 275
viral exanthems, 272t
Respiratory distress syndrome (RDS), 229
Respiratory syncytial virus (RSV), 275
Respiratory tract cancer
epidemiology of, 46
parenchymal lung cancer, 46, 47t
superior sulcus tumor, 46–49, 48f
Restless leg syndrome, 372
Restrictive lung disease, 42, 44t
diagnosis and treatment of, 43t
Retina, 442–444
age-related macular degeneration, 442
diabetic retinopathy, 442, 443f
physical findings of, 444
retinal detachment, 444
retinitis pigmentosa, 444
Retinal detachment, 444, 448t
Retinitis pigmentosa, 444
Retinoic acid, birth defects due to, 219t
Retrobulbar hemorrhage, 449t
Retrobulbar Neuritis, 434
Retropharyngeal abscess, 314–316
Rett's syndrome, 509
Reye syndrome, 289
RF. See Rheumatoid factor
Rhabdomyosarcoma, 295, 446
Rheumatoid arthritis (RA), 38, 97–98, 97f
Rheumatoid factor (RF), 98
Rhubarb, 552
Rickets, 93
causes of, 93
signs and symptoms of, 93
Right atrial enlargement (RAE), 27
Right bundle branch block (RBBB), 26
Right lower quadrant (RLQ), 158, 162t
Right upper quadrant (RUQ), 67, 158, 161t
Right ventricular hypertrophy (RVH), 27
Rimexolone, 449t
Ring enhancement, 452
Rinne's test, 312
Risperidone, 354t
RLN. See Recurrent laryngeal nerve
RLQ. See Right lower quadrant
Rocker Bottom Feet, 291
Rocky mountain spotted fever, 424
ROM. See Rupture of membranes
Rorschach, 363
Roseola infantum (Exanthem subitum), 272t
Rotator cuff injury, 334
Roth spots, 36, 444
Rotor syndrome, 60t
Roux-en-Y gastric bypass, 187, 188f
RSD syndrome. See Reflex sympathetic
dystrophy syndrome
RSV. See Respiratory syncytial virus
RTA. See Renal tubular acidosis
Rubella (German measles), 272t
Ruptured globe (open globe injury), 448t
Rupture of membranes (ROM), 221
RUQ. See Right upper quadrant
RVH. See Right ventricular hypertrophy

S
Salicylates, 289
Salpingitis, 162t
Sarcoidosis, 104–106
signs and symptoms of, 104
stages of, 105f
Sarcoptes scabiei, 424
SBO. See Small bowel obstruction
SBP. See Spontaneous bacterial peritonitis
Scabies, 424, 425f
Scaphoid fracture, 336–337, 338f
Scarlet fever, 399
Schafer's disease, 509
Schindler's disease, 509
Schirmer test, 437t
Schizoaffective disorder, 353t
Schizoid personality disorders, 359t
Schizophrenia, 352, 353t
Schizotypal personality disorders, 359t
Schmidt's syndrome, 509
Schwannoma, 446
Sclerodactyly, 104
Scleroderma, 103–104, 103f
Sclerosing cholangitis, 61
Sclerotic bone lesions, 455t, 462f
Sclerotic lesion, 452
Scombroid, 473t–474t
Scrofula, 51
Scrotal emergencies, 198–200
Scurvy, 93
causes of, 93
signs and symptoms of, 93
Sea fan neovascularization, 444
Seborrheic dermatitis, 403, 403f
Seborrheic keratosis, 408, 412f
Seizures, 382, 383t
anti-seizure medications, 384t–385t
presentation of, 382
status epilepticus, 385
terminology, 382
therapy, 383t
treatment of, 383
Selective serotonin reuptake inhibitors (SSRI), 354
Selenium, 346t
Sengstaken–Blakemore tube, 68
Senile dementia of Alzheimer type, 383,
385–386
Sentinel loop, 164
Separation anxiety, 364. See also Child and
adolescent psychiatry
Septic arthritis, 108, 127t, 284t
Septic shock, 127t
Seronegative spondyloarthropathy, 100–103
ankylosing spondylitis, 102
inflammatory bowel disease, 103
osteoarthritis, 100–102
psoriatic arthritis, 103
reactive arthritis, 102–103
Serotonin norepinephrine reuptake inhibitor
(SNRI), 354
Serpiginous threadlike lesion, 428
Sertoli-Leydig cell tumor, 258t
Serum protein electrophoresis (SPEP), 95
Settlement, 487t

Sexual abuse, 301
Sexuality and gender identity disorders, 368–369
Sexually transmitted disease (STD), 324,
        325t–327t, 428. See also Urogenital
        complaints
Sézary syndrome, 124
SFA. See Superior femoral arteries
SH. See Social history
Shock
    defect in, 153t
    diagnosis of, 153t
Shoulder injuries, 333–335. See also Sports
        medicine complaints
    dislocation, 334–335, 334f
    shoulder rotator cuff injury, 335
Shuffling gait, 386
SIADH. See Syndrome of inappropriate
        antidiuretic hormone
Sickle cell anemia, 115–116, 115f
Sideroblastic anemia, 112–114
Sigmoid volvulus, 163t, 469f
Sinusitis, 313, 314t
    acute bacterial, 314t
    chronic bacterial, 314t
    fungal, 314t
Sinus tachycardia, 45
Sipple's syndrome, 92t
Sister Mary Joseph sign, 167
Sjögren's syndrome (SS), 100, 554
Skilled nursing facilities (SNF), 493
Skin cancer, 414t–415t, 415f–417f
SLE. See Systemic lupus erythematosus
Sleep, 370–372
    apnea, 371
    disorders, 370–372
    NREM, 370, 370t
    REM, 370
    stages, 370t
    walking, 372 (See also Parasomnias)
Slipped capital femoral epiphysis, 285t
Small bowel neoplasms, 177
    signs and symptoms of, 177
Small bowel obstruction (SBO), 175–177, 176f
    causes of, 175
Small cell (oat cell) carcinoma, characteristics
        of, 47t
Small intestine, 57–59
    carcinoid syndrome, 59
    Crohn's disease, 58–59, 58t
    duodenal ulcer, 57–58
    surgery, 175–177
        small bowel neoplasms, 177
        small bowel obstruction, 175–177
Smoking
    and CAD, 2
    and duodenal ulcer, 57
Snake bite, 475t
SNF. See Skilled nursing facilities
SNRI. See Serotonin norepinephrine reuptake
        inhibitor
Social history (SH), 489
Social Security Act, 493
Somatoform disorder, 360–362
    body dysmorphic disorder, 362

conversion disorder, 362
    definition of, 360
    hypochondriasis, 362
    somatization disorder, 361–362
Somatostatinoma, 175
Somnambulism. See Sleepwalking
Sorafenib, 169
Spastic cerebral palsy, 388
SPEP. See Serum protein electrophoresis (SPEP)
Spaghetti and meatball appearance, 429t
Spastic cerebral palsy, 388
Speckled irises (Brushfield spots), 293
Spherocytosis, 118t
Sphingomyelin, 229
Spinal stenosis, 332t, 333
Spironolactone, 31
Splenic rupture, 163t
Splinter hemorrhages, 36
Spongiosis, 389
Spontaneous bacterial peritonitis (SBP), 63, 127t
Sports medicine complaints, 331–343
    ankle injuries, 343
    clavicle fracture, 335
    elbow injuries, 335–336
    hip problems, 338–339
    knee problems, 339–341
    low back pain, 331–333
    plantar fasciitis, 331
    shoulder injuries, 333–335, 334f
    wrist injuries, 336–338, 337f
Squamous cell carcinoma, 47t, 414t
SS. See Sjögren's syndrome
SSRI. See Selective serotonin reuptake inhibitors
Stable angina pectoris, 2–4
    causes of, 2
Staccato cough, 278
Staphylococcus aureus, 35, 278, 320, 377t,
        396, 435
Statistical values, calculation of, 480–485, 481t.
        See also Ethics and law
    likelihood ratios, 482–485
    post-test probability of disease, 482
    sensitivity, defined, 481
    specificity, defined, 481
    test accuracy, 481–482
    two-by-two table, 480–481
STD. See Sexually transmitted disease
Steeple sign, 459t
ST-elevation myocardial infarction (STEMI),
        4, 7–10
ST elevations, diagnosis of, 27
Steroids (topical), 449t
Stevens–Johnson syndrome, 421
Strawberry tongue, 399
Streptococcus agalactiae, 275, 377t
Streptococcus pneumoniae, 271, 376, 377t, 435
Streptococcus pyogenes, 396, 435
Stress echocardiogram, 8t
Stress incontinence, 261
Stress treadmill, 8t
Striae, 84, 85f
Stridor, 280–282, 280f, 281f
    biphasic, 280
String of beads on renal arteriogram, 460t

String sign on barium swallow, 459t
Stroke, 373–374
    diagnosis of, 374
    presentation of, 373–374, 373t
    prognosis, 374
    terminology, 373
    treatment of, 374
Stromal cell tumor, 265t
Sturge–Weber syndrome, 407, 418t
Subacute thyroiditis, 89–90
Subarachnoid hemorrhage, 306, 307t
Subclavian steal syndrome, 216
Subconjunctival hemorrhage, 434, 438t, 440f
Sublimation, 360
Subperiosteal abscess, 275
Substance abuse, 303
Suicide, 303
Sulfonylureas, 83t
Superficial thrombophlebitis, 225
Superior femoral arteries (SFA), 213
Superior sulcus tumor, 46–49, 48f
Superior vena cava (SVC) syndrome, 46–49
Supraglottitis, 279f, 280
Supraventricular tachycardia (SVT), 29
    definition of, 29
    etiology of, 29
Surgery, 138–217
    abdomen, 158–159, 158f–160f
    bariatric surgery, 186–189
    blood product replacement, 142–144
    breast, 189–198
    burns, 154–155
    colon, 177–184
    esophagus, 159–166
    exocrine pancreas, 172–175
    fluid and electrolytes, 138–141
    gallbladder, 169–172
    gastric tumors, 166–167
    hepatic tumors, 169
    hernia, 167–168, 167t
    neck mass differential diagnosis, 156t–157t
    neurosurgery, 202–208
    perioperative care, 145–148
    rectum and anus, 182f, 184–186
    small intestine, 175–177
    trauma, 148–153
    urology, 198–201
    vascular diseases, 208–217
SVC syndrome. See Superior vena cava syndrome
Sweet's syndrome, 509, 509f
Swinging flashlight test, 431
Syndrome of inappropriate antidiuretic hormone
    (SIADH), 72–73
Syndrome X, 509
Syphilis (Treponema pallidum), 326t
Systemic diseases, 74t
Systemic lupus erythematosus (SLE), 36,
    98–100, 99f, 481
    drug-induced, 100

T
Tachycardia, 229–231
Takayasu's arteritis, 215
Tanner stages, 269t

Tardive dyskinesia, 355t
Tay–Sachs disease, 382, 509
TB. See Tuberculosis
TBG. See Thyroid-bonding globulin
TBW. See Total body water
Tear duct inflammation. See Dacryocystitis
Telangiectasias, 104
Temazepam, 557
Temporal arteritis, 306, 307t
Temporal bone fractures, 204
Temporal mandibular joint (TMJ), 307t
Tendonitis. See Epicondylitis
Tennis elbow, 335
Tensilon test, 111
Tension headache, 307t
Teratogens, 219t
Term delivery, 218
Testicular appendage, appendix testis torsion
    of, 200
Testicular feminization syndrome, 87t
Testicular torsion, 198
Tetracaine, 449t
Tetrahydrozoline hydrochloride, 450t
Tetralogy of fallot, 297–299, 298f
Tetrodotoxin, 474
Thalassemia, 114–115, 114t–115t
Theophylline, 473t
Thiabendazole, 428
Thiamine deficiency, 381
Thiazide diuretic, 3t
Thiazolidinediones, 83t
Thimerosal, 364
Third-trimester bleeding, 243
Thompson's test, 343
Thrombin time (TT), 143
Thrombocytopenia, 117
    causes of, 117, 119t
    lab values, 120t
Thromboembolic disease, pregnancy with,
    224–225
Thrombophlebitis, 314
Thrombosed external hemorrhoid, 185
Thrombotic thrombocytopenic purpura (TTP),
    119t
Thumb sign, 459t
Thyroglossal duct cyst, 156t
Thyroid adenoma, 89
Thyroid-bonding globulin (TBG), 223
Thyroid disorder, 87–91
    hyperthyroidism, 87–90
    hypothyroidism, 90–91
Thyroid malignancy, 91–92
    anaplastic CA, 92
    follicular CA, 92
    medullary CA, 92
    papillary CA, 92
    radioactive iodine cold nodule, 92
    radioactive iodine hot nodules US, 92
    solitary dominant thyroid nodule, 91–92
Thyroid-stimulating immunoglobulin (TSI), 89
Thyroid storm, 90
TIA. See Transient ischemic attack
TIBC. See Total iron binding capacity
Tietze syndrome, 190

Tinea, 429t
Tinea pedis (Athlete's foot), 429t
Tinea versicolor, 429t
Tinel's sign, 338
Tinnitus, 310
Tissue plasminogen activator (tPA), 8, 374, 538
TLC. See Total lung capacity
TM. See Tympanic membrane
TMJ. See Temporal mandibular joint
TM perforation, 476t
TNF. See Tumor necrosis factor
TOA. See Tubo-ovarian abscess
Tobramycin, 450t
Tocodynamometer, 236
Togavirus, 272t
Tonic seizure, 382
Topical steroids, usage of, 396t
Topiramate, 385t
ToRCHS, 270t–271t
Torticollis, 156t
Total body water (TBW), 138
Total iron binding capacity (TIBC), 112, 541
Total lung capacity (TLC), 40
Total parenteral nutrition (TPN), 172, 345
Tourette's disorder, 365–366. See also Child
        and adolescent psychiatry
Toxicology, 471t–473t
    acetaminophen, 471t
    alkali agents, 471t
    anticholinergic, 471t
    arsenic, 471t
    aspirin, 471t
    β-blockers, 471t
    benzodiazepine, 471t
    carbon monoxide, 471t
    cyanide, 472t
    digoxin, 472t
    ethylene glycol, 472t
    heparin, 472t
    iron, 472t
    isoniazid, 472t
    lead, 472t
    mercury, 472t
    methanol, 472t
    opioids, 472t
    organophosphate, 472t
    phenobarbital, 472t
    quinidine, 473t
    theophylline, 473t
    tricyclics, 473t
    warfarin, 473t
Toxic synovitis, 284t
Toxoplasma encephalitis, 324
Toxoplasmosis, 206t, 270t, 379t, 455t
tPA. See Tissue plasminogen activator
TPN. See Total parenteral nutrition
Transfusions, 143–144, 144t
Transient ischemic attack (TIA), 216, 373
Transposition of great arteries, 297
Transurethral resection of prostate (TURP), 329
Traube's sign, 32
Trauma, 148–153, 150f, 299–303. See also
        Pediatrics
    child abuse, 299–303, 300f

    poisonings, 302–303
    primary surgery, 148–152
    secondary surgery, 152–153
    shock, 153
Trauma, orbital, 447t–449t
    blowout fracture, 448t
    chemical burns, 447t
    eyelid laceration, 447t
    foreign body, 447t
    hyphema, 448t
    ocular melanoma, 449t
    retinal detachment, 448t
    retrobulbar hemorrhage, 449t
    ruptured globe (open globe injury), 448t
    traumatic optic neuropathy, 448t
Traumatic optic neuropathy, 448t
Trench fever, 423
Treponema pallidum, 413
Triamcinolone, 396t
Triceps skin fold, 344. See also Nutrition
Trichomonas, 253, 253t
Trichotillomania, 370
Tricuspid regurgitation, 33t
Tricuspid stenosis, 33t
Tricuspid valve disease, 35
Tricyclic antidepressants (TCA)
    depression treated with, 350t
    panic disorder treated with, 355
Tricyclics, 473t
Trifluridine, 450t
Trigeminal neuralgia, 306, 307t
Trisomy 13, 291
Trisomy 18, 292
Trisomy 21, 292
Trochanteric bursitis, 338. See also Sports
        medicine complaints
Tropical spastic paraparesis, 510
Trousseau's syndrome, 175
Truncal obesity, 84, 85f
TSI. See Thyroid-stimulating immunoglobulin
TT. See Thrombin time
TTP, See Thrombotic thrombocytopenic purpura
Tuberculosis (TB)
    classic chronic extrapulmonary reactivation
            syndromes, 51–52
    Dx and Tx, 52–53
    miliary TB, 51, 51f
    primary TB, 49
    secondary TB, 49–51, 50f
Tuberous sclerosis, 295, 296f, 418f, 418t.
        See also Genetic and congenital
        disorder, pediatrics
Tubo-ovarian abscess (TOA), 162t
Tumor, 332t
Tumor necrosis factor (TNF), 59
Tumors of kidney, 78–79
    renal cell cancer, 78
    Wilms tumor, 78–79
Turcot's syndrome, 178, 510
Turner's Syndrome, 293, 295f
TURP. See Transurethral resection of prostate
T-wave inversions, 4
Twin-twin transfusion syndrome, 247
Tympanic membrane (TM), 268

U

UA. *See* Unstable angina; Urinalysis
Ulcer, *459t*
Ulcerative colitis, *58t*, 59
Ulnar fracture, *336*
Ultrasound, *453t*
Umbilical cord compression, *229*
Unconjugated hyperbilirubinemia, *288*
Unilateral cleft lip, *291*
Unilateral cystic renal mass, *460t*
Unilaterally elevated diaphragm, *458t*, *468f*
United States Medical Licensing Examination
   (USMLE), *348*
Unstable angina (UA), *4–5*
   causes of, *4*
   risk stratification of, *7t*
UPEP. *See* Urine protein electrophoresis
Upper respiratory disorders, pediatric,
      276t–277t
   bacterial tracheitis, *277t*
   croup (laryngotracheobronchitis), *276t*, *278f*
   epiglottitis, *277t*, *279f*, 280
   foreign-body aspiration, *277t*
   pertussis, *276t*
Upper respiratory infection (URI), 38
Up-slanted palpebral fissures, *293*
Uremia, 73
Urethritis, *103*, *126t*
Urge incontinence, *261*, *261f*
URI. *See* Upper respiratory infection
Urinalysis (UA), *145*, 323
Urinary incontinence, *261*, *373t*
   stress incontinence, *261*
   types of, *261*, *261f*
   urge incontinence, *261*, *261f*
Urinary tract infection (UTI), *77*, *223*, 320–324
   bacterial prostatitis, *324*
   epidemiology of, *320*
   signs and symptoms of, *320*
   treatment of, *323*
   urinalysis, *323*
Urinary tract obstruction, *77–78*
   characteristics of, *77*
   nephrolithiasis, *78*
Urination, burning during, *320*
Urine protein electrophoresis (UPEP), *95*
Urogenital complaints, *320–331*
   acquired immunodeficiency syndrome,
      324–328
   hematuria, *328*
   impotence, *330–331*
   prostate, *328–329*
   sexually transmitted disease, *324*,
      325t–327t
   urinary tract infection, *320–324*
Urogram, *328*
Urogynecology, *260–262*
   definition of, *260*
   pelvic relaxation, *260*
   signs and symptoms of, *261*
   urinary incontinence, *261*
Urology surgery, *198–201*
   prostate cancer, *200–201*
   scrotal emergencies, *198–200*

Urticaria, *404*, *404f*
US Food and Drug Administration Drug
      Categories, *220t*
Usher syndrome, *510*
USMLE. *See* United States Medical Licensing
      Examination
Uterine activity, monitoring of, *235*
Uterine atony, *239*. *See also* Postpartum
      hemorrhage
Uterine bleeding, *256*, 262
Uterine hyperstimulation, *229*
Uterine infection, postpartum, *240–241*
Uterine leiomyomas, *264*
Uteroplacental insufficiency, *229*
UTI. *See* Urinary tract infection
Uveitis, *438t*, *441f*

V

Vaginal bleeding, *221*
Vaginal cancer, *266*
Vaginal contraceptive ring contraception,
      252t
Vaginitis, *253*, *254f*
   Candida, *254f*
   diagnosis of, *253t*
   Trichomonas, *254f*
Valproate
   bipolar disorder treated with, *351*
   birth defects due to, *219t*
   seizure therapy with, *383*
Valproic acid, *384t*
Valvular disease
   aortic regurgitation, *32–34*
   aortic stenosis, *35*
   endocarditis, *35–37*
   hypertrophic cardiomyopathy, *35*
   mitral stenosis, *32*
   mitral valve prolapse, *31–32*
   mitral valve regurgitation, *32*
   rheumatic fever/heart disease, *37*
   tricuspid and pulmonary valve diseases, *35*
Vancomycin-resistant enterococci (VRE), *37*
Varicella (chickenpox), *272t*
Vascular diseases, surgery, *208–217*
   aneurysms, *208–209*, *210f*, *211f*
   aortic dissection, *209–212*
   carotid vascular disease, *215–216*
   mesenteric ischemia, *217*
   peripheral vascular disease, *212–214*
   renovascular hypertension, *216–217*
   subclavian steal syndrome, *216*
   vessel disease, *214–215*, *214f*, *215f*
Vasoactive intestinal peptide (VIP), *175*
Vector–borne diseases, *423–424*
   bacillary angiomatosis, *423–424*
   lyme disease, *423–424*
   rocky mountain spotted fever, *424*
Veno-occlusive disease, *70*
Ventricular aneurysm, *27*
Ventricular fibrillation (v-fib), *25*, 30
Ventricular septal defect (VSD), *296–297*
Ventricular tachycardia (V-tach), *29–30*
   definition of, *29*
Verner–Morrison syndrome, *510*

Verrucae, 413
   human papilloma virus, 413
   verruca plana (flat wart), 413
   verruca vulgaris, 413
Verruca plana (flat wart), 413
Verruca vulgaris, 413
Vertical sleeve gastrectomy, 188, 189f
Vertigo, causes of, 310t
Vesicle, 389, 393f
Vessel disease, 214–215, 214f, 215f
Vidarabine, 450t
VIN. See Vulvar intraepithelial neoplasia
VIP. See Vasoactive intestinal peptide (VIP)
Viral conjunctivitis, 437t
Viral exanthems, 272t
Viral labyrinthitis, 310t
Virchow's node, 166
Virchow's triad, 45
Virilization, 257, 258t
Visceral hernia, 168
Vitamin A, 346
Vitamin C, 346
Vitamin D, 346
Vitamin E, 346
Vitamin K, 346
Vitamins/minerals, 345–347
   B_1 (thiamine), 345
   B_2 (riboflavin), 345
   B_3 (niacin), 345
   B_5 (pantothenate), 345
   B_6 (pyridoxine), 346
   B_{12} (cyanocobalamin), 346
   biotin, 346
   chromium, 346
   copper, 346
   folic acid, 346
   iodine, 346
   iron, 346
   selenium, 346
   vitamin A, 346
   vitamin C, 346
   vitamin D, 346
   vitamin E, 346
   vitamin K, 346
   zinc, 347
Vitiligo, 404–405, 405f
Volvulus, 183
von Hippel–Lindau syndrome, 78, 418t
Von Recklinghausen's disease, 510
von Willebrand factor (vWF), 120, 142
VSD. See Ventricular septal defect
Vulvar cancer, 266
Vulvar intraepithelial neoplasia (VIN), 266
vWF. See von Willebrand factor

W
Wandering pacemaker, 18f, 26
Warfarin, 142, 225, 473t

Warts. See Verrucae
Wasp sting, 475
Water-bottle-shaped heart on PA plain film,
   456t
Water hammer pulse, 32
Waterhouse–Friderichsen, 84
Watershed infarct, 373
Weber's test, 311–312
Wechsler Adult Intelligence Scale-Revised
   (WAIS-R), 363
Wechsler Intelligence Scale for Children- Revised
   (WISC-R), 363
Wechsler Preschool and Primary Scale of
   Intelligence (WPPSI), 363
Wenckebach block, 25
Wermer's syndrome, 92t
Wernicke–Korsakoff's encephalopathy, 65
Wernicke's aphasia, 373
Wernicke's encephalopathy, 381
Wharthin–Starry silver stain, 424
Wheal, 389, 393f
Whipple's disease, 36
Whipple's procedure, 175
Wide-Range achievement Test (WRAT), 363
Wilms tumor, 78–79
Wilson's disease, 66–67, 381
Wiskott–Aldrich syndrome, 510
Withdrawal headache, 307t
Wolff–parkinson–White syndrome, 26
   causes of, 26
Wrist injuries, 336–338. See also Sports
         medicine complaints
   Carpal tunnel syndrome, 337–338
   fractures, 336–337, 337f
Wrongful death, 487t

X
Xanthelasma, 408
Xanthoma, 408, 409f
Xeroderma pigmentosa, 511
Xerophthalmia, 437t
XYY syndrome, 87t

Y
Yellow eye (icterus), 440
Yellow vision, 440
Yersinia enterocolitis, 162t

Z
Zenker's diverticulum, 165
Zinc, 346
Ziprasidone, 354t
Zollinger–Ellison syndrome, 175
Zolpidem, 557